The EMDR Coloring Book

The EMDR Coloring Book
A Calming Resource for Adults
Featuring 200 Works of Fine Art
Paired With
200 Positive Affirmations

Mark Odland - MA, LMFT, MDIV

Bilateral Innovations
Minnesota

Published in the United States by Bilateral Innovations
www.bilateralinnovations.com
mark@bilateralinnovations.com

Artwork of Alphonse Legros printed with permission from the National Gallery of Art.

Names: Odland, Mark, author.
Title: The EMDR Coloring Book: A Calming Resource for Adults Featuring 200 Works of Fine Art Paired with 200 Positive Affirmations
Description: First American edition. Minnesota: Bilateral Innovations, an assumed name of North Woods Christian Counseling, LLC, [2017]
BISAC: Medical / Mental Health

ISBN-13: 9781540523907
ISBN-10: 154052390X

Content available as a Paperback Book.

PRINTED IN THE UNITED STATES OF AMERICA

10 9 8 7 6 5 4 3 2 1

First American Edition

PREFACE

Who this Book is for

While this book could be enjoyed by almost anyone, it's designed specifically for those receiving EMDR therapy. If you're in this process, your therapist may have already helped you develop resources like a "safe place," "calm place," or "container." Often used before or after EMDR therapy, these resources can also be a wonderful way to practice emotional regulation between sessions. The EMDR Coloring Book is designed to complement these strategies, providing you with another resource for the journey.

Whether you choose to use crayons, markers, colored pencils, or paint, this "coloring book" will help you practice being in the moment. A break from past hurts and future worries, this book provides an opportunity to reclaim the curious and playful parts of yourself. Paired with positive self-statements (*some of which are "positive cognitions"*), each work of art invites thoughtful meditation on the truths so many of us hope to believe as the healing process unfolds.

When to Use this Book

This book could be useful in situations where you would like to:

1) Center yourself before, during, or at the end of an EMDR therapy session.
2) Practice emotional regulation between EMDR therapy sessions.
3) Relax at home or on the road.
4) Enjoy beautiful and thought-provoking artwork.
5) Meditate on positive self-statements.
6) Rediscover the the playful and curious side of yourself.

How to Use this Book

Choose your medium to create with

You may use crayons, colored pencils, markers, watercolor paints, or any other creative medium that feels right for you. Some find it helpful to journal or jot down ideas next to the images. Others will create a collage. There are no rules with this book, so feel free to "color outside the lines."

Stage your environment

When used at home, you might consider eliminating distractions and arranging your environment to be visually beautiful and emotionally peaceful (*light candles, play soothing music, etc.*). When used outside the home, this may not be possible. However, when on the move, this book's portability allows it to be used in a therapist's office, at a park, on a bus, or anywhere you see fit.

Use as part of a larger self-care plan

While this book is helpful to use as needed for practicing mindfulness and relaxation, you might also consider using it as part of a larger self-care plan. With busy schedules, taking care of ourselves can be challenging. However, taking even small steps to add beauty, love, and peace into our lives can make a big difference over time. By investing just a few minutes a day, coloring and journaling could become an enjoyable addition to your daily or weekly routine.

Select a page to interact with and begin

As you begin to color or paint, consider being mindful of how the image and positive statement associated with it impacts you. If thinking about the positive statement leads to pleasant emotions, simply notice these feelings and continue. If this focus leads to unsettling emotions that are tolerable, you can either choose to color, paint, or journal your way "through them," or instead redirect your focus back to your surroundings and to the creative process… simply noticing the weight of the object in your hand, the texture of the paper, and the various colors as they emerge. Let yourself go with the flow, allowing yourself to simply respond rather than overthinking it. Of course, you are free to finish at any time.

Disclaimer

* This book is designed to be relaxing. It may provide you with a much needed break from the stress of life, and an opportunity to be more fully-present in the moment. For most, the tactile nature of the creative process tends to be grounding. However, if for some reason the process becomes upsetting or leads to emotions that are too difficult to manage, you can always stop. Simply stand-up, take deep breaths, move your body, engage your senses, and utilize your coping skills. While the book can be used as a resource during the EMDR therapy process, it is not to be confused with EMDR therapy itself, which should only be provided by a trained EMDR therapist. When using this book, make sure to talk with your therapist and make sure that it aligns with your treatment goals.

How the Positive Affirmations were Selected

The positive self-statements in this book were inspired by the positive "cognitions" listed in EMDR therapy basic trainings. These core affirmations and their variants are familiar to EMDR therapists around the world because they depict the types of statements clients want to believe as they heal from their trauma. While some of these statements might not technically meet the definition of a "cognition," they've been included because of their potential to be helpful and encouraging.

How the Artwork was Edited

Each piece of artwork was digitally transformed to black and white. In addition, subtle details and gray tones were often reduced or eliminated in order to create the white space necessary for coloring or painting. Whenever possible, editing was kept to a minimum in order to honor the artist's original intent.

How the Artwork was Chosen

Each work of art in this book was created by the famous French printmaker, Alphonse Legros. The crisp lines of his etchings, drypoint, lithographs, and drawings provide a striking canvas for your creative expression. The content of his artwork falls into two broad categories: 1) landscapes, and 2) human emotion.

His landscapes convey a simple, yet noble beauty. The relative neutrality of these scenes promotes calm, and guards against emotional escalation. They provide a type of emotional "blank slate" upon which your calm and creativity can flow.

His depictions of humanity capture the deep emotions that transcend time and culture. While not as emotionally-neutral as his landscapes, these images are refreshingly honest. They validate how challenging life can sometimes be, and remind us that we're not alone. As such, they may evoke more emotion. However, the process of observing and creating helps ensure that these emotions are either contained or safely processed, keeping you grounded firmly in the present. I sincerely hope that you enjoy using this book, and that it plays some small role in your process of healing.

Blessings,

Mark Odland - MA, LMFT, MDIV

CONTENTS

40   I can choose to let it out
Near the Mill (Pres du moulin) - etching and drypoint (photo process?)

41   I can learn to take care of myself
Peasant Woman Seated near a Hedge (Paysanne assise pres d'une haie) - etching and drypoint

42   I am important
Plain near a Lake (La plaine pres du lac) - etching and drypoint

43   I can make my needs known
Two Studies of Hands - graphite

44   I can choose whom to trust
Return from the Woods (Le retour du bois) - etching

45   I can be real
Roman Ruin (Ruine romaine) - etching and drypoint

46   I am okay
Rope-yards (Les corderies) - etching and drypoint

47   I now have choices
Salmon Fisher (Le pecheur de saumon) - etching

48   I can take care of myself
Sleeping Shepherd (Le repos du berger) - etching

49   I did the best I could
Small Boat in Peril (Barque en peril) - drypoint

50   I can learn from it
Solitude (Solitude (Paysage) - drypoint

51   I am lovable
Storm (Un orage) - etching? and drypoint

52   I am beautiful
Breton Peasant (Paysan breton) - drypoint

53   I am significant
Wash-house, called "The Washerwomen" (Le lavoir, dite "Les Laveuses") - etching

54   I learned from it
Antique Dealer - etching and drypoint

55   I can safely show my emotions
Archeologist (L'archeologue) - etching and drypoint

56   I deserve good things
Head of an Old Man with a Wide-Brimmed Hat - pen and brown ink on laid paper

57   I can be whole
Beggar with Hat in Hand (Mendiant avec son chapeau a la main) - etching and drypoint

58   I can express myself
Beggars of Brussels (Les mendiants de Bruges) - etching

59   I can safely feel my emotions
Black Cat (Le chat noir) - etching

60   I can grow
Broken Cart (La charrette brisee) - etching

61   I am worthy
Desperate Man (Le desespere) - drypoint and etching

62   I am worthwhile
Desperate Young Girl (La jeune desesperee) - etching and drypoint

63   I am radiant
Distributor of the Holy Water (Le donneur d'eau benite) - etching and drypoint?

64   I survived
Donkey Upset by Storm (L'ane renverse par la foudre) - etching

65   I matter
Egg-sellers, 2nd plate (Les marchandes d'oeufs) - etching and drypoint

66   I can trust my judgment
Fording a River (Le gue) - etching

67   I am safe now
Harvesters Surprised by the Storm (Moissonneuses surprises par l'orage) - etching

68   I deserve love
Head of a Young Girl (Tete de jeune fille) - etching and drypoint

69   I am now in control
Hurricane (L'ouragan) - etching

70   I can learn to trust myself
Job, 2nd plate - drypoint and etching?

71   I deserve to live
Little Beggar (Le petit mendiant) - etching

72   I am not alone
Man and Wife Seated by the Road with a Basket (Homme et femme assis au bord de la rou te aven un panier) - etching

73   I am able to succeed
Man Foraging (L'homme au fourrage) etching and drypoint

74   I am worthy of love
Meditation (La meditation) - etching? and drypoint

75   I can be trusted
Old man, Old Tree (Vieil homme, vieil arbre) - etching and drypoint

76   I am honorable
Paralytic (Le paralytique) - etching and drypoint?

77   I have dignity
Peasant in a Round Hat (Paysan avec chapeau rond) - etching

78   I am valuable
Peasant Woman of Boulogne (Paysanne des environs de Boulogne dite La femme au panier) - etching

79   I am able to learn
Poor Man (Pauvre homme) - drypoint and (etching?)

80   I am fine as I am
Egg-sellers, 1st plate (Les marchandes d'oeufs) - etching and drypoint

81   I am only human
At the Foot of the Cross (Au pied de la croix) - lithograph

82   I am smart
Study of a Man's Head (Etude de tete d'homme) - etching

83   I am whole
Seated Beggar (Mendiant assis) - etching and drypoint

84   I can handle it
Shadow (Ombre) - etching

85   I am enough
Siesta of a Laborer (Sieste d'un ouvrier) - drypoint

86   I can be myself
Sinbad the Sailor (Sinbad le marin) - etching and drypoint?

87   I can make mistakes
Sleeper (Un dormeur) - etching

88   I am intelligent
Supper of the Poor (Le souper chez misere) - etching? and drypoint

89   I am strong now
The Fire, 2nd plate (L'incendie) etching

90   I can be healthy
The Prodigal Son, 2nd plate (L'enfant prodigue) - etching and drypoint

91   I am a work in progress
Man Climbing a Wall (L'escalade) - etching and drypoint?

92   I do the best I can
The Prodigal Son, 3rd plate (L'enfant prodigue) etching and drypoint

93   I am a good person
The Prodigal Son, 6th plate (L'enfant prodigue) - etching and drypoint

94   I am okay just the way I am
The Tree of Salvation (L'arbe de salut) - drypoint and etching?

95   I am strong
Thunder (Un coup de foudre) - etching

96   I can do it
Tornado (Le typhon) - drypoint

97   I am forgiven
Two Beggars (Les deux mendiants) - etching

98   I have what it takes
Victims of the Lightning (Victimes de la foudre) - etching and drypoint

99   I am okay as I am
Woman Seated against a Wall, Child with His Head in Her Lap (Femme assis, muraille au fond, enfant la tete dans son giron) - etching and drypoint

100   It is okay to be me
Woman Seated against a Wall, Child with His Head in Her Lap (Femme assise, muraille au fond, enfant la tete dans son giron - etching and drypoint

101   I can accomplish my goals
Woodcutters, 3rd plate (Les bucherons) - etching

102   I am unforgettable
Abandoned Village (Le village abondonne) - etching and drypoint?

103   I am worthy of joy
Along the River (Le long de la rive) - etching and drypoint

104   I have mastery
Along the Thames (Sur la Tamise) - etching? and drypoint

105   I did enough
Angler (Le pecheur a la ligne) - etching

106   I can be free
Avenue of Poplars (L'allee de peupliers) - drypoint

107   I can make good decisions
Banks of the Adour (Bord de l'Adour) - etching

108   I am alright
Banks of the Liane (Les bords de la Liane) - etching

109   I am lovely
Banks of the Marne (Bord de la Marne) - drypoint and etching?

110   I am remarkable
Banks of the Somme near Amiens (Bord de la Somme pres d'Amiens) - etching

111   I was just a kid
Banks of the Venelle (Bord de la Venelle) - etching? and drypoint

112   I am excellent
Banks of the Yanne (Les bords de la Yanne) - drypoint and etching?

113   I can move on
Beggar (Un mendiant) - drypoint

114   I am able
Bend in the River (Un coin de riviere) - etching

115   I can conquer my fears
Birch Trees: Water's Edge Seen in Morning Light (Les bouleaux: Bord de l'eau, effet du matin) - etching and drypoint?

116   I am a masterpiece
Blacksmith (Le forgeron) - drypoint and etching

117   I am a person of integrity
Bohemien Encampment (Campement de bohemiens) - etching

118   I am priceless
Castle in Spain (Chateau en Espagne) - drypoint and etching

119   I am respectable
Chickweed Merchant (Marchand de mouron) - etching? and drypoint

120   I am a work of art
Contre-bass Player (Le joueur de contre-basse) - etching

121   I deserve to thrive
Convalescent (Le convalescent) - drypoint and etching?

122   I am desirable
Cottage with a Cart (Chaumiere a la charette) - etching

123   I am okay in my imperfection
Curious Man (Un curieux) - etching and drypoint

124   I am tough
Digger (Le piocheur) - etching

125   I am secure
Edge of a Brook (Bord de ruisseau) - drypoint

126   I can manage it
Edge of a Forest in Bourgogne (Un coin de foret en Bourgogne) - etching and drypoint

127   I am praiseworthy
Edge of the Water (Au bord de l'eau) - etching

128   I am bright
Farm on a Hill (La ferme sur la colline) - etching

129   I am faithful
Plate made for an Exhibition at the Dunthorne Home (Planche faite pour une exposition chez Dunthorne) - etching and drypoint

130   I am justified
Gust of Wind (Le coup de vent) - etching

131   I can achieve
Harvesters (Les moissoneurs) - etching

132   I am worthy of respect
Peddler (Le colporteur) - drypoint and etching?

133   I can let go
Near the Woods (Pres du bois) - drypoint and (etching?)

134   I lived
Meadow in Sunshine (Le pre ensoleille) - drypoint and etching?

135   I am unique
Traveler Reclining on the Grass (Le voyageur etendu sur le gazon) - etching and drypoint

136   I can hold it together
Horse-driven Mill (Le manege) - etching

137   I can go with the flow
Returning with the Hay (Rentrant le foin) - etching and drypoint

138   I deserve to be treated well
Landscape (Paysage) - drypoint and etching

139   I am powerful
Young Peasant (Jeune paysanne) - lithograph

140   I can believe in myself
Travelers Resting (Les voyageurs fatigues) - drypoint

141   I am worthy of love
Study of Woman Praying - pen and brown ink over graphite on laid paper

142   I am precious
Sunrise, Woods of Clamard (Lever du soleil, bois de Clamard) - drypoint and etching?

143   I am admirable
Young Peasant Seated in a Church (Jeune paysanne assise dans une eglise) - etching and drypoint?

144   I am well
Landscape (Paysage) - etching and drypoint

145   I can fulfill my purpose
Wheelwright (Un charron) - drypoint

146   I am worthy of peace
Village of Wimille, near Boulogne (Village de Wimille, pres Boulogne) - etching

147   I am competent
Landscape (Paysage) - etching

148   I can discover my purpose
View of Reeds (Coin de roseau) - drypoint

149   I can live with uncertainty
Remembrance of a Valley in Bourgogne (Souvenir d'une vallee en Bourgogne) - etching and drypoint

150   I can be flexible
Landscape: Sunrise (Paysage: Lever du soleil) - etching and drypoint

151   I am free
Traveler Resting (Repos du voyageur) - etching and drypoint

152   I can hold on
Valley in Bourgogne (Une vallee en Bourgogne) - drypoint and etching

153   I deserve to exist
Village (Un village) - etching and drypoint

154   I am acceptable
Squaring Logs (Homme que fend des buches) - etching and drypoint

155   I am a person of character
Landscape (Paysage) - etching

156　I can change
Valley of Dunes (La vallee des dunes) - etching and drypoint

157　I am complete
Peasant at the Source - pen and ink over touches of graphite on laid paper

158　I am worthy of good relationships
Tower (La tour) - drypoint

159　I am wise
Poplars near Amiens (Pres d'Amiens, les tourbieres) - drypoint and etching

160　I am meaningful
The Plow (La charrue) - etching

161　I am secure now
Landscape (Paysage) - etching and drypoint

162　I can be authentic
The House of the Well (La maison du puits) - etching and drypoint

163　It is finished
Siesta of a Harvester (Sieste d'un faucheur) - drypoint

164　I can just notice
Study for the Prodigal Son (Etude pour L'enfant prodigue) - etching and drypoint?

165　I am wholesome
Landscape: Near Chailleux (Paysage: Pres Chailleux) - etching and drypoint?

166　I can be imperfect
Rectory Wall (Le mur du presbytere) - etching and drypoint

167　I can be present
Thatched Cottage (Chaumiere) - etching and drypoint

168　I am stronger than I used to be
Woodcutter (Le bucheron) - etching

169　I can find meaning
Old Village (Ville vieille) - etching and drypoint?

170　My situation is different now
Mushroom Gatherers (Les ramasseurs de champignons) - drypoint and etching?

171　I do not need to have all the answers
Valley in Bourgogne (Une vallee en Bourgogne) - etching

172   I can be transformed
Vagabond Moving along a Lane (Un vagabond passant dans une ruelle) - etching

173   I did what I could
Near Nordkerque (Pres de Nordkerque) - etching? and drypoint

174   What happened does not define me
In the Forest of Fontainebleau (Dans le foret de Fontainebleau) - etching? and drypoint

175   I can learn to make my needs known
Riverbank (Bord de la riviere) - drypoint and (etching?)

176   I can live with paradox
Willows (Les saules) - drypoint

177   I now have better judgment
Man Watering a Horse (Homme abreuvant un cheval) - etching

178   I can learn to be honest
Man with a Punt, Figure to the Right (Pecheurs des truites) - etching and drypoint?

179   I know enough
Hovel on a Hillside (Masure sur la colline) - etching and drypoint?

180   I am worth it
Head of a Young Girl (Tete de jeune fille) - drypoint

181   My heart was in the right place
Prospect (Le point de vue) - etching and drypoint

182   I can be transformed
Landscape (Paysage) - etching and drypoint

183   I am one of a kind
Siesta in the Country (Sieste dans la capagne) - drypoint and etching?

184   I can do what I need to do
Return of the Peasants (Le retour des paysans) - transfer lithograph?

185   I can be honest
Old Chateau (Un vieux chateau) - etching

186   I am just right
Landscape with a Boy in a Tree (Paysage avec un garcon grimpe sur un arbre, dite "Le denicheur d'oiseaux") - etching and drypoint

187 I can be healthier
Little Burner of Grass (Le petit bruleur d'herbe) - etching and drypoint

188 I am special
Study of the Head of a Man Reading (Etude de tete d'homme lisant) - etching and drypoint?

189 I now have more choices
Valley in Bourgogne (Une vallee en Bourgogne) - etching and drypoint?

190 I am full of heart
Man in Punt - etching

191 I can learn to be myself
Woman of the Marketplace (Femme du marche) - etching and drypoint

192 I have been made new
Head of a Man (Tete d'homme) - drypoint

193 I can learn to succeed
Landscape with Roller (Le paysage au rouleau) - etching and drypoint

194 I am better now
Return to the Farm (Le retour a la ferme) - etching

195 I am a person of principle
Pigeon Tower (La tour aux pigeons) - etching and drypoint

196 The worst is over
The Gate (L'entree du champ) - drypoint and etching?

197 I am transformed
Plain (La plaine) - etching and drypoint

198 I now have more control
Trees at Water's Edge (Les arbres au bord de l'eau) - drypoint and etching?

199 I am being reshaped
Shepherd's Hut on a Hillside (Bergerie sur le coteau) - etching and drypoint

200 I am a soulful person
Orphans (Les orphelins (?)) - etching and drypoint?

201 I can be transformed
Rest along the Banks of the River (Repos au bord de la riviere) - etching and drypoint?

202 I have a good heart
Head of Souliote (Tete de Souliote) - etching and drypoint?

203   I am calm
Peasants (Paysannes) - etching and drypoint

204   I have soul
Head - black chalk

205   I am able to reach my goals
View of a Farm (La ferme de Beauchamp) - etching

206   I deserve healthy relationships
Small Hill (Le coteau) - etching

207   I am valuable the way I am
Stand of Trees (Bouquet d'arbres) - etching? and drypoint

208   I am a survivor
Study for Head of a Man (Etude de tete d'homme) - etching and drypoint?

209   I am not defined by my past
In the Forest of Fontainebleau (Dans la foret de Fontainebleau) - etching and drypoint

210   I am acceptable the way I am
Sleeping Beggar (Mendiant endormi) - etching and drypoint

211   I am dignified
Head of a Man Facing Left - graphite

212   I am able to become healthy
Woman Reading: Lesson under the Trees (La liseuse: La lecture sous les arbres) - etching and drypoint?

213   I am stronger now
Valley in Bourgogne (Une vallee en Bourgogne) - etching and drypoint?

214   I am a person of faith
Peasant Women of Boulogne (Paysannes des environs de Boulogne) - etching and drypoint?

215   I am resilient
The Hand of the Artist's Daughter - black crayon

216   I am safe
Thinker (Le penseur) - etching and drypoint

217   I know more now
Burning Grass (Le bruleur d'herbes) - etching and drypoint

218   I am a person of strength
Mme. Kemp, 4th plate - etching

219 I am redeemed
Study of Cupid (Head of a Girl) - metalpoint on prepared paper

220 I am worthy the way I am
Finding the Sheep (Le mouton retrouve) - etching

221 I am a new creation
Brick-works (La Briqueterie) - drypoint

I am...

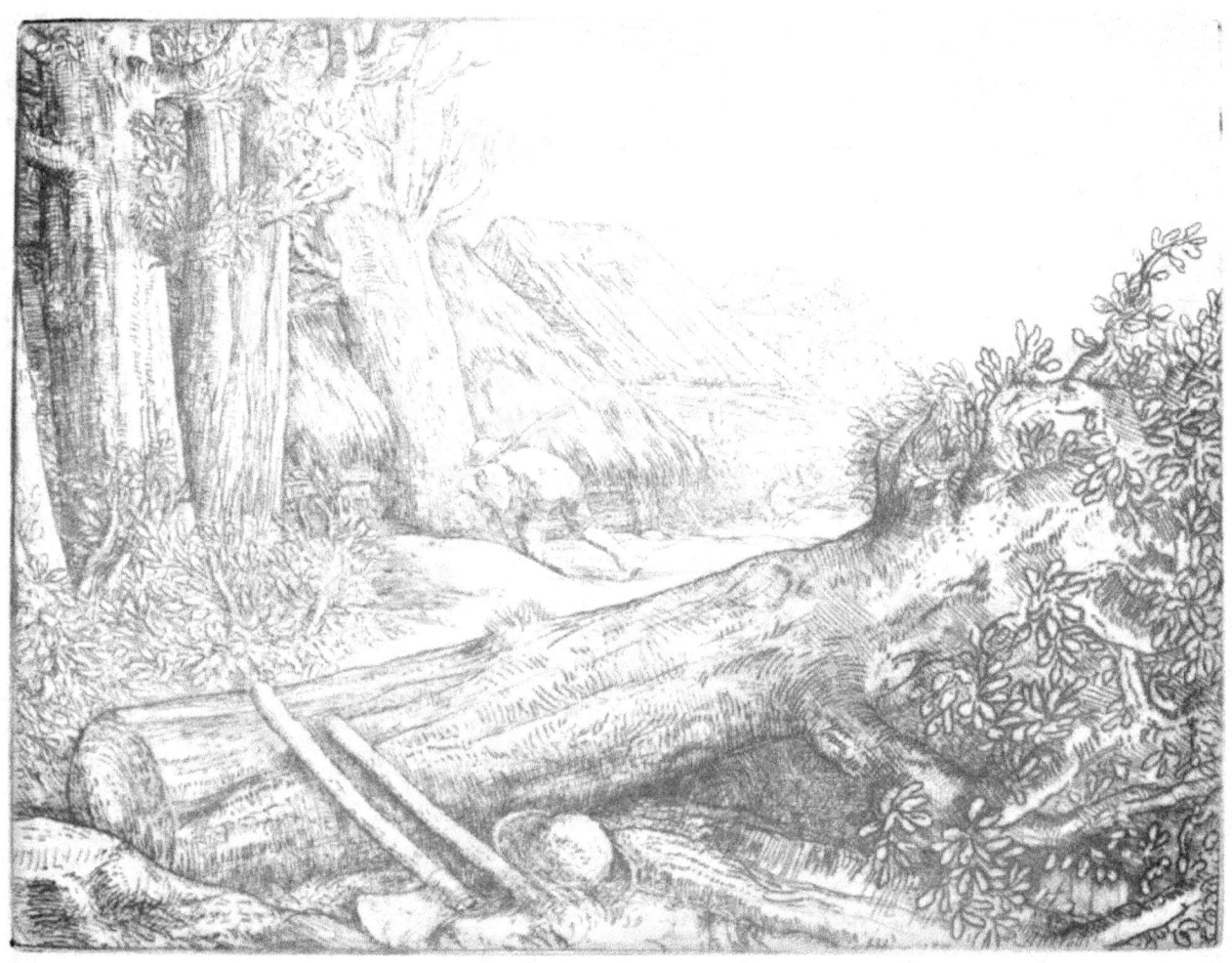

I am loved

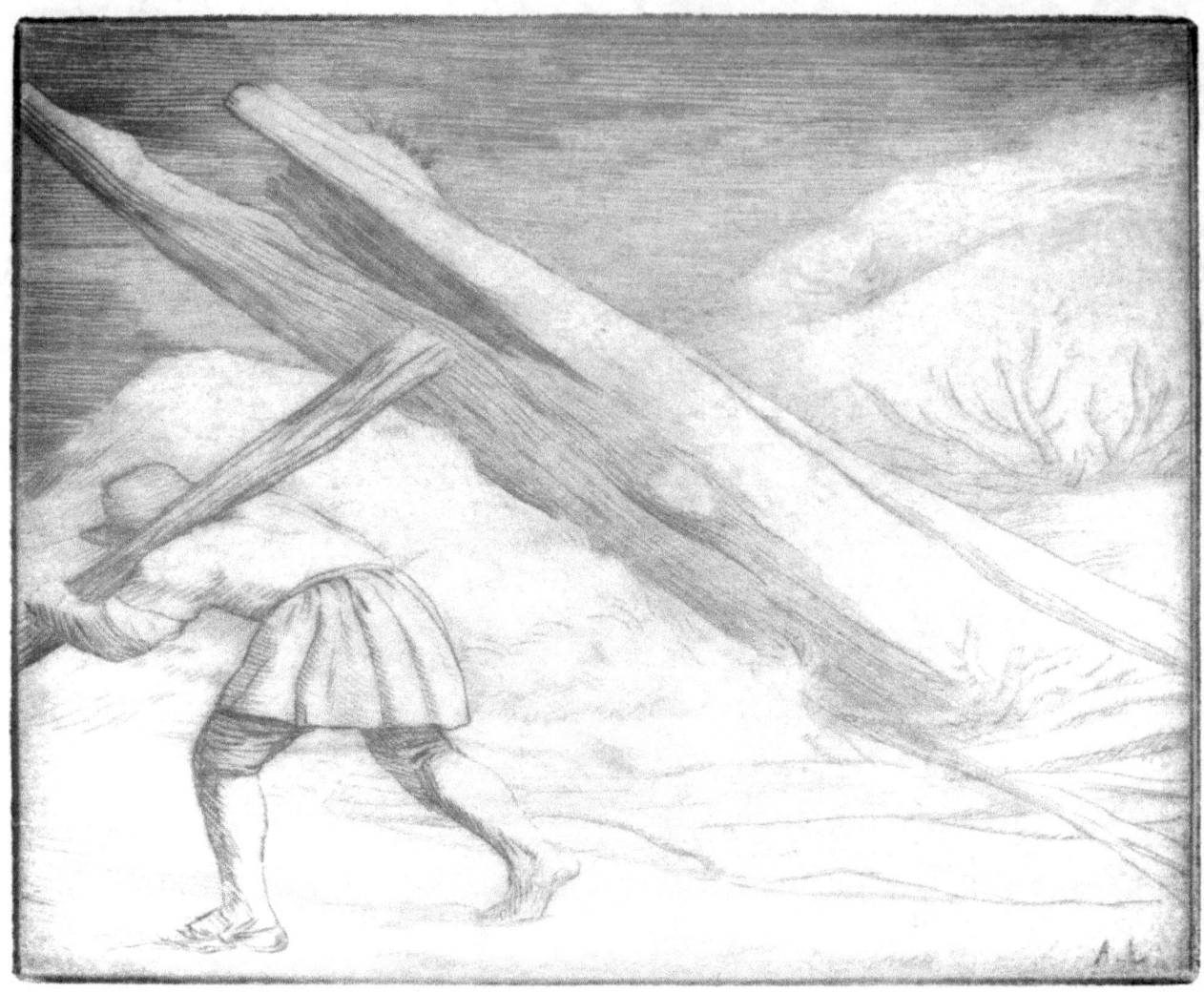

I am free

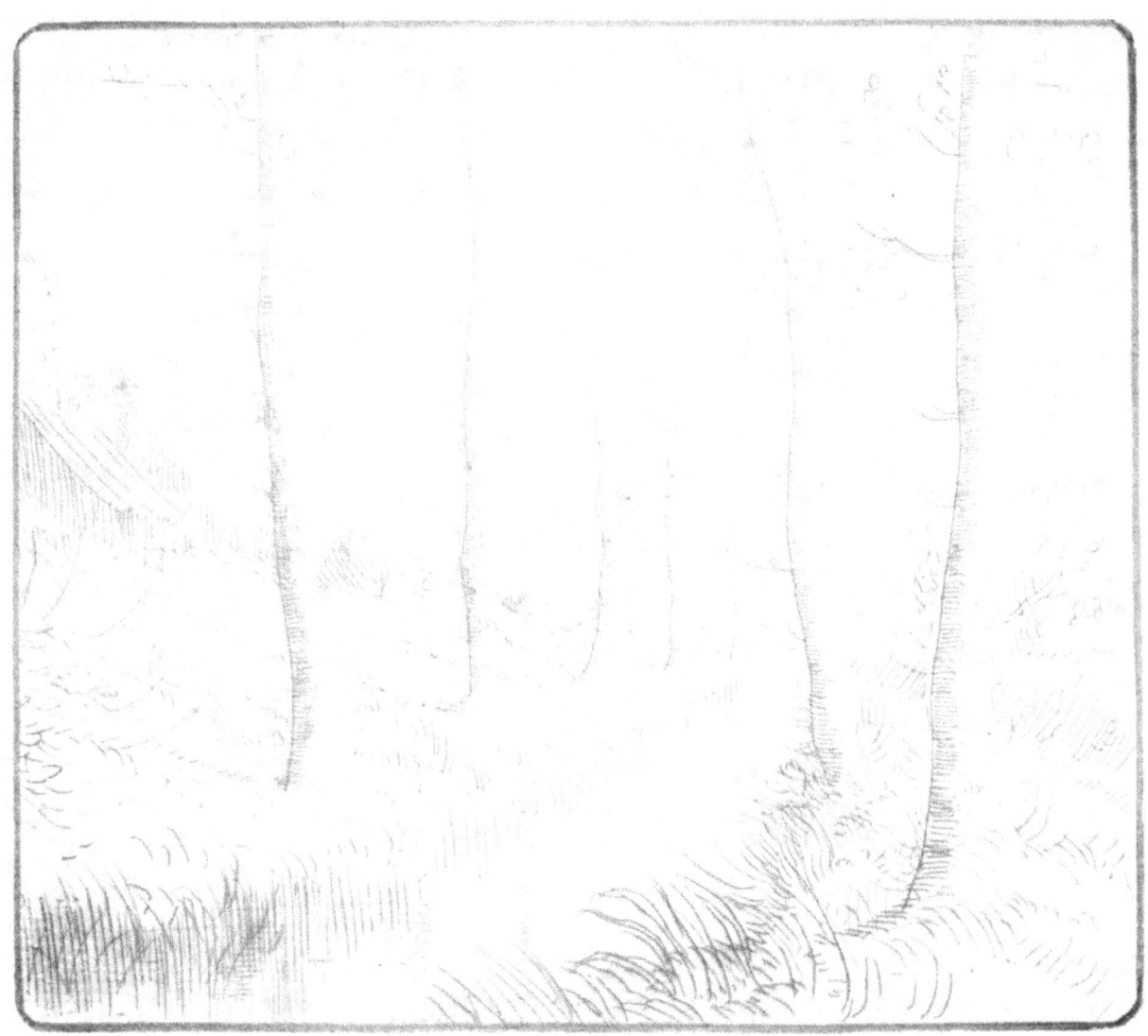

I am stronger now

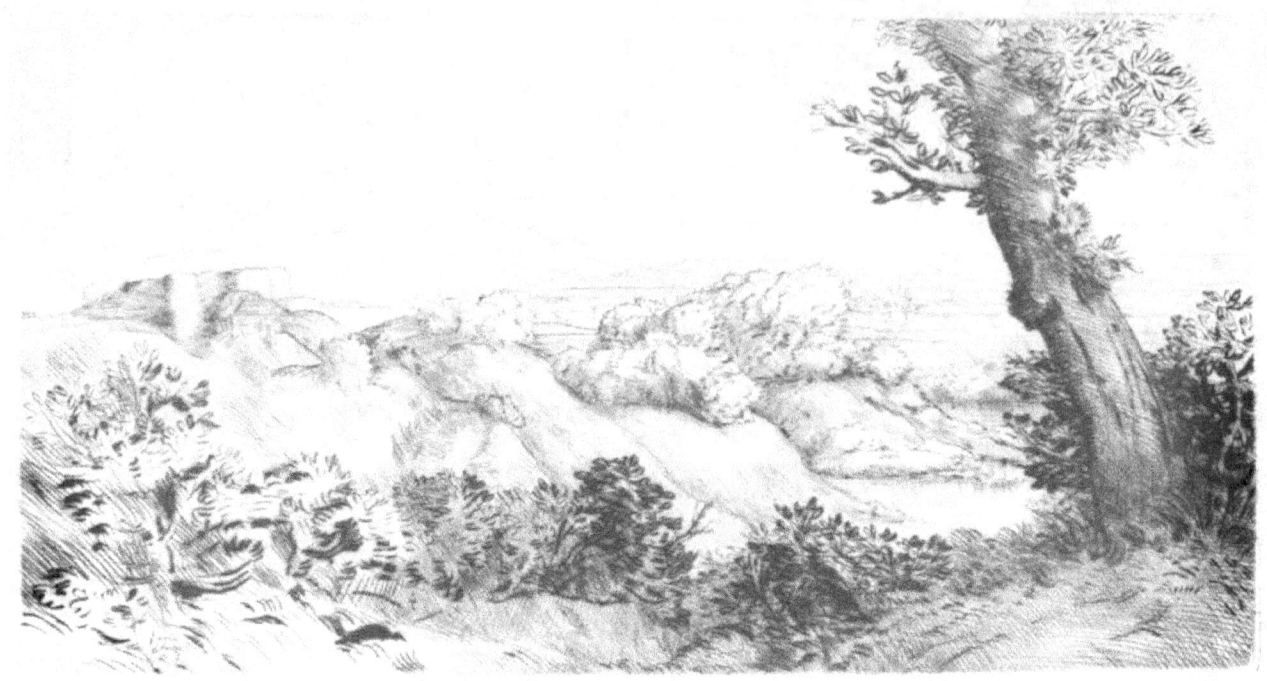

I am a treasure

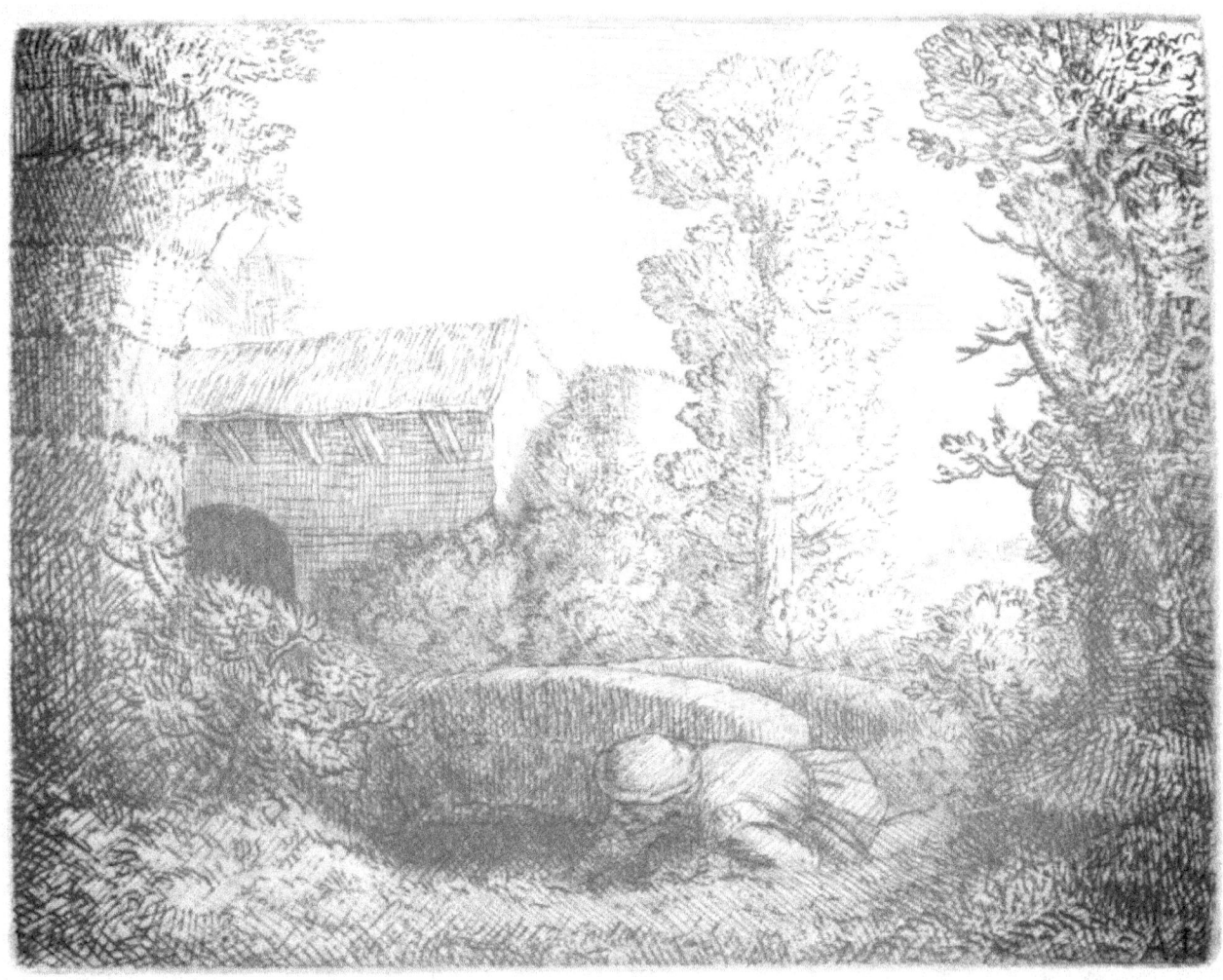

I am capable

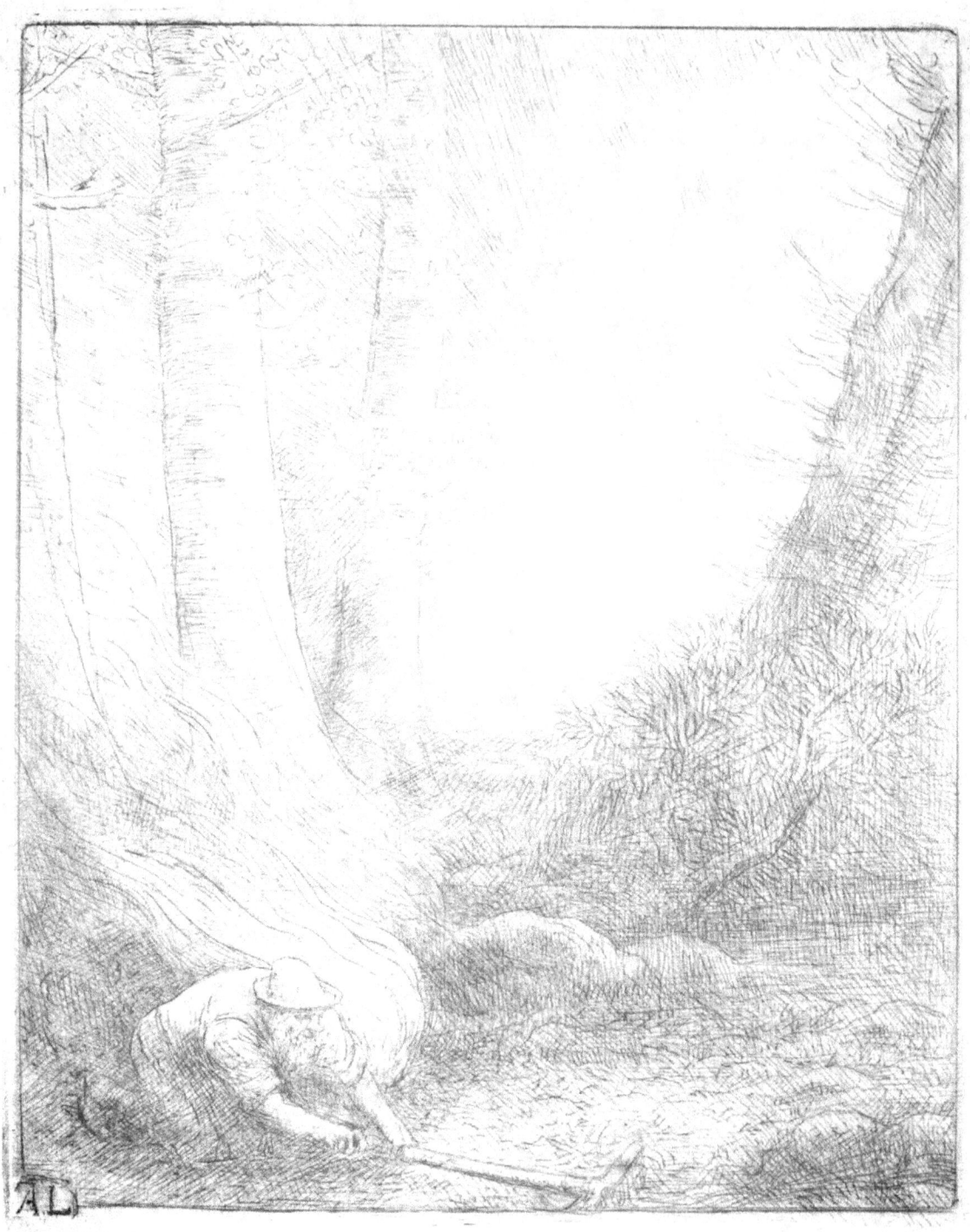

I can have love

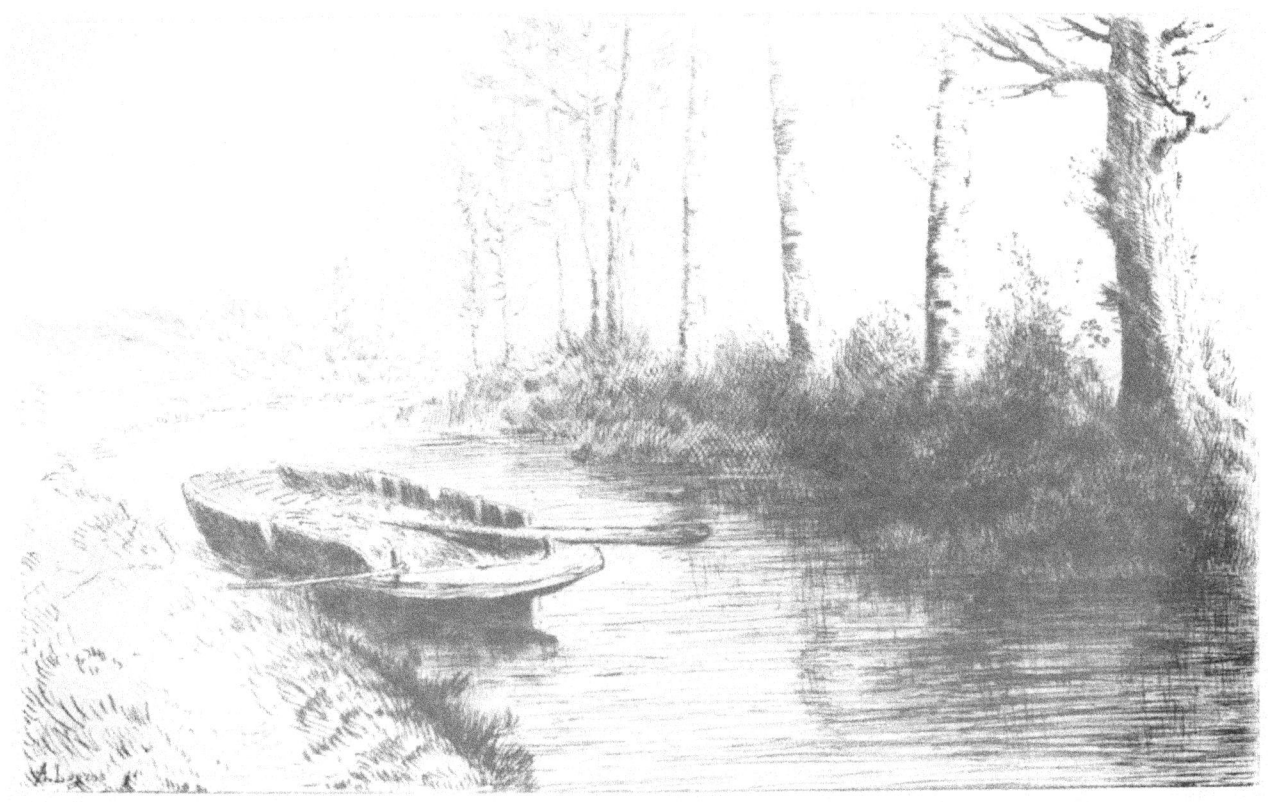

I am attractive

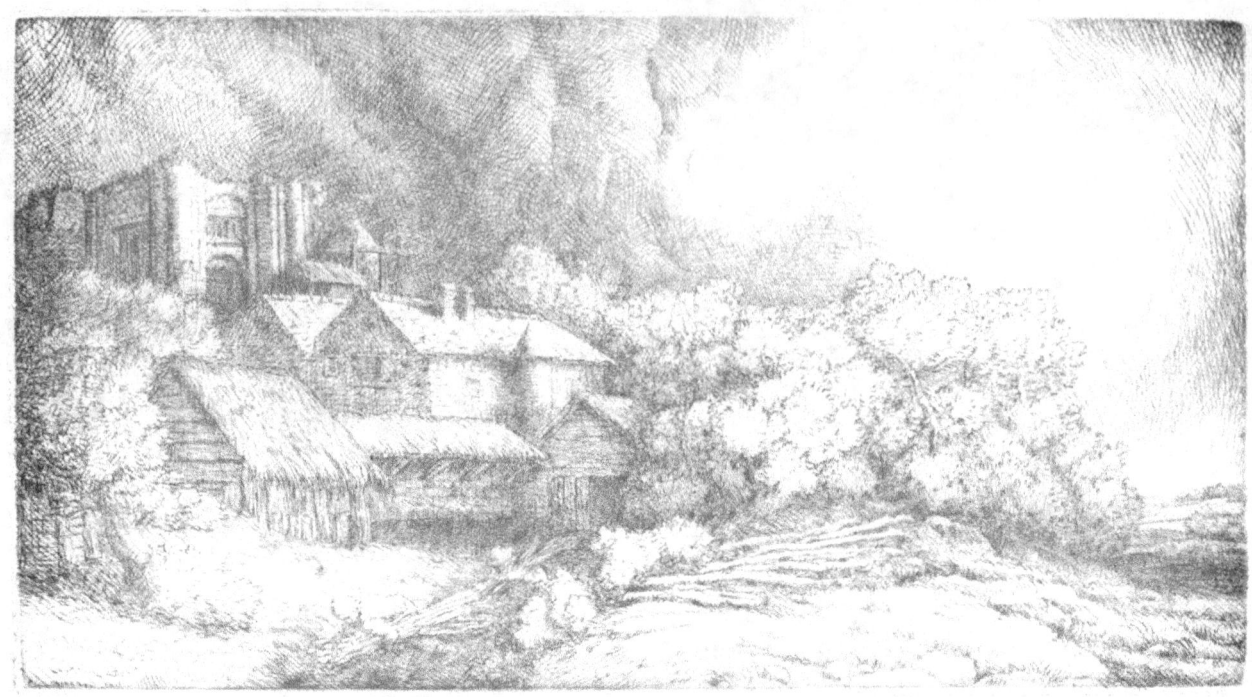

I am fine

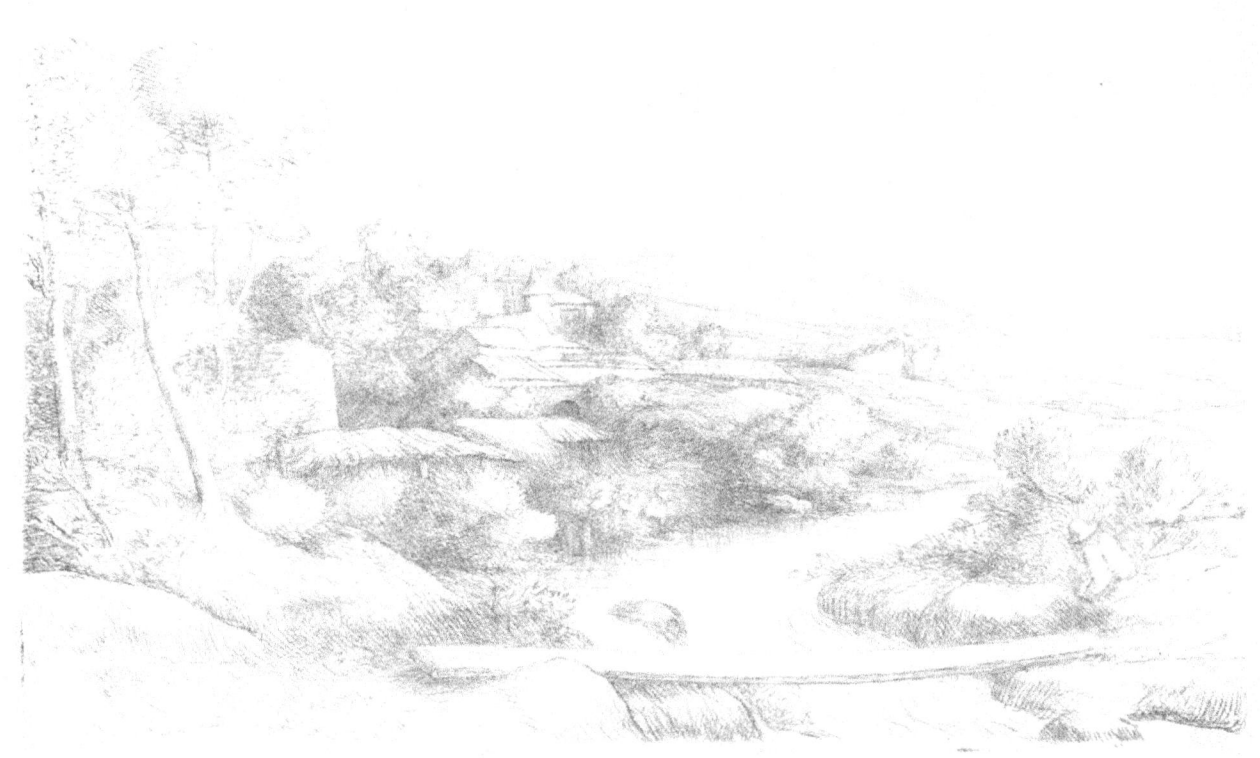

It is over

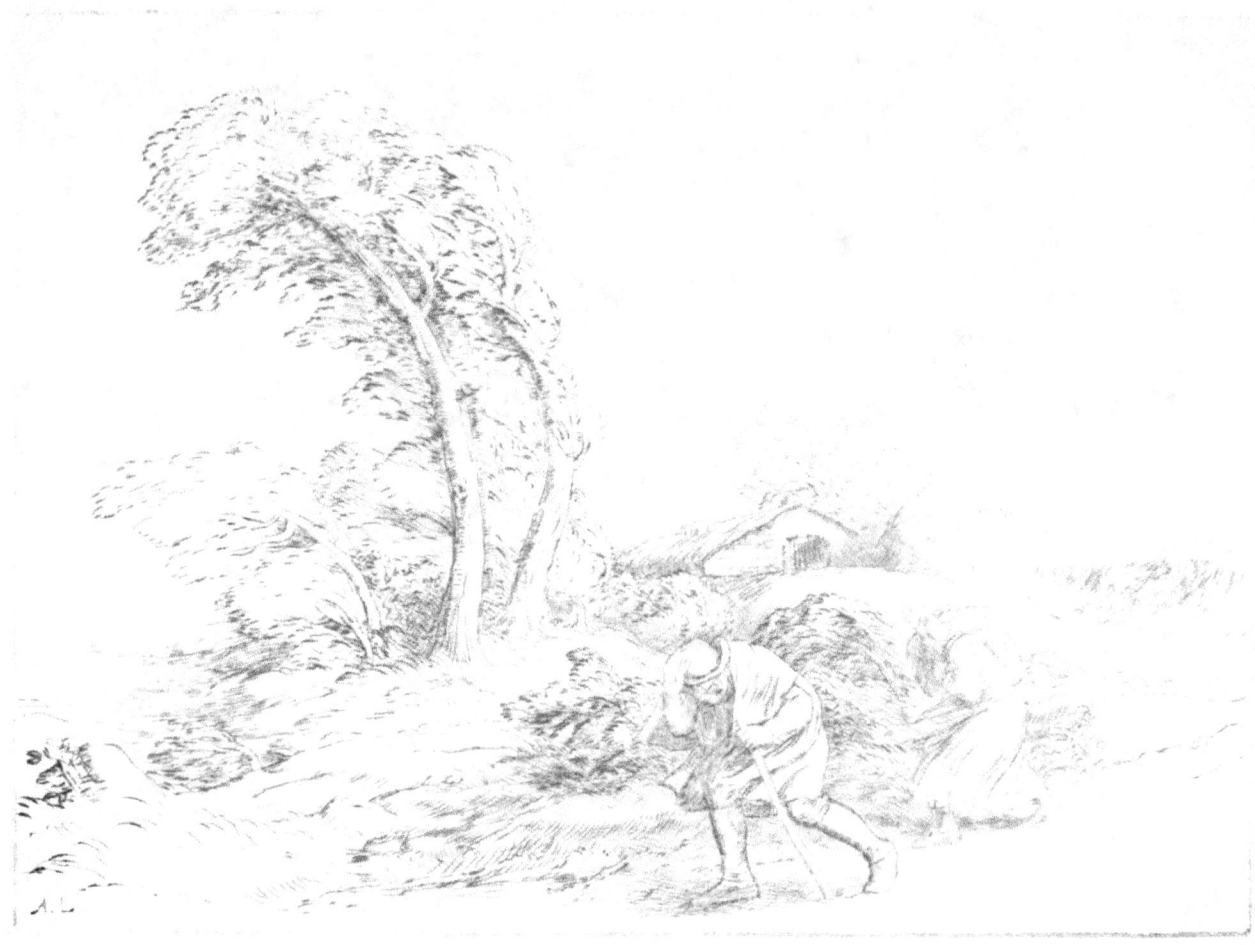

I am a loving person

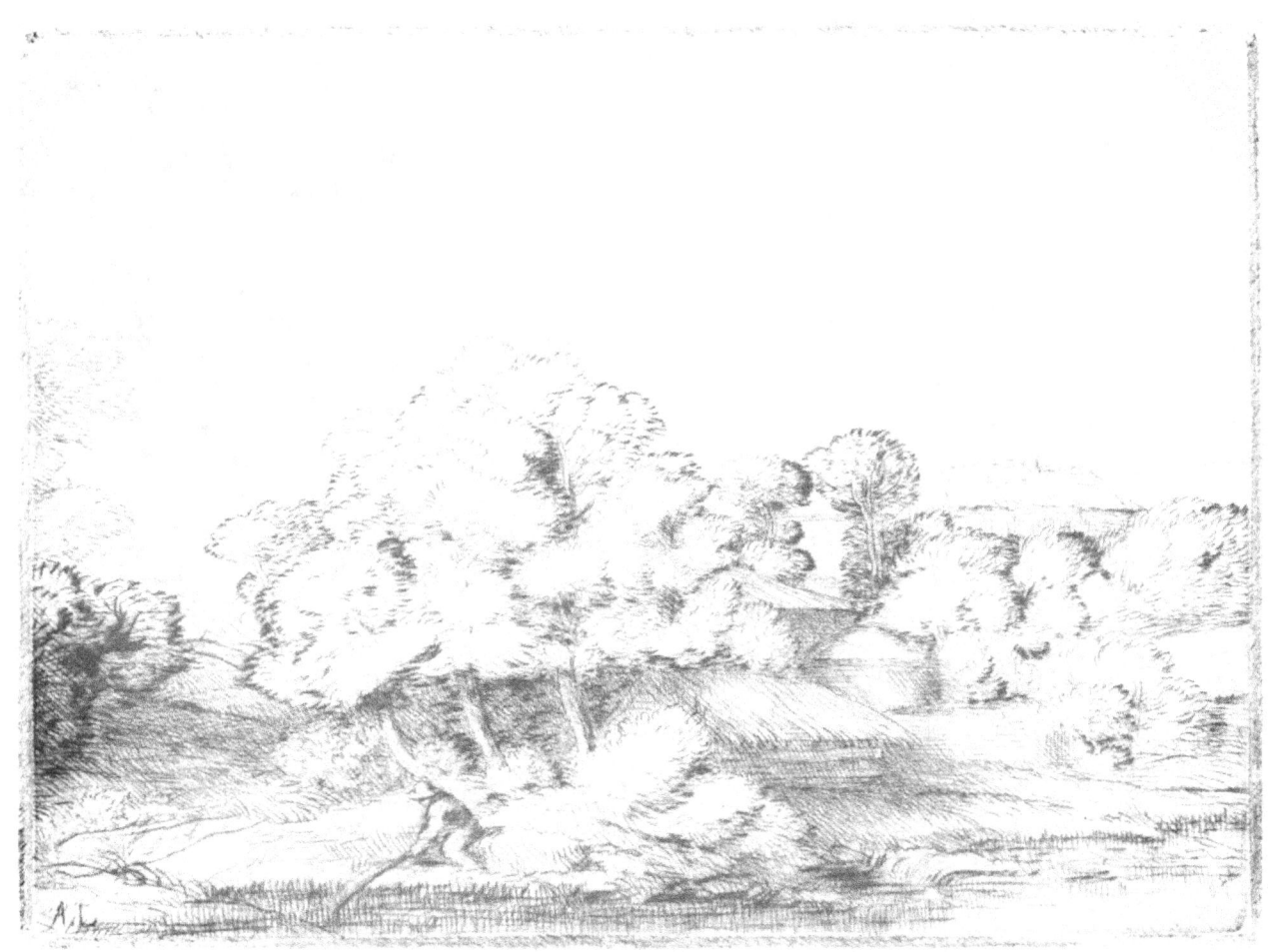

I am deserving

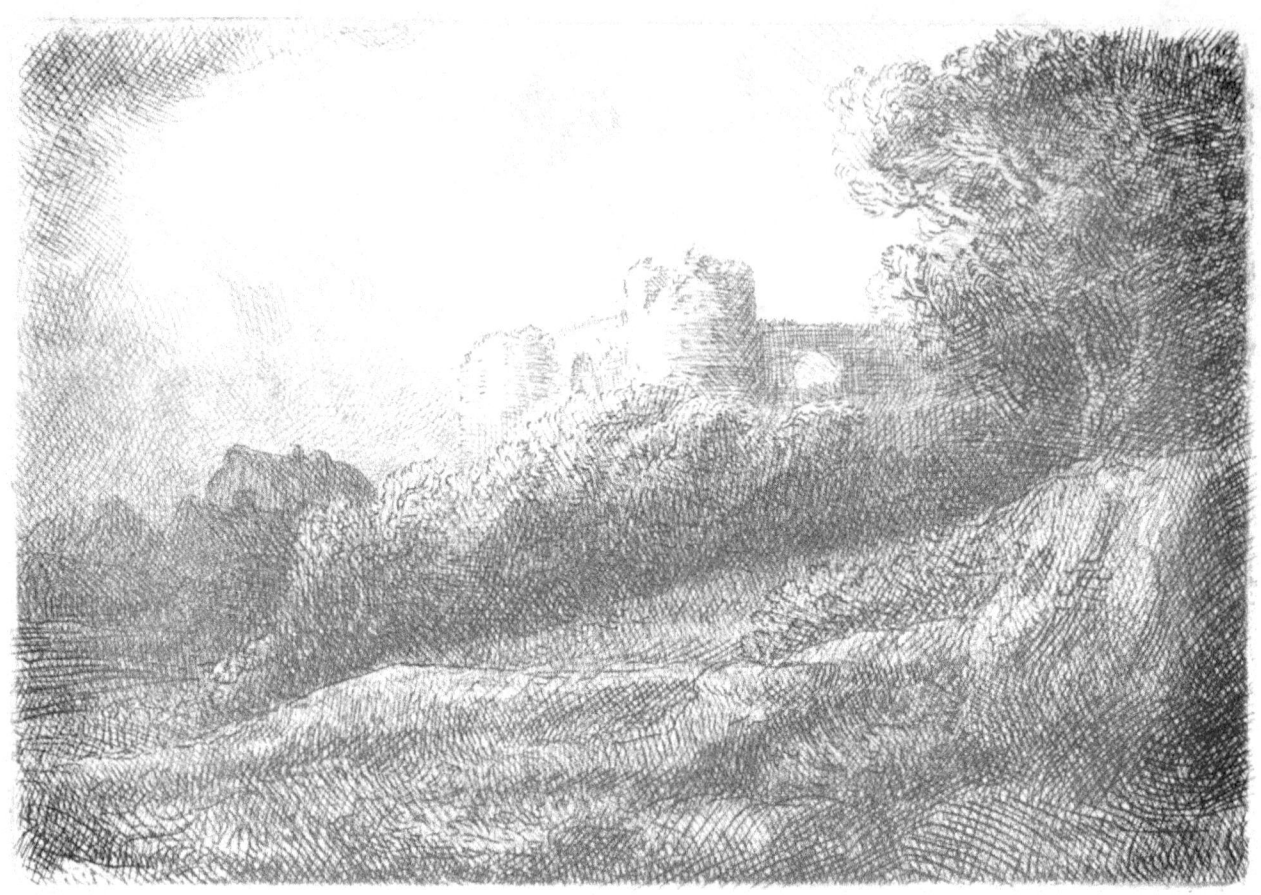

I am healthy

I deserve to be happy

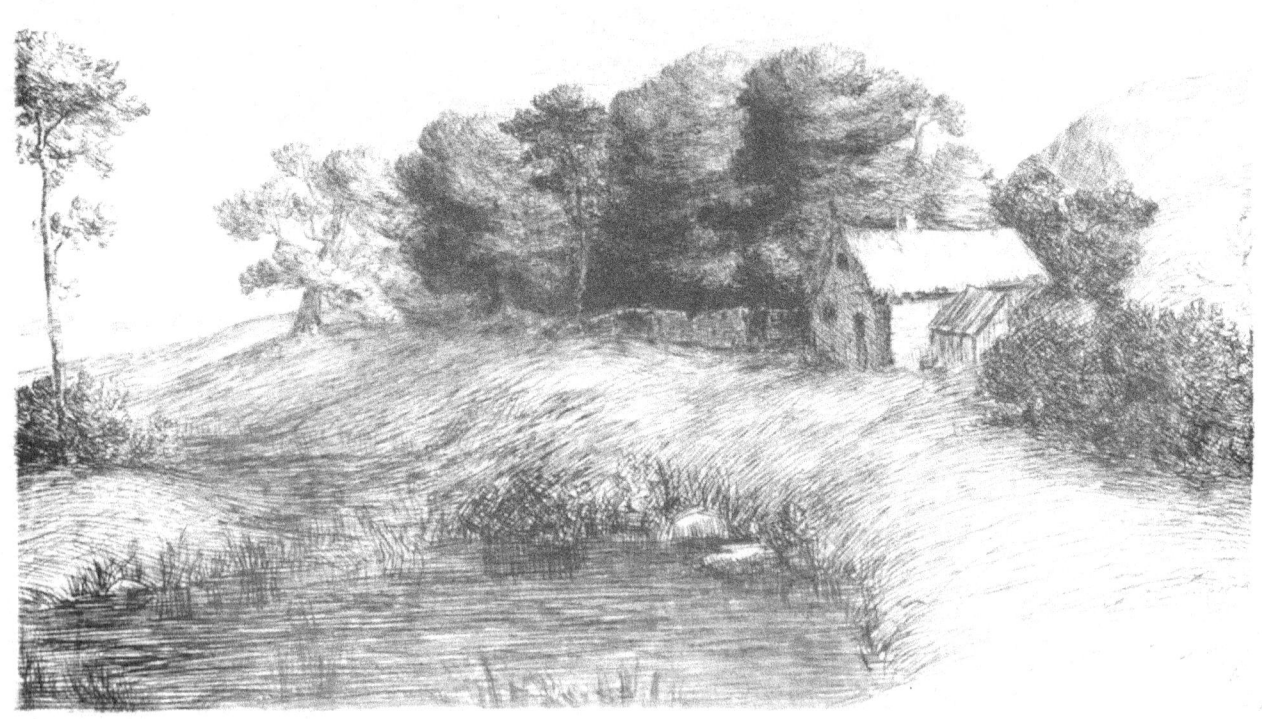

I can become stronger

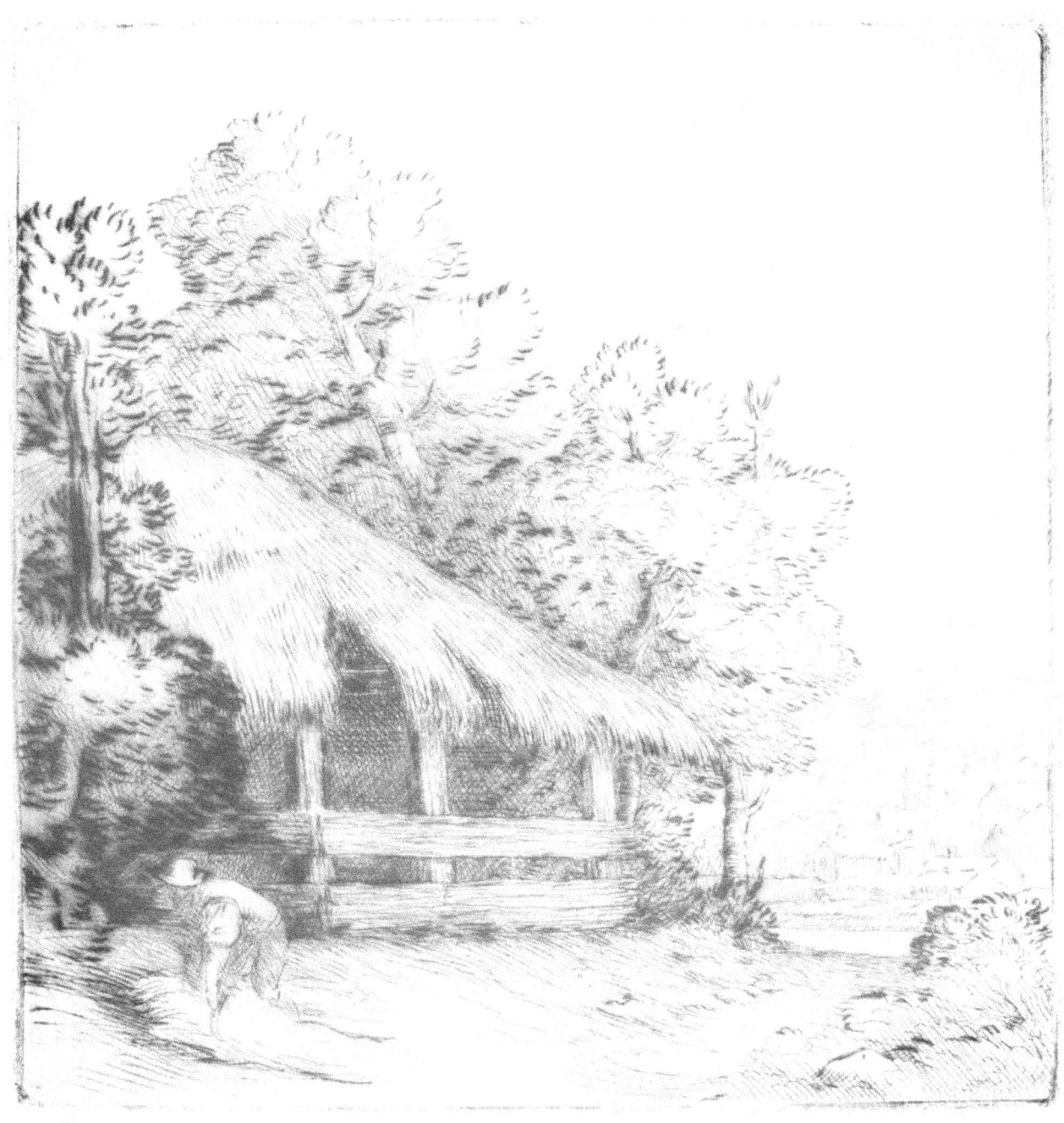

I can trust myself

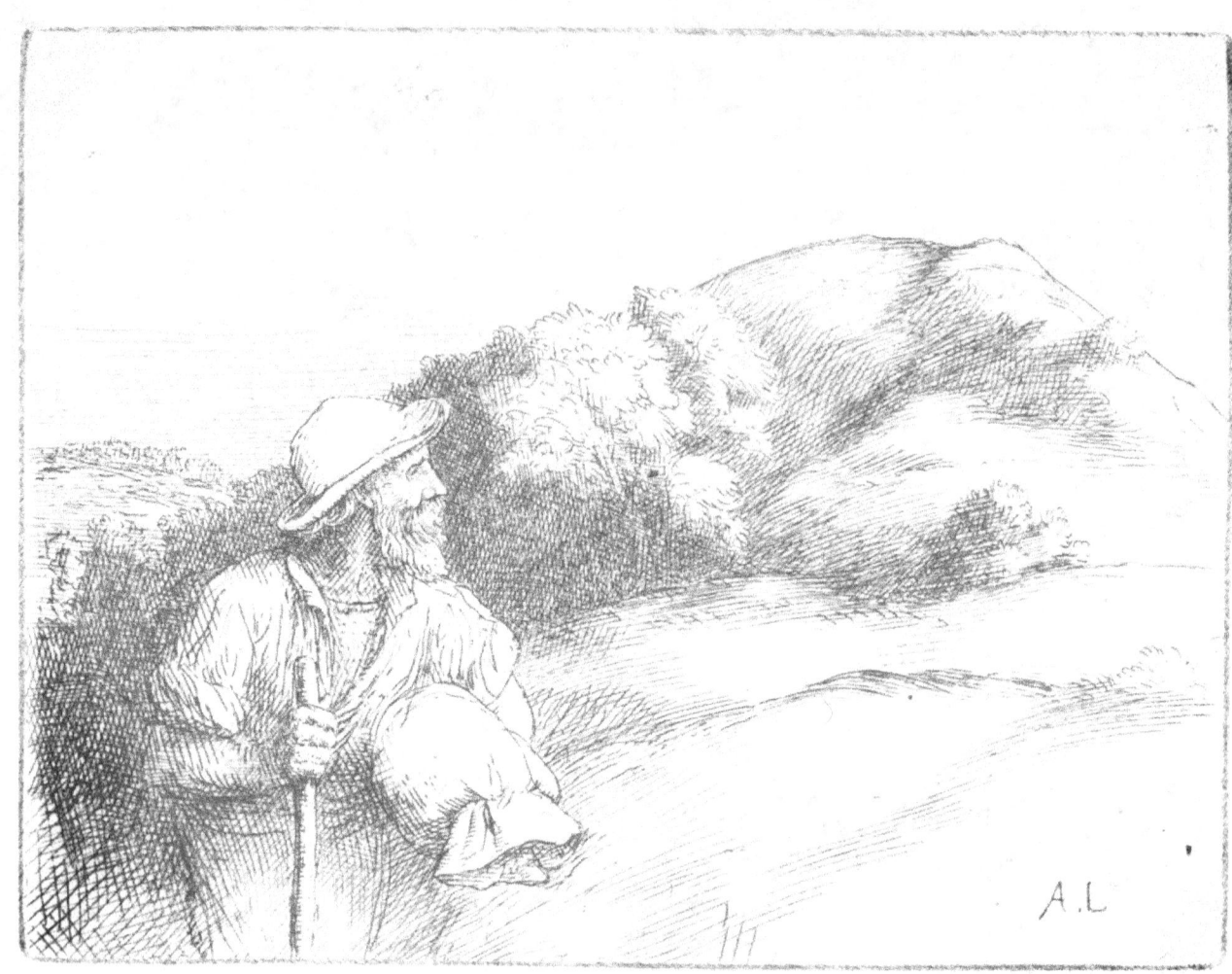

I can succeed

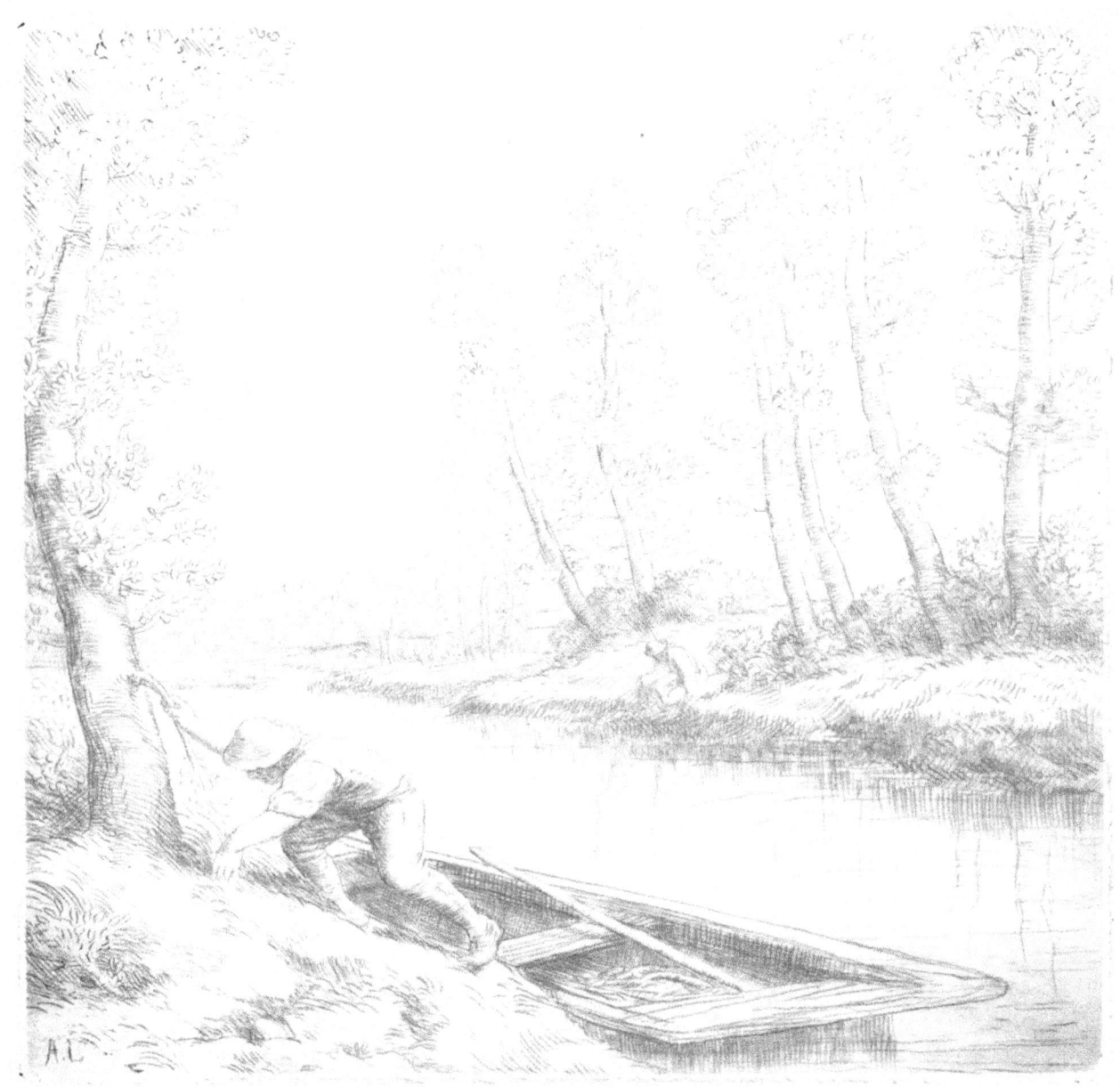

I can choose to let it out

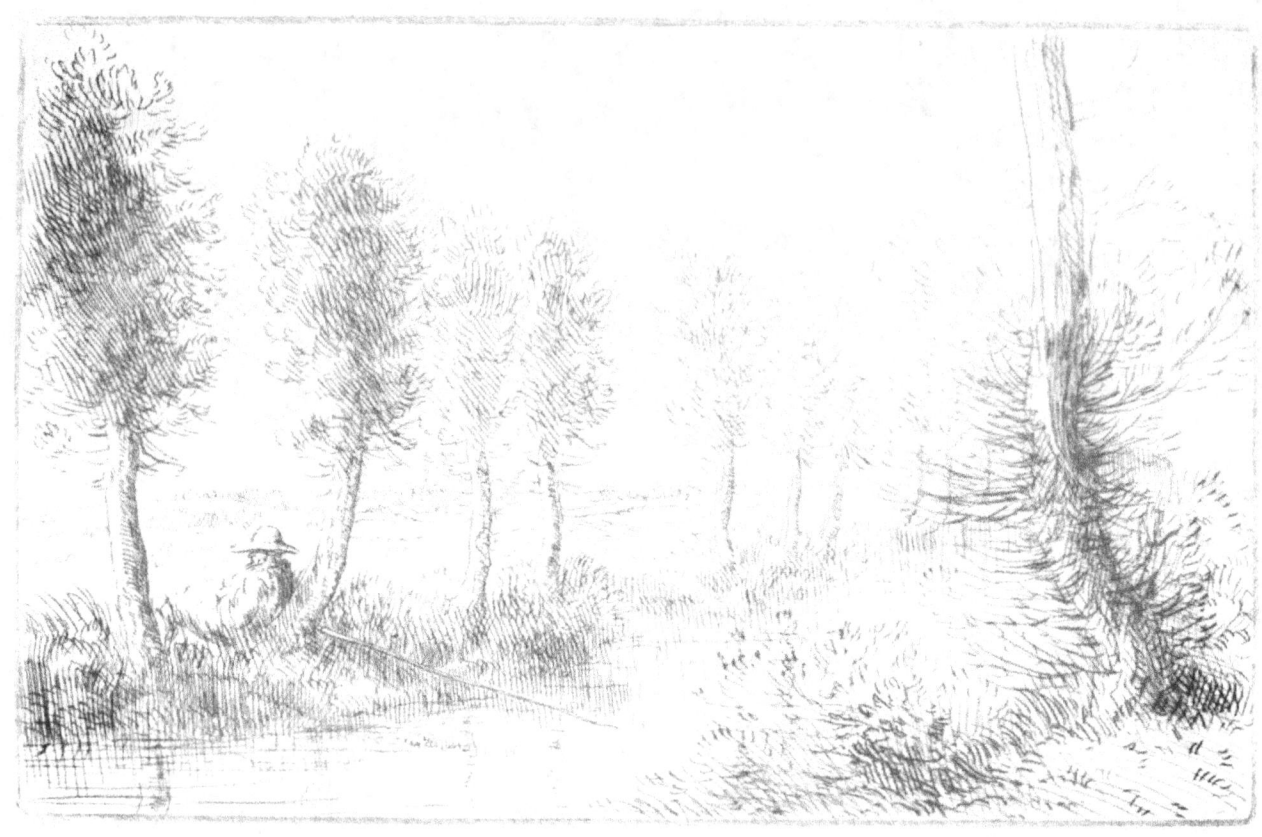

I can learn to take care of myself

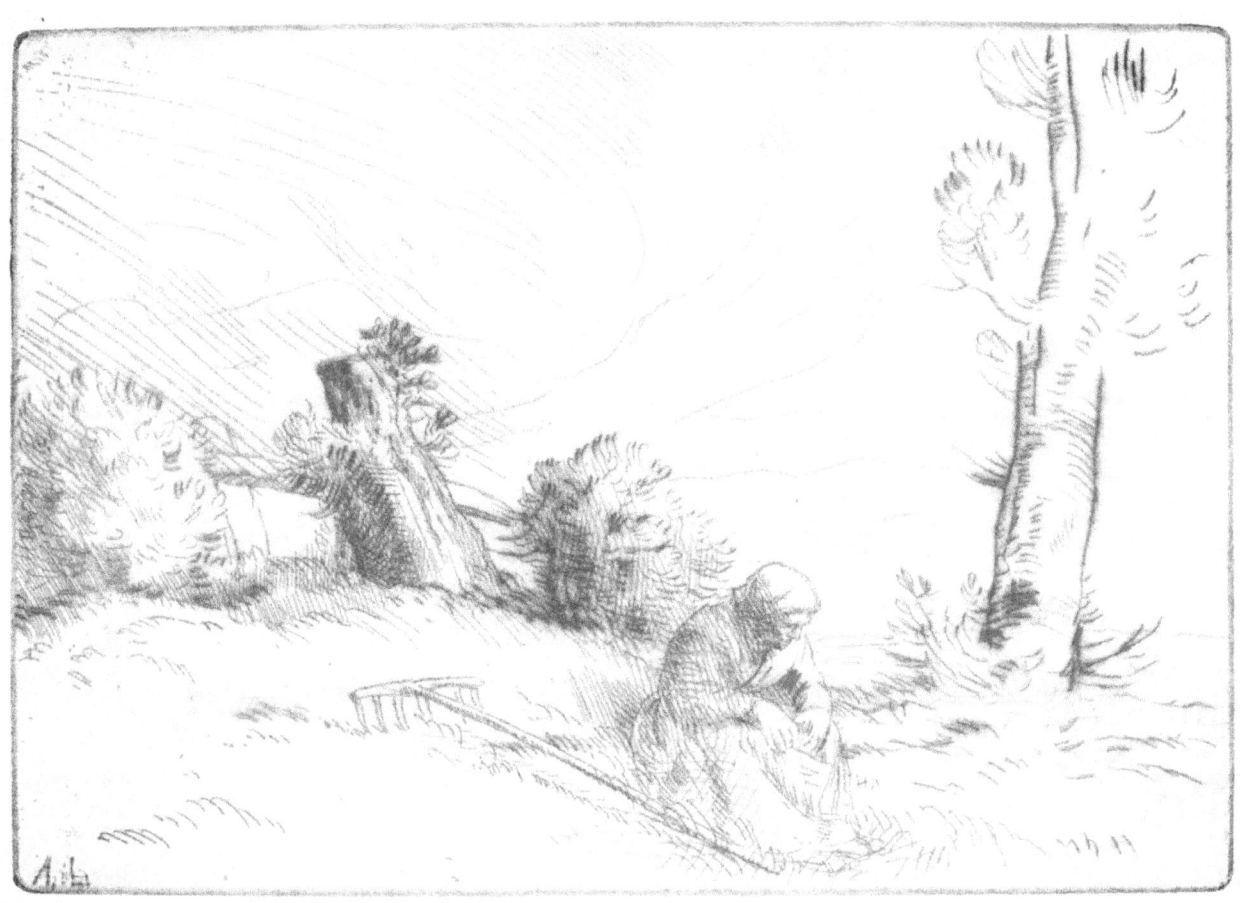

I am important

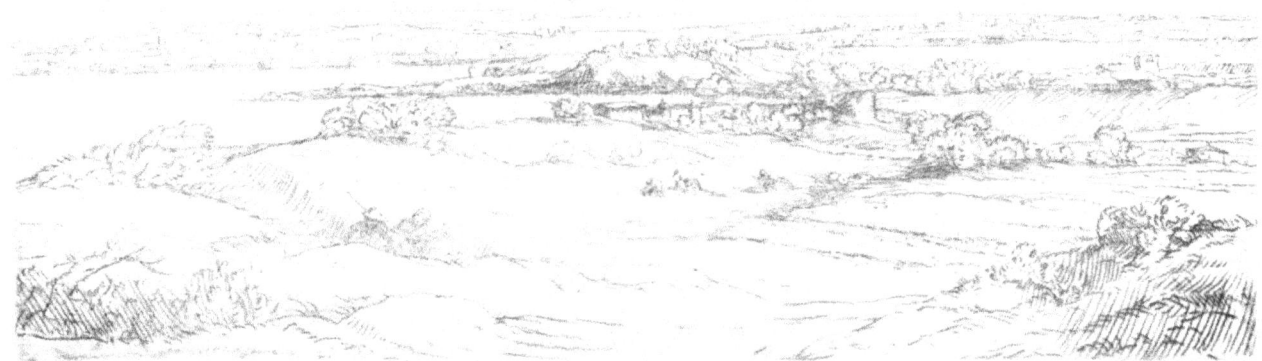

I can make my needs known

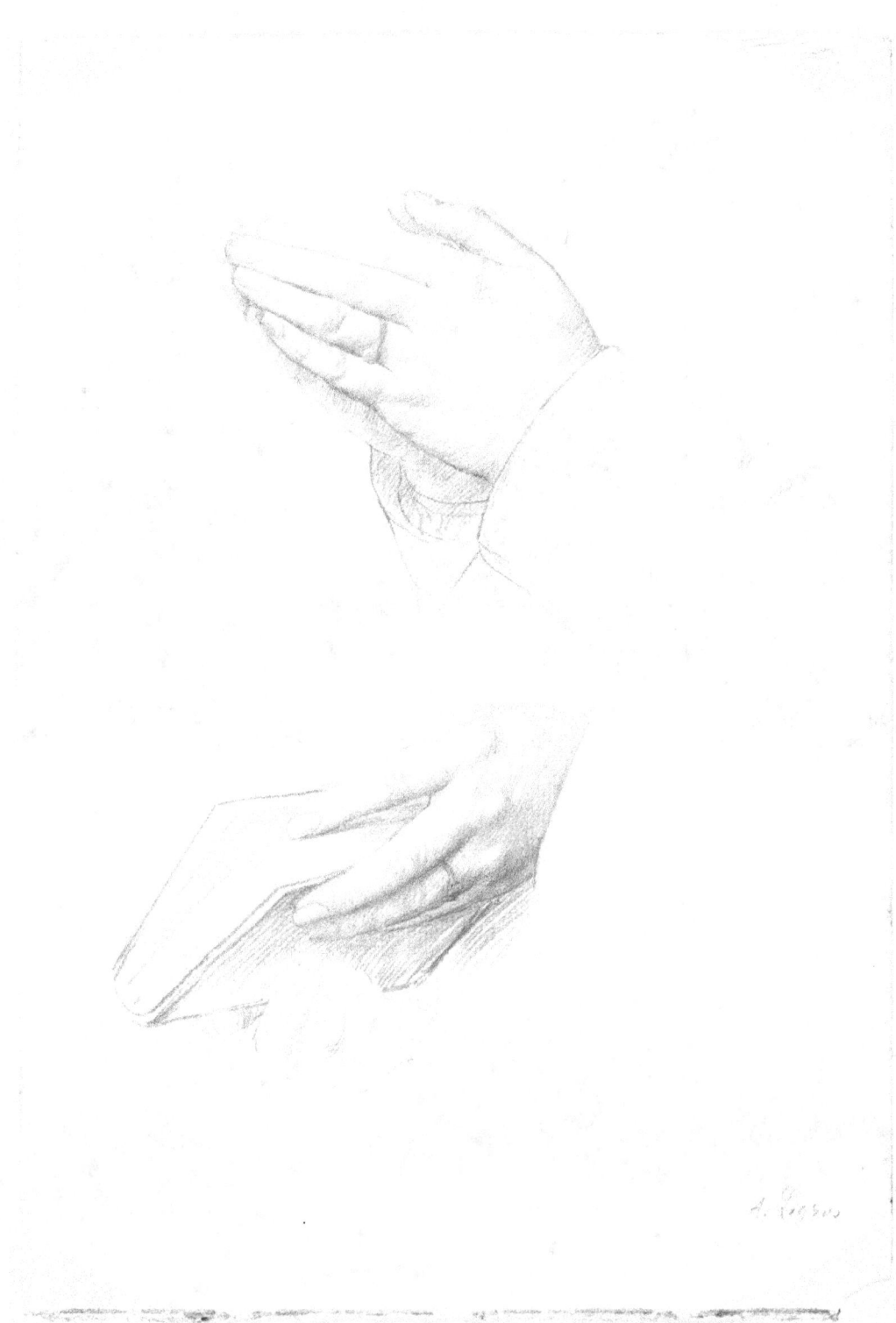

I can choose whom to trust

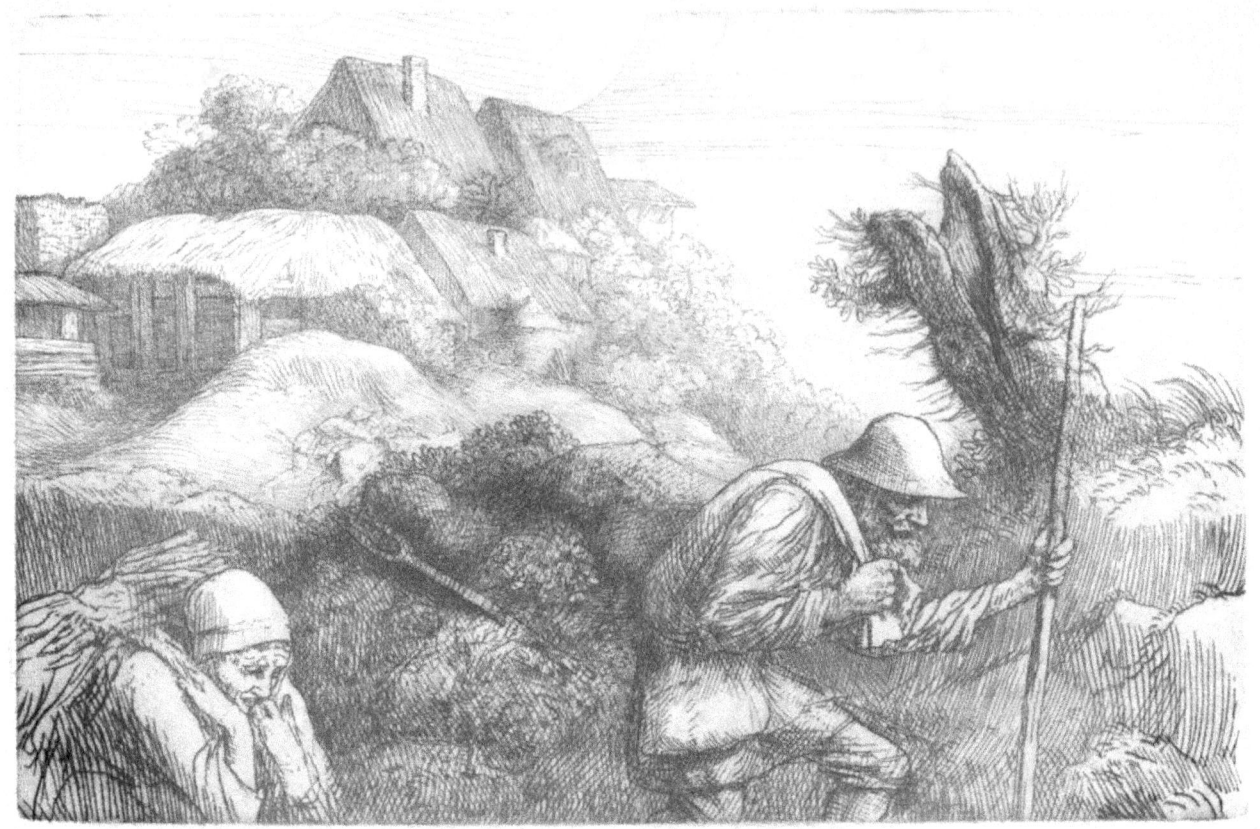

I can be real

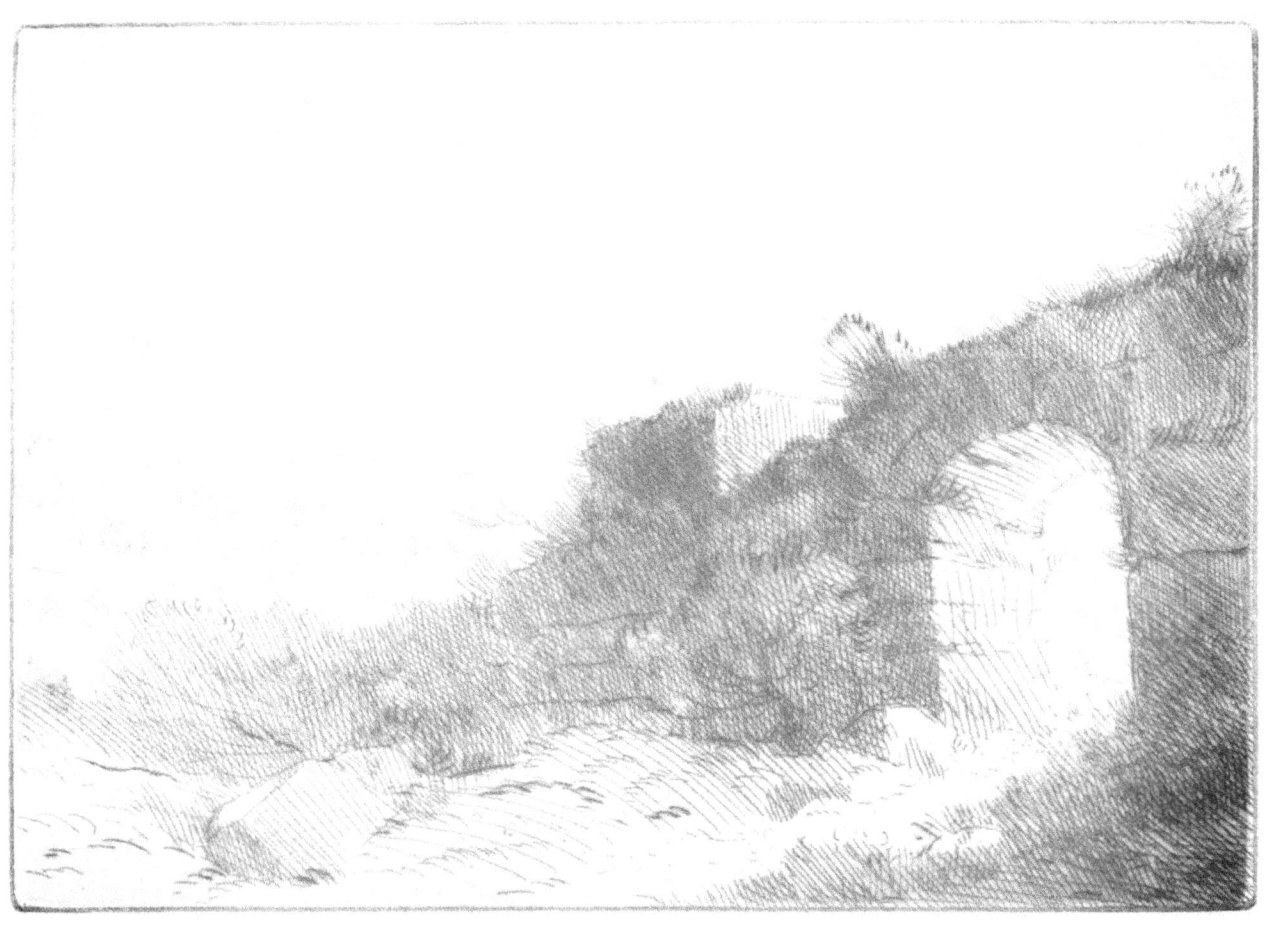

I am okay

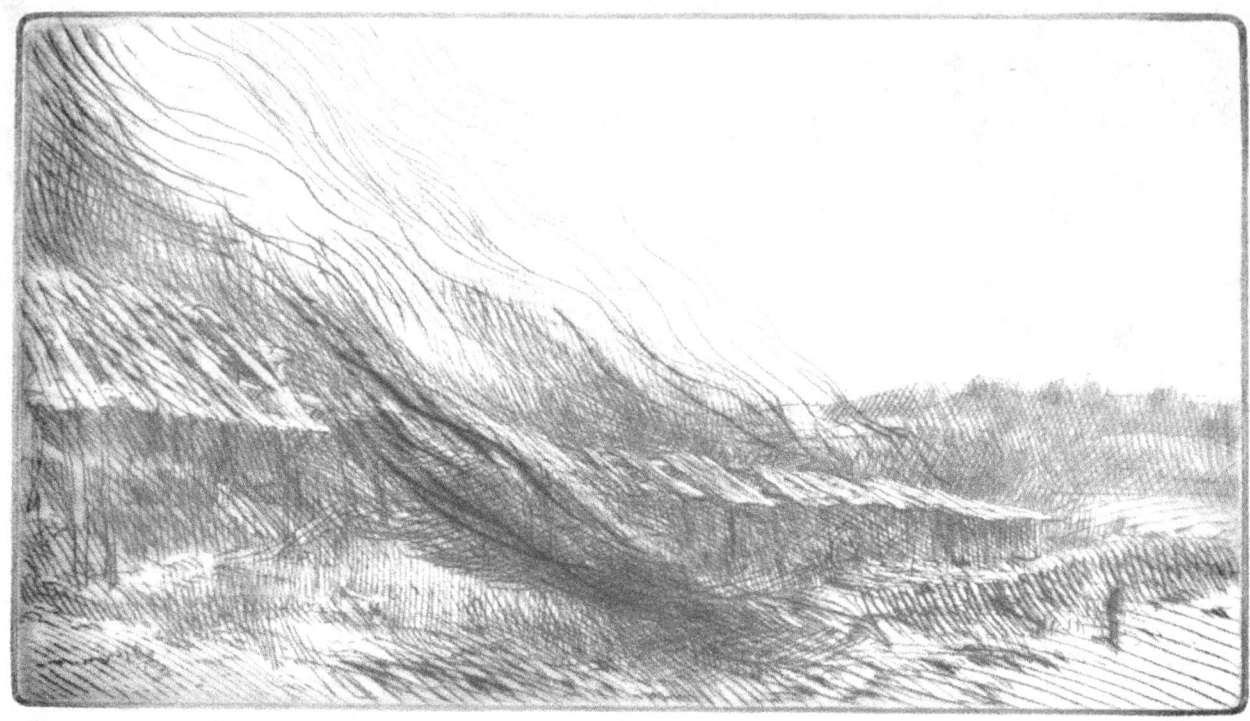

I now have choices

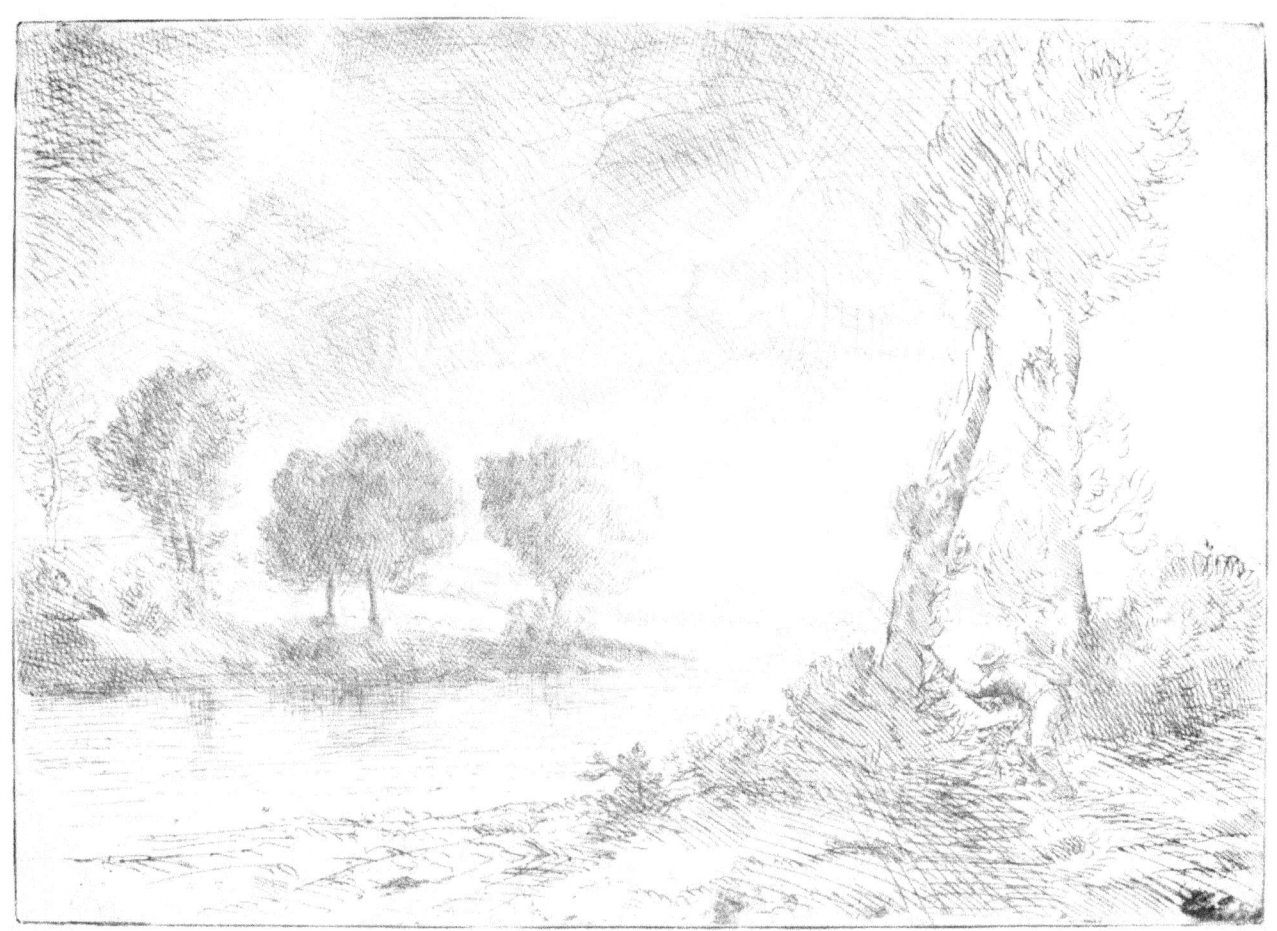

I can take care of myself

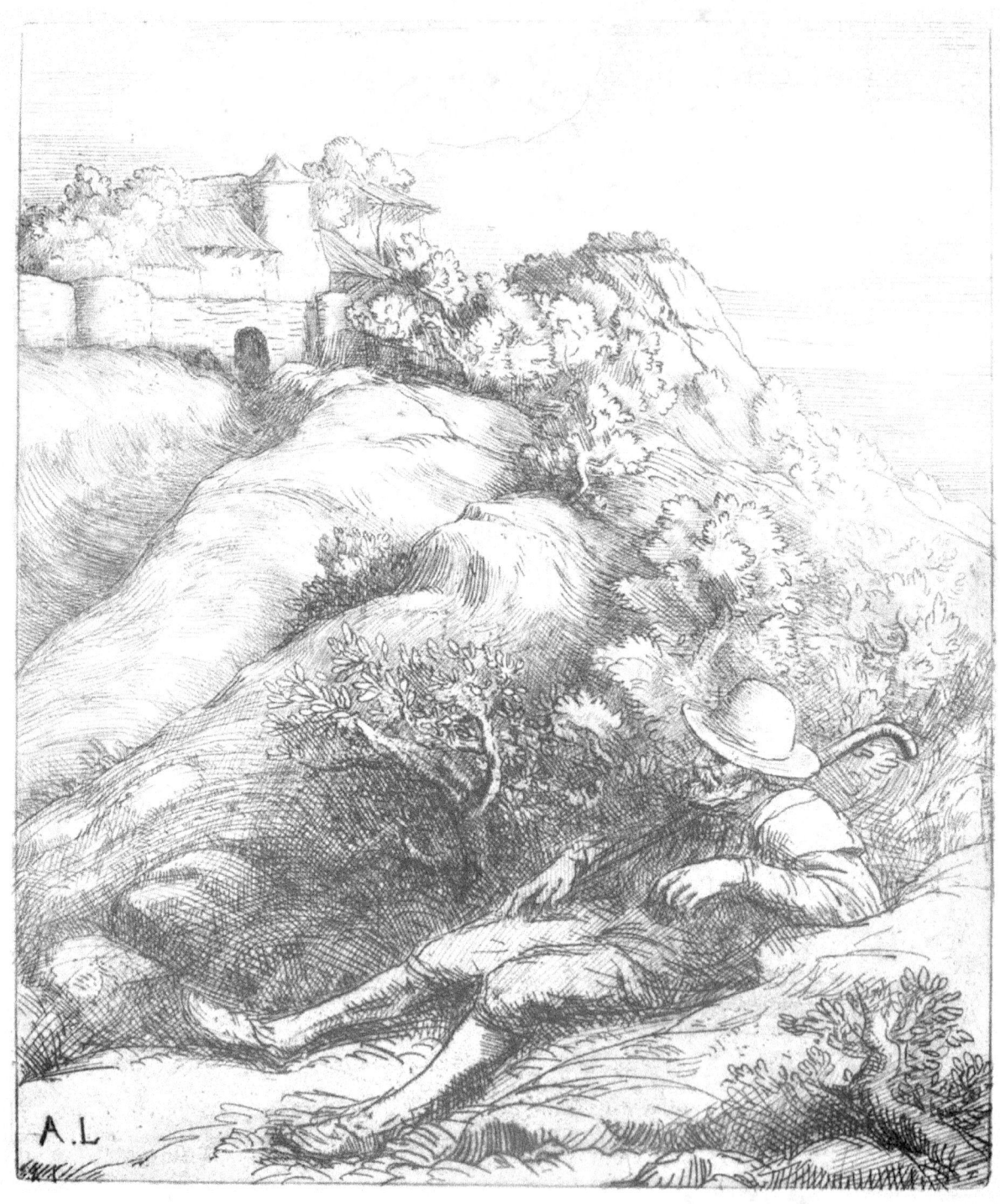

I did the best I could

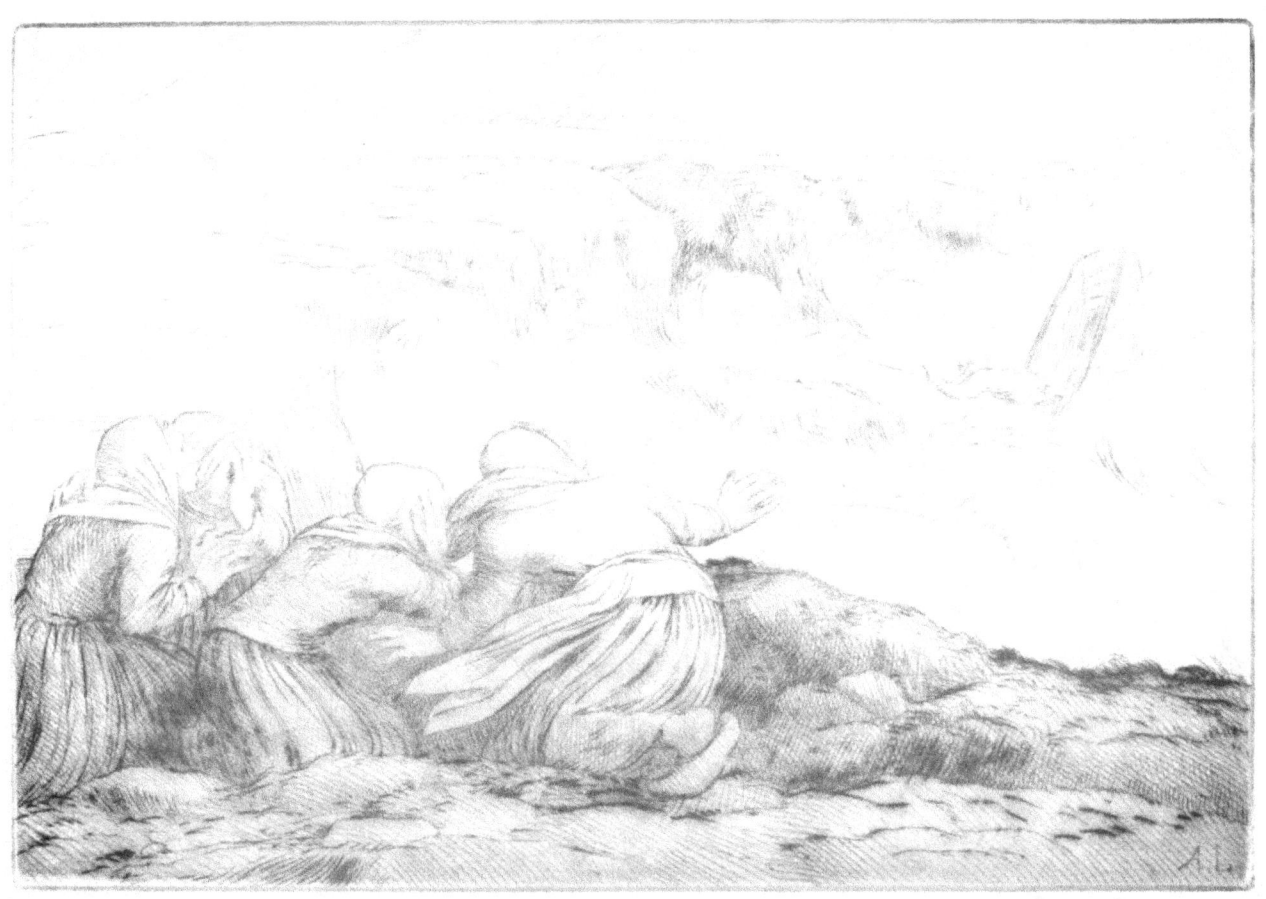

I can learn from it

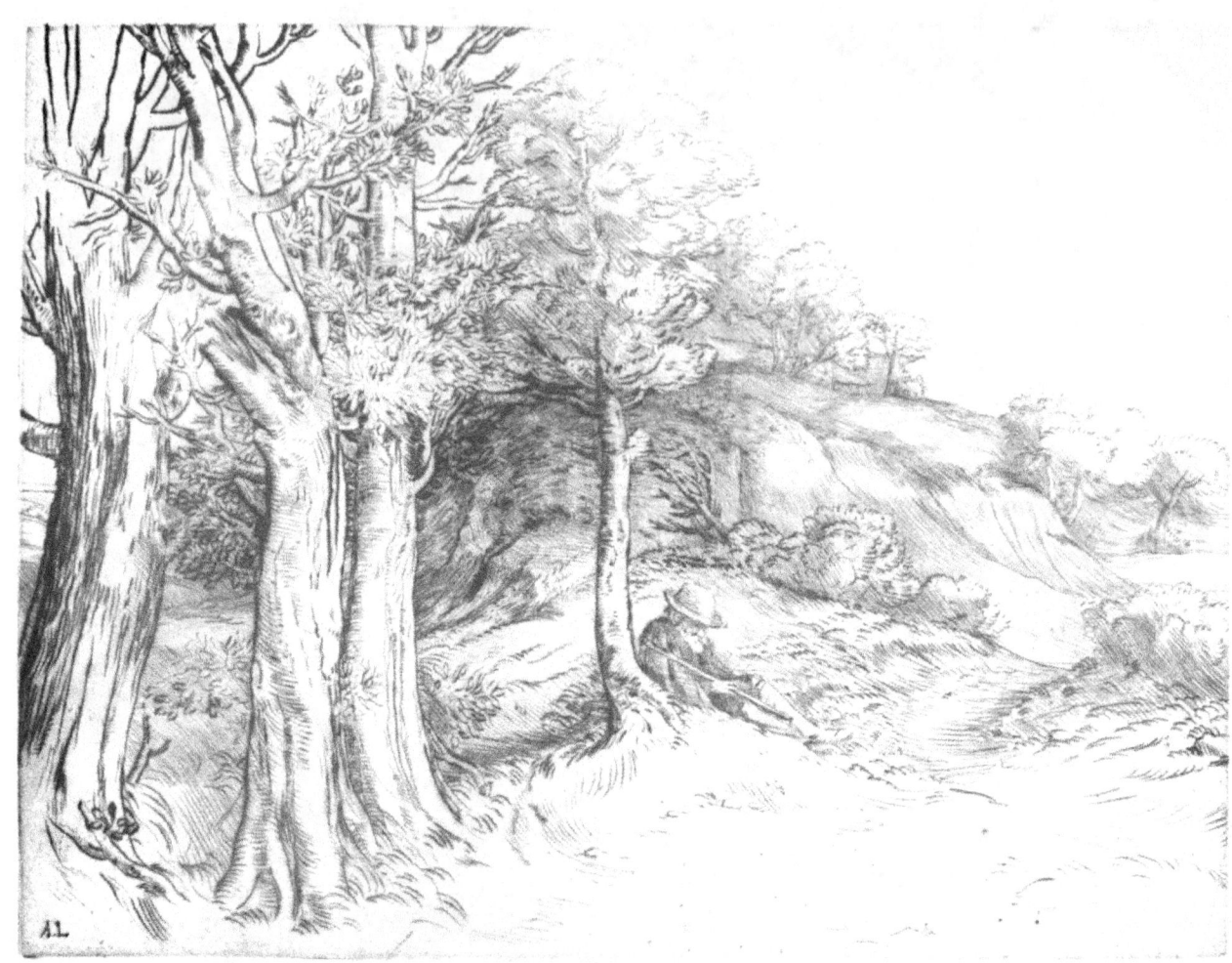

I am lovable

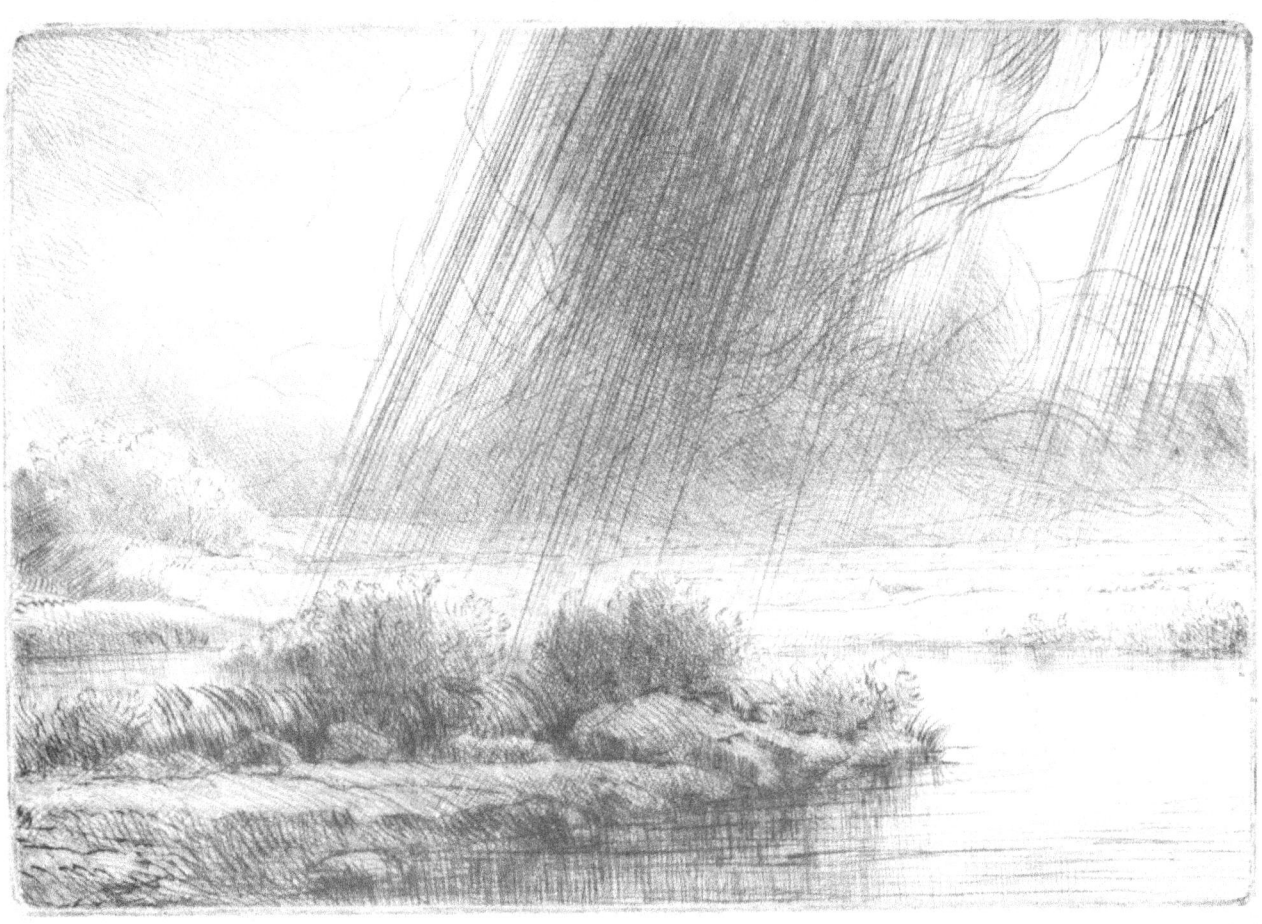

I am beautiful

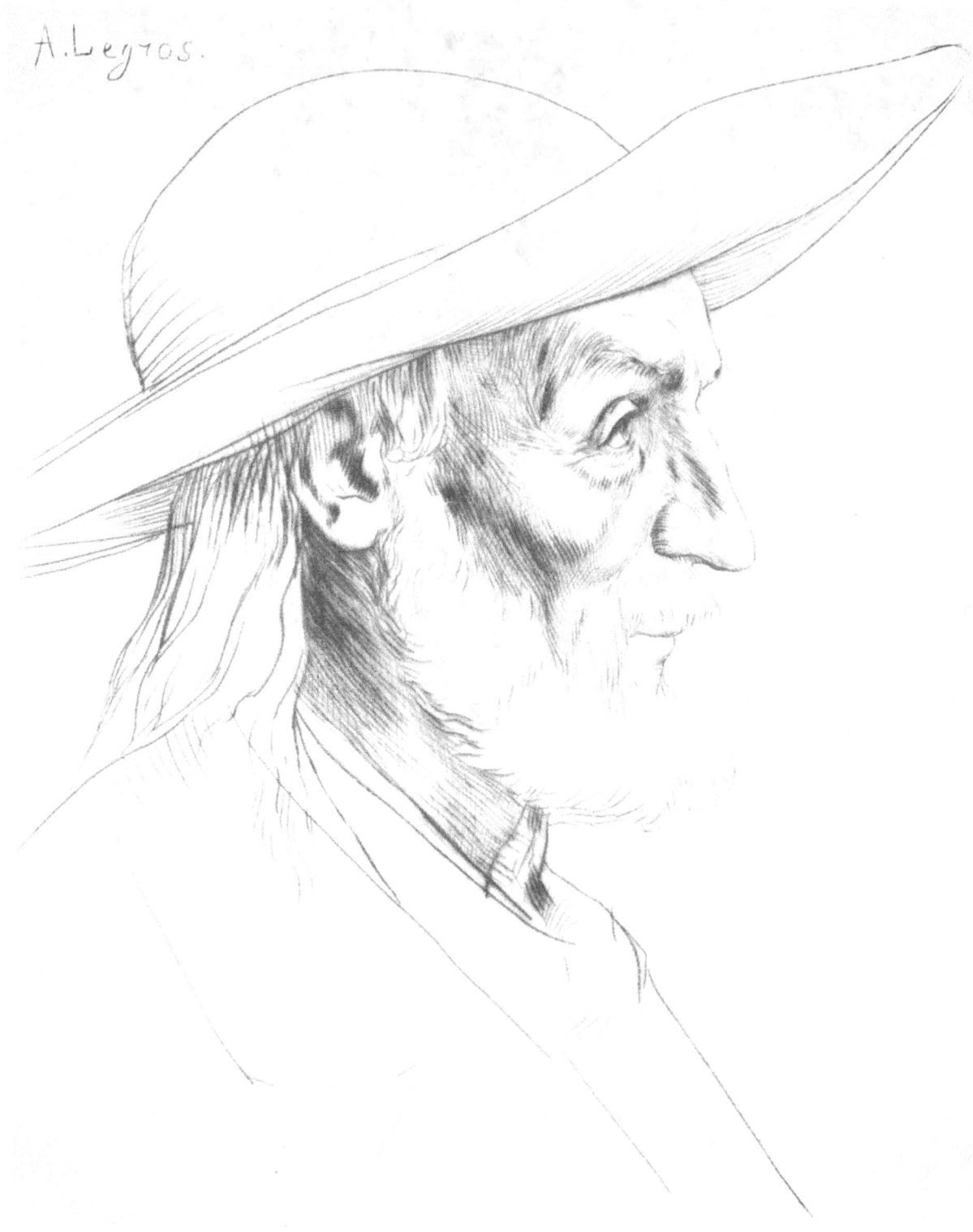

I am significant

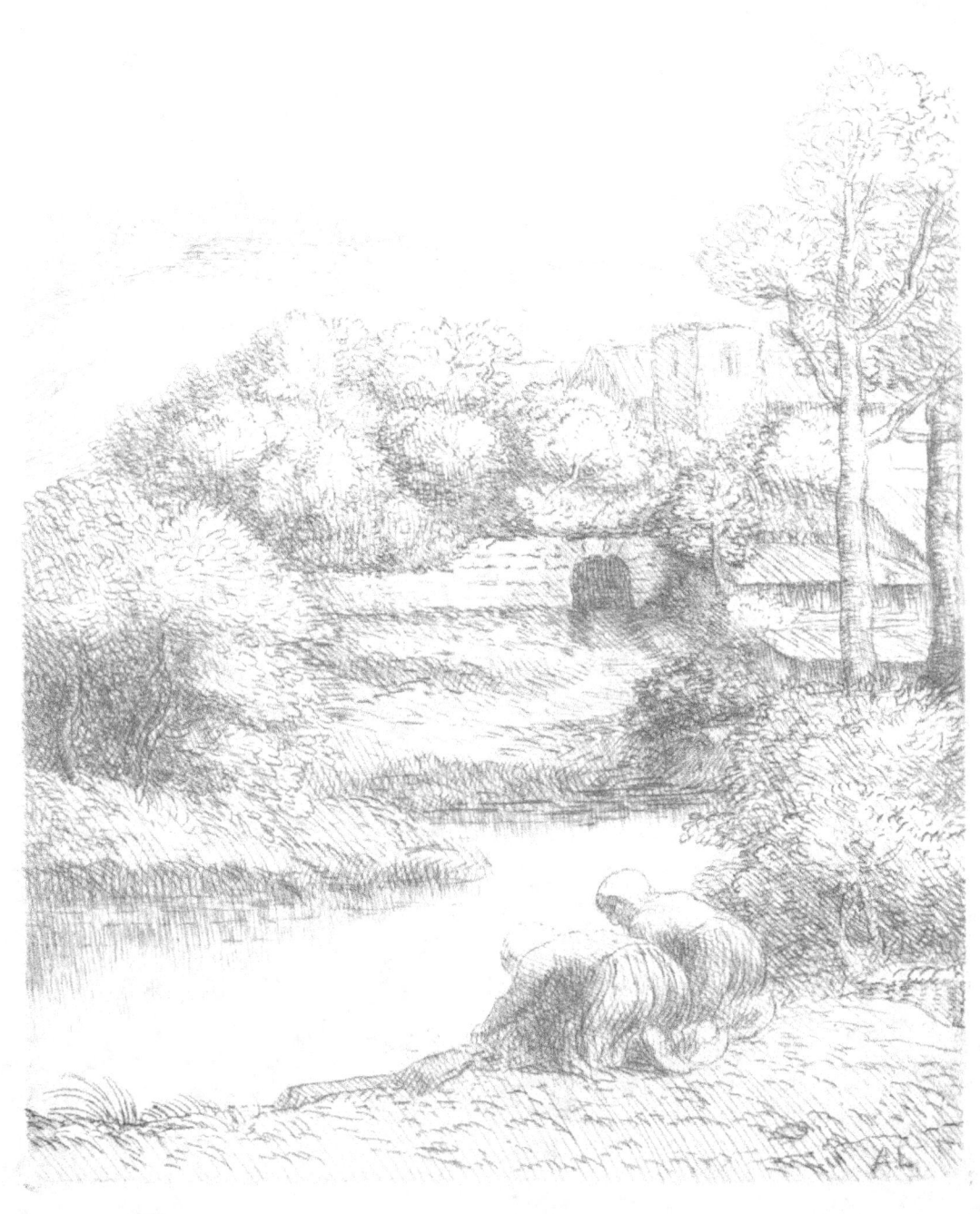

I learned from it

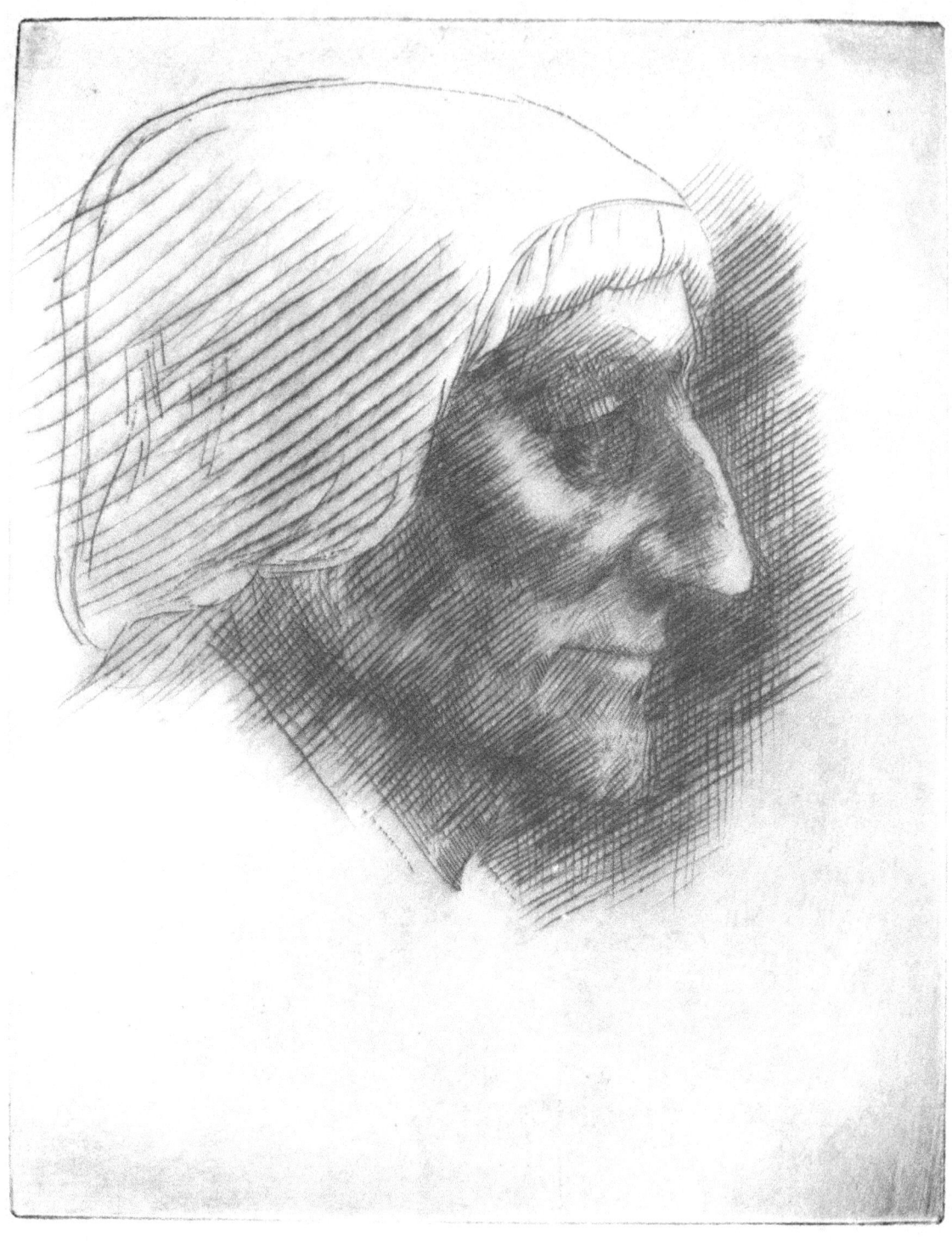

I can safely show my emotions

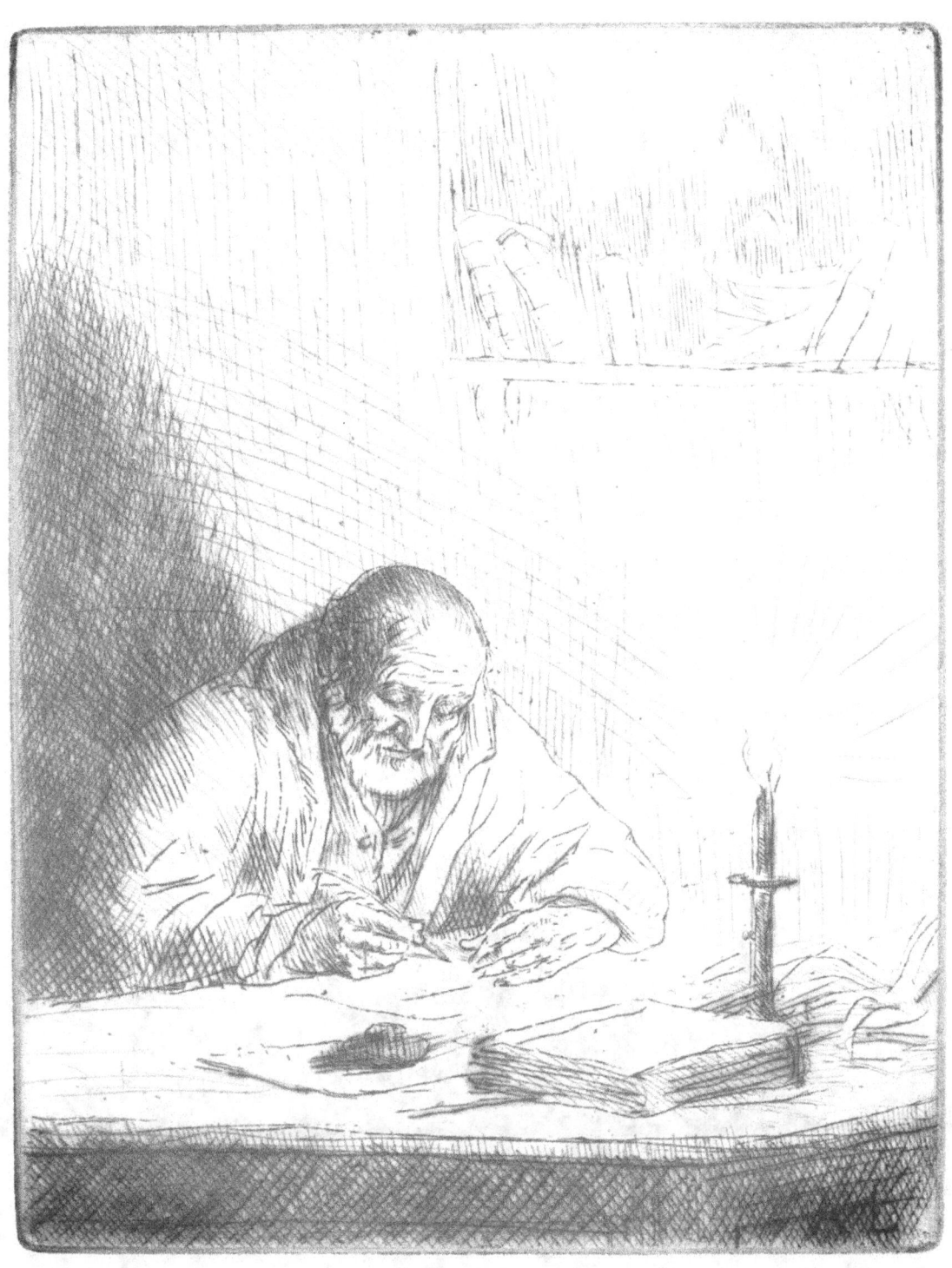

I deserve good things

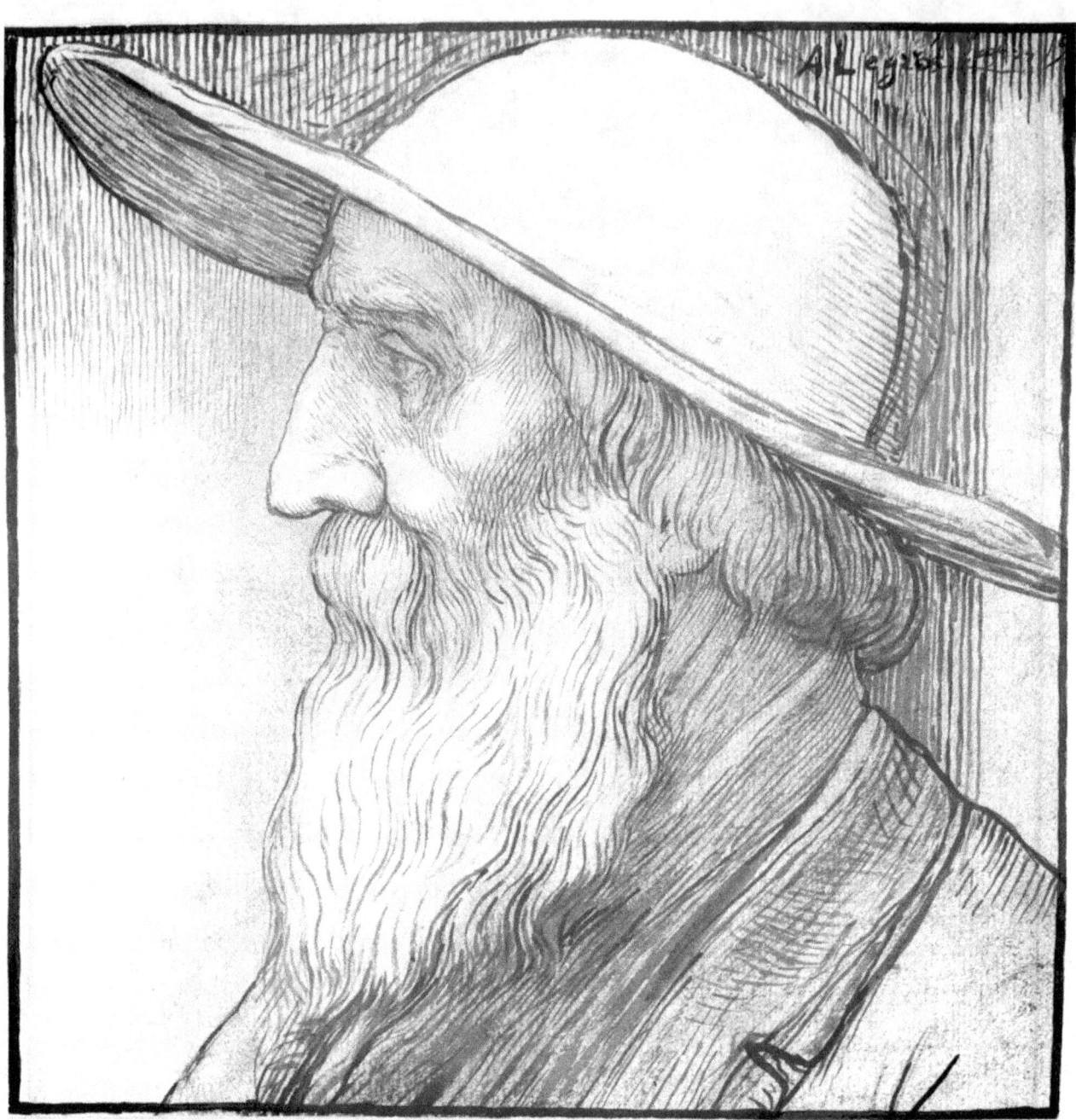

I can be whole

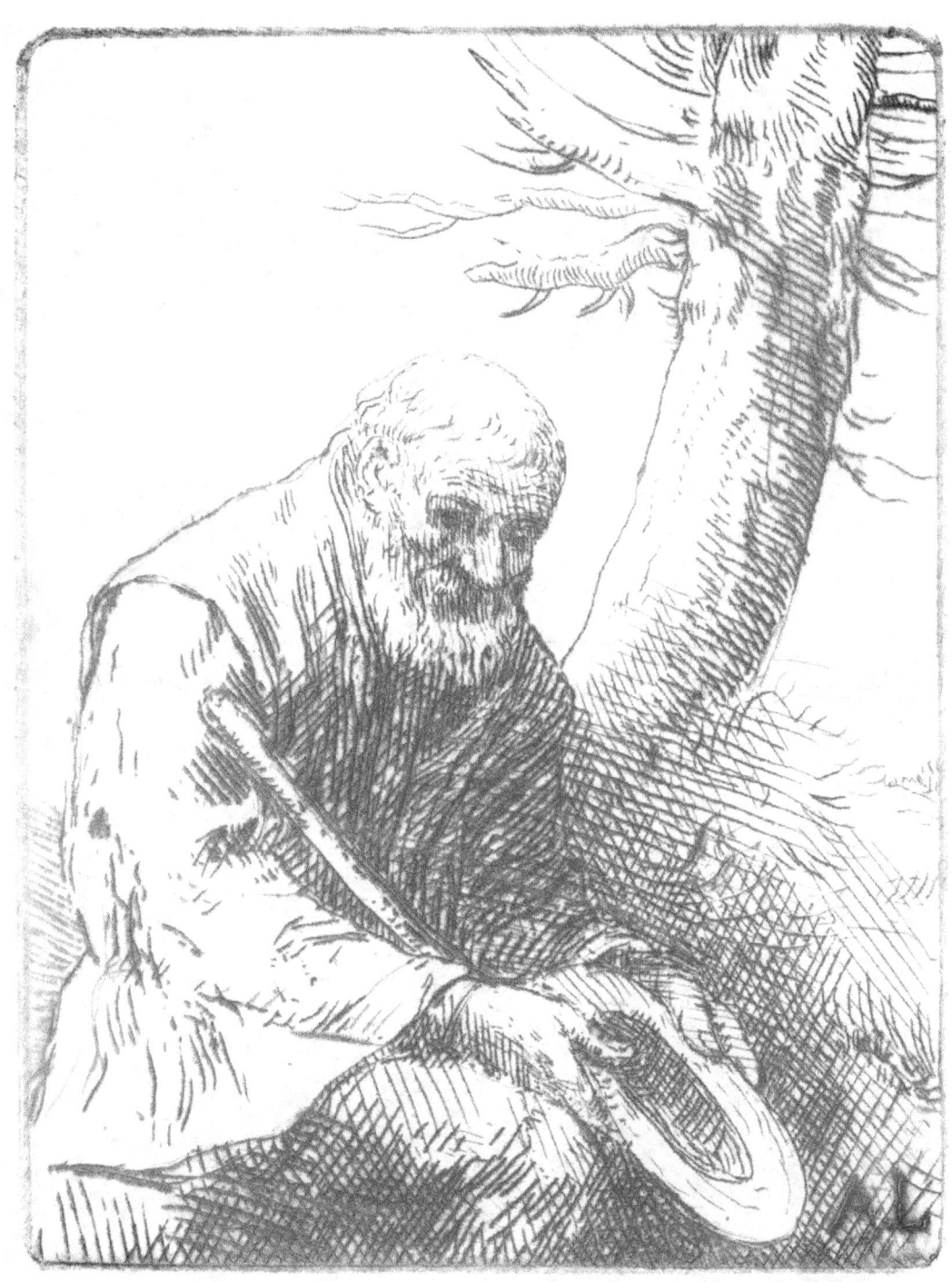

I can express myself

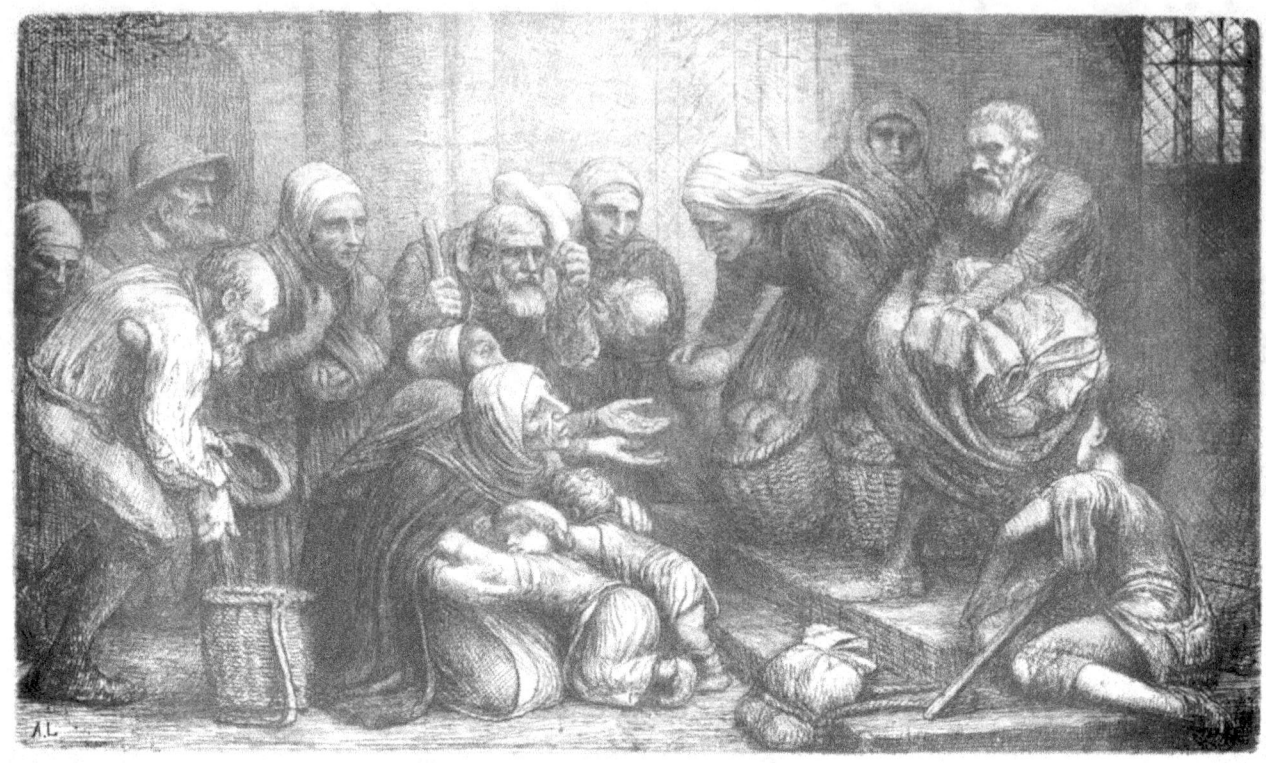

I can safely feel my emotions

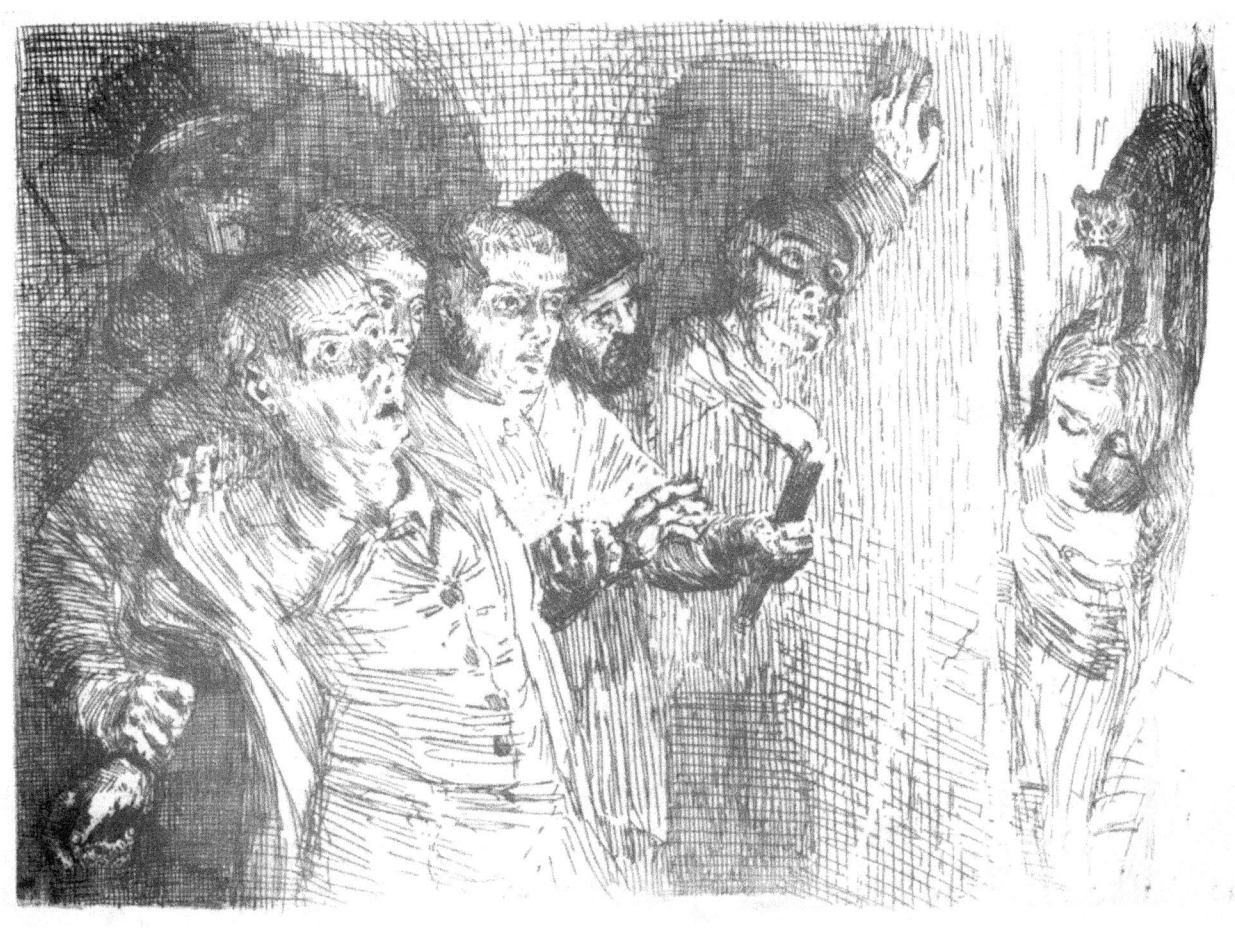

I can grow

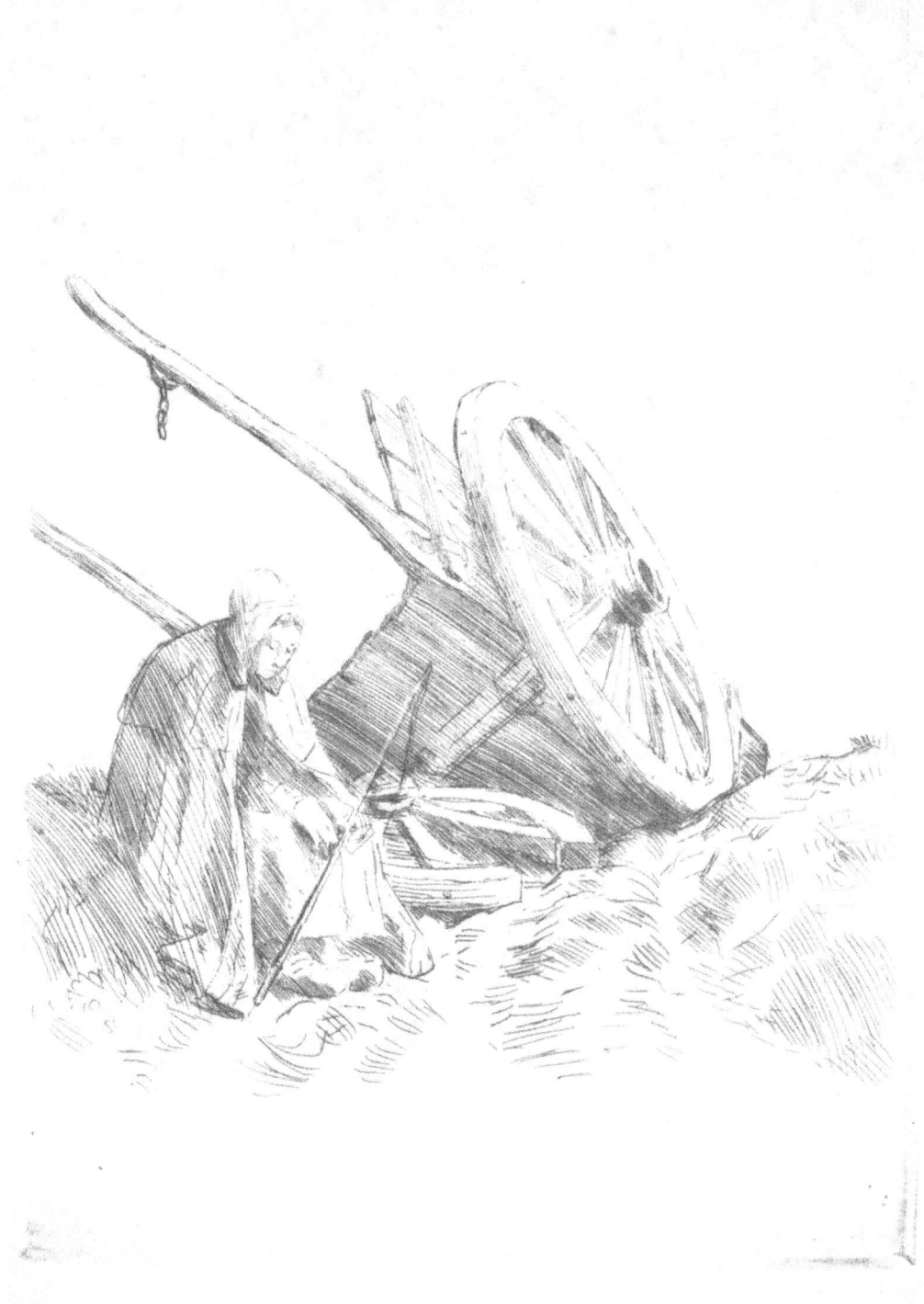

I am worthy

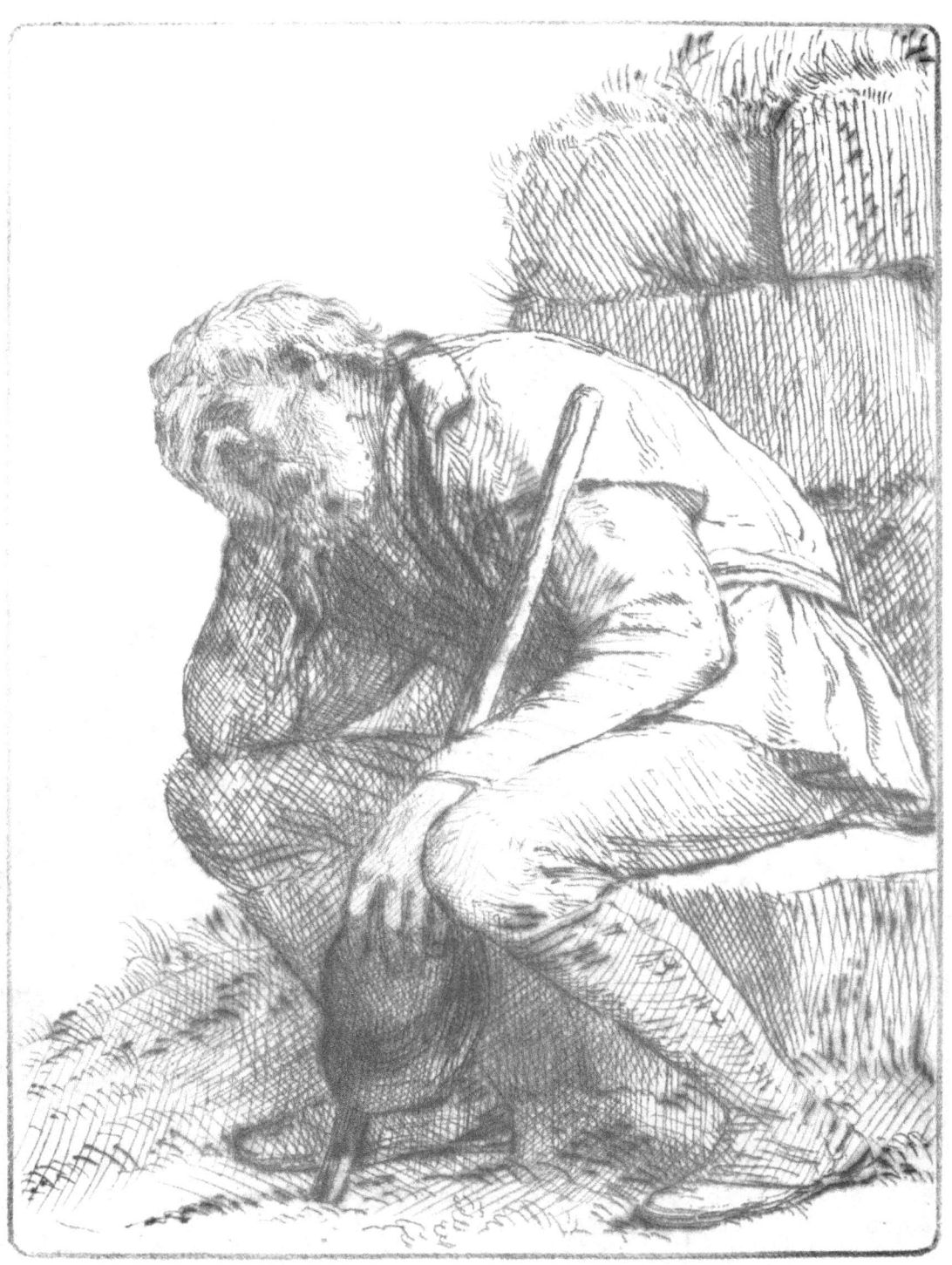

I am worthwhile

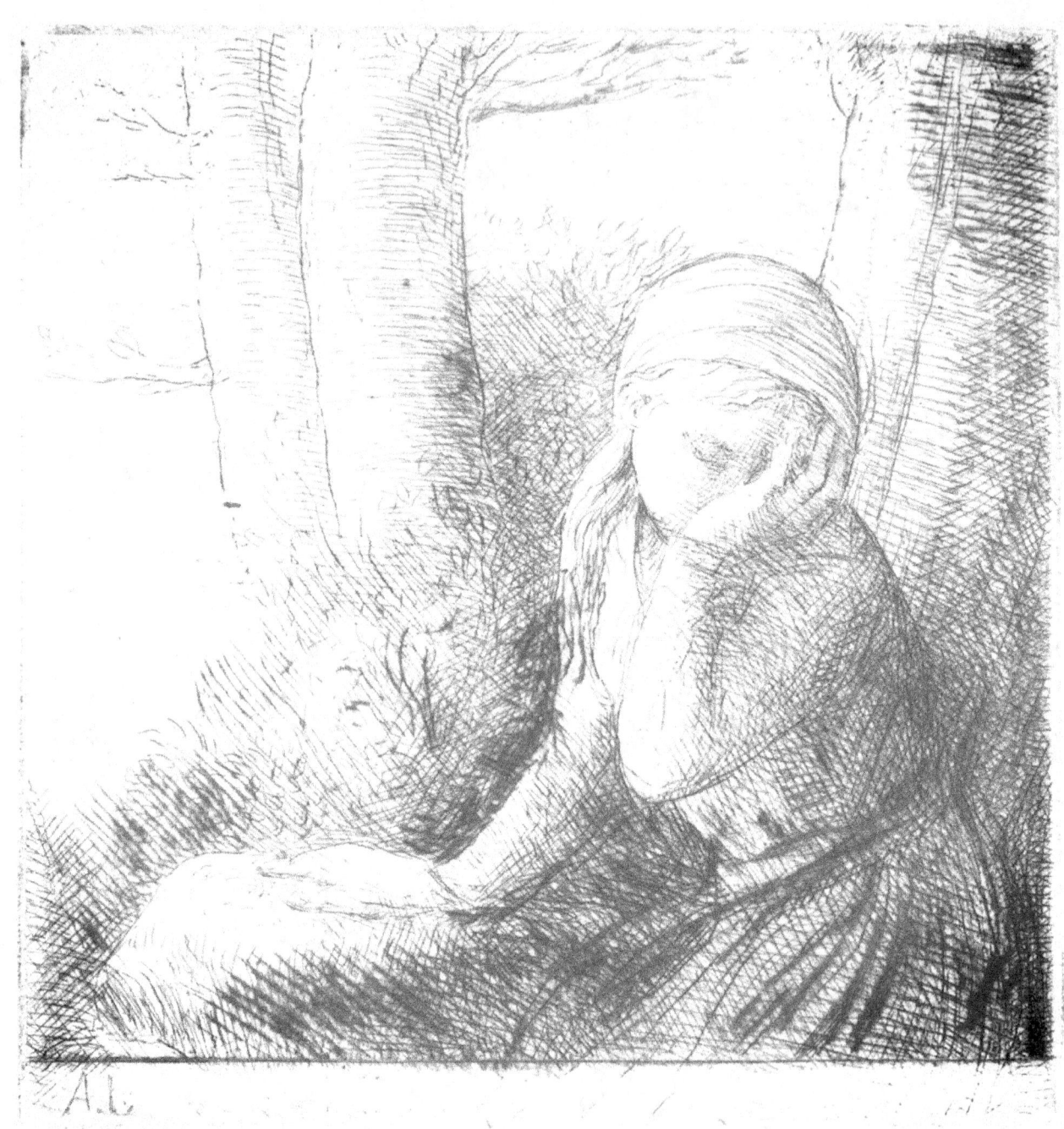

I am radiant

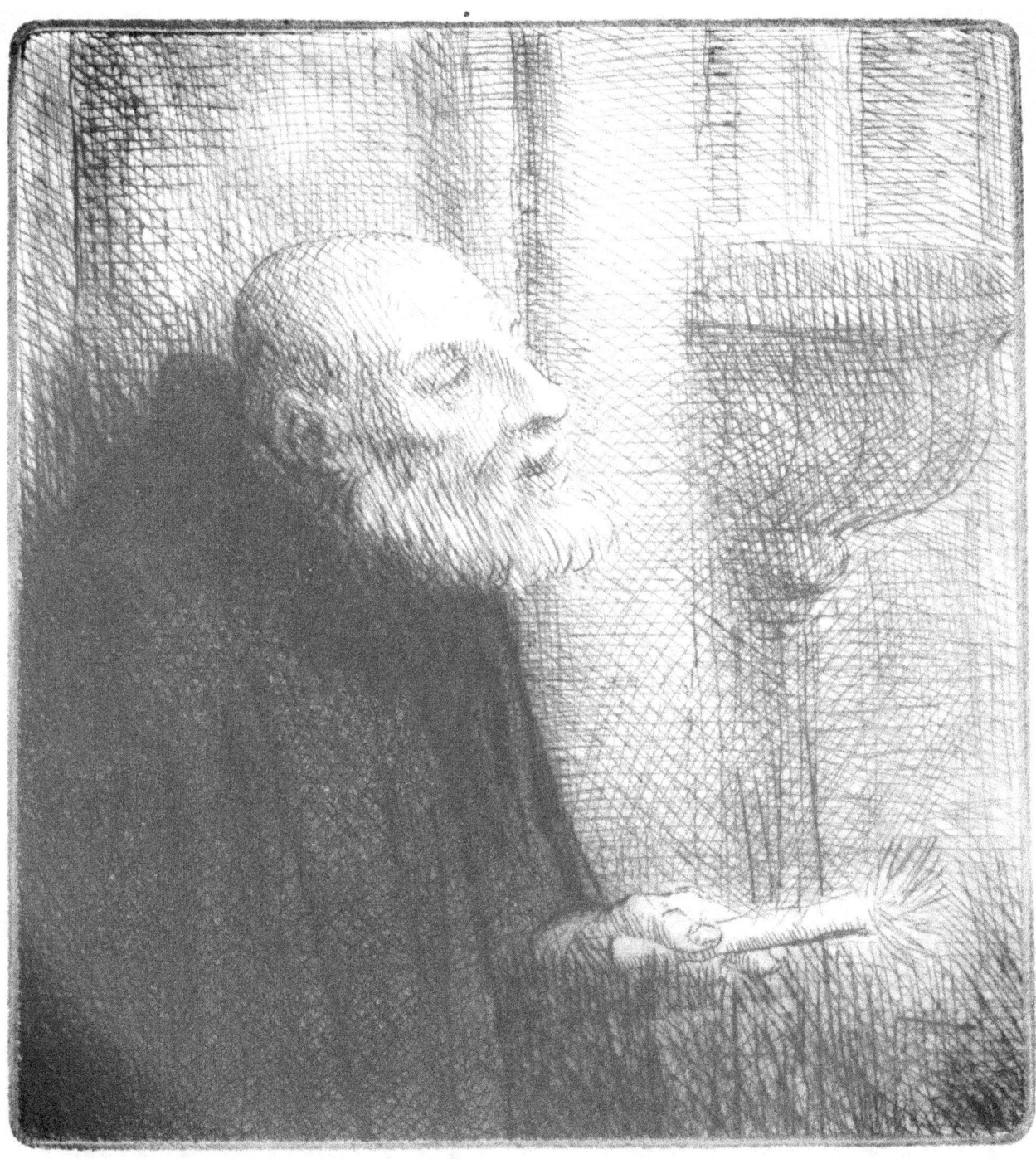

I survived

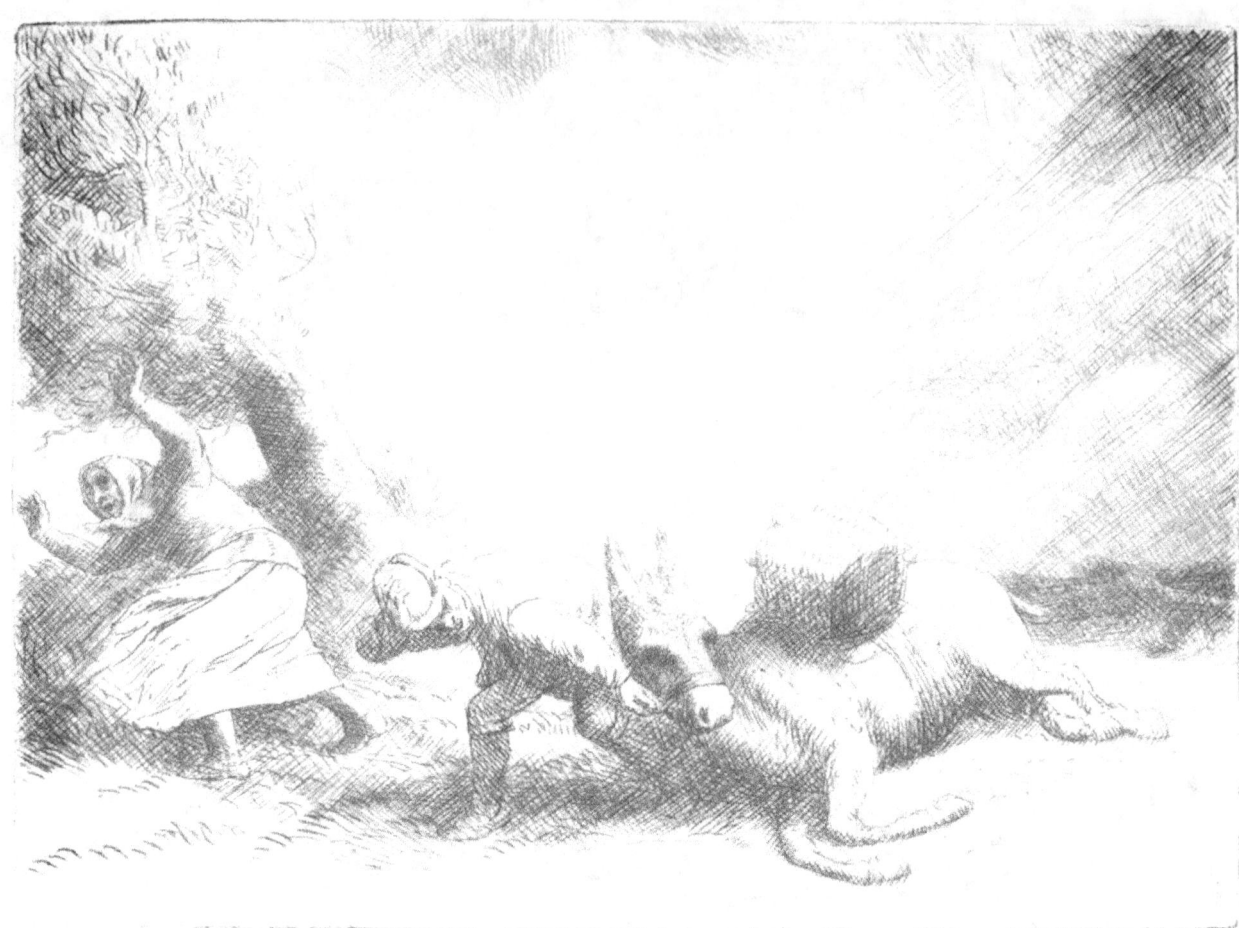

I matter

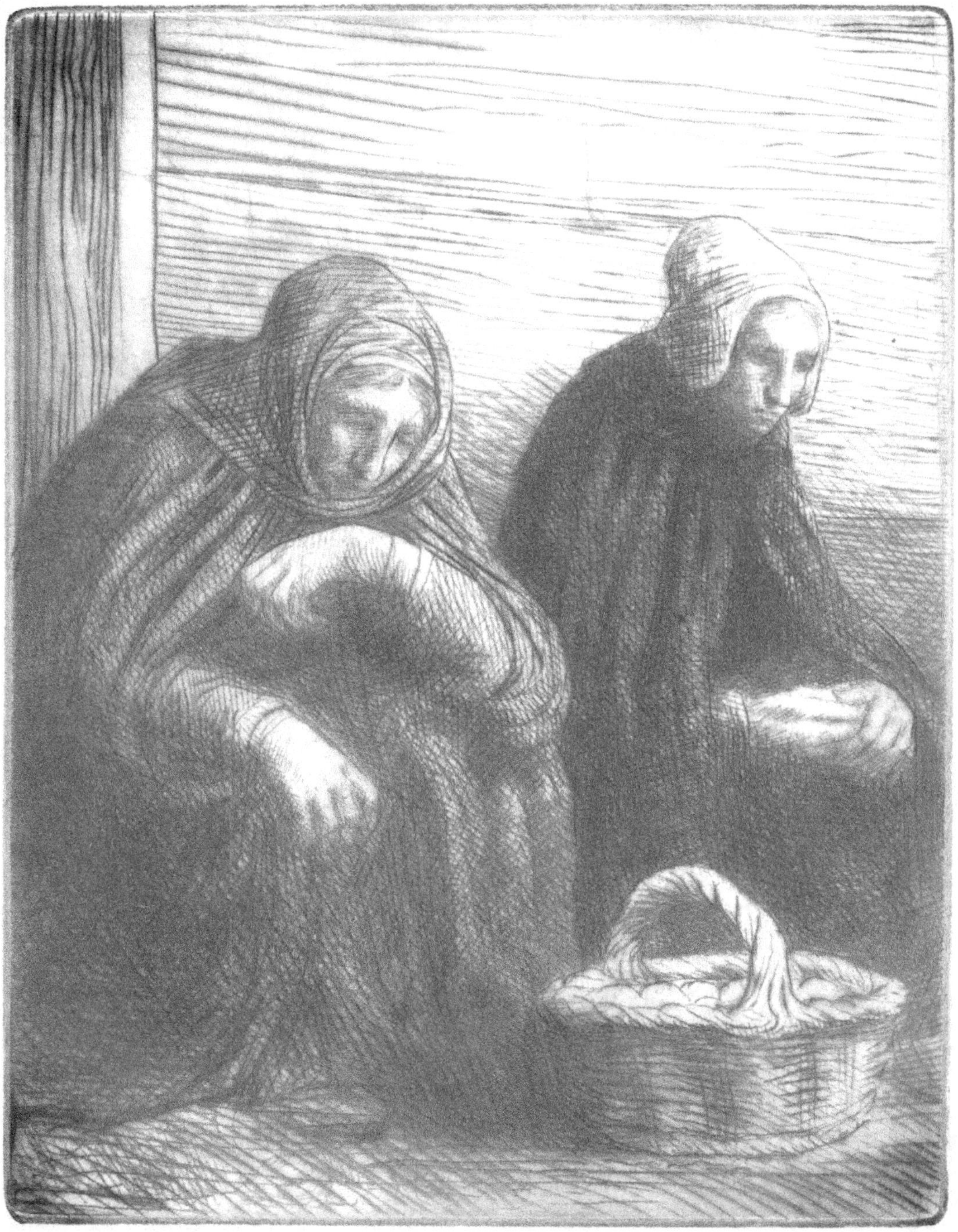

I can trust my judgment

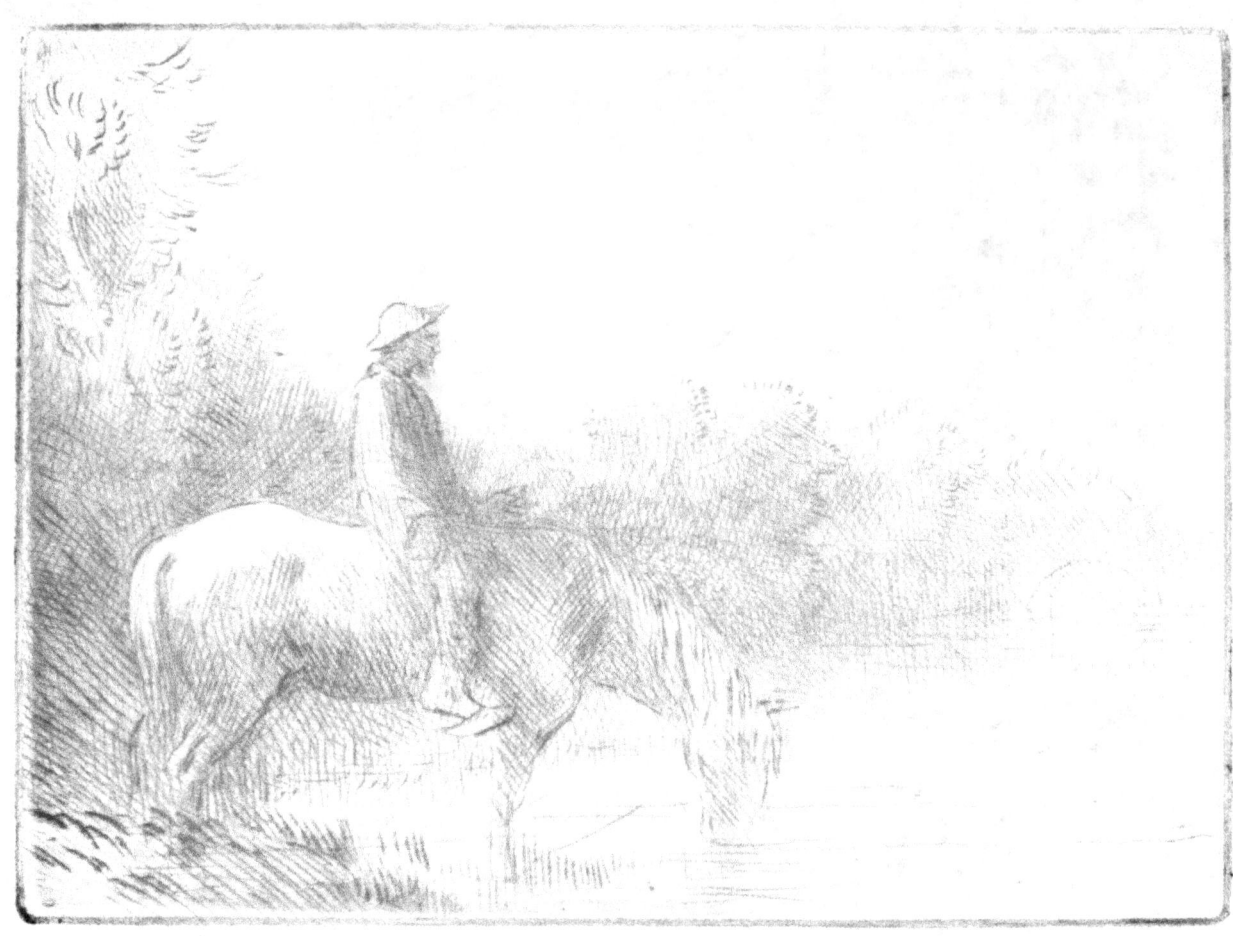

I am safe now

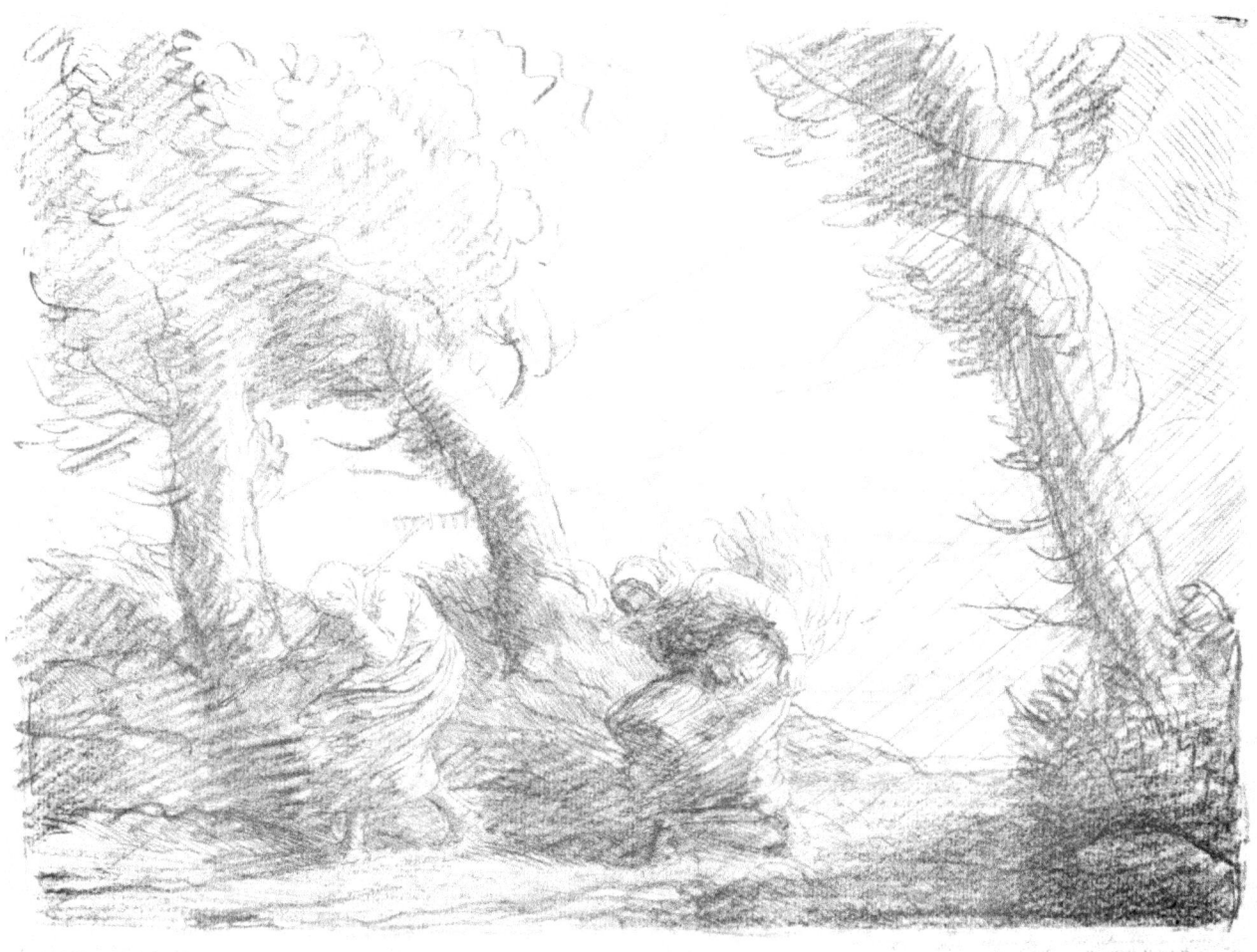

I deserve love

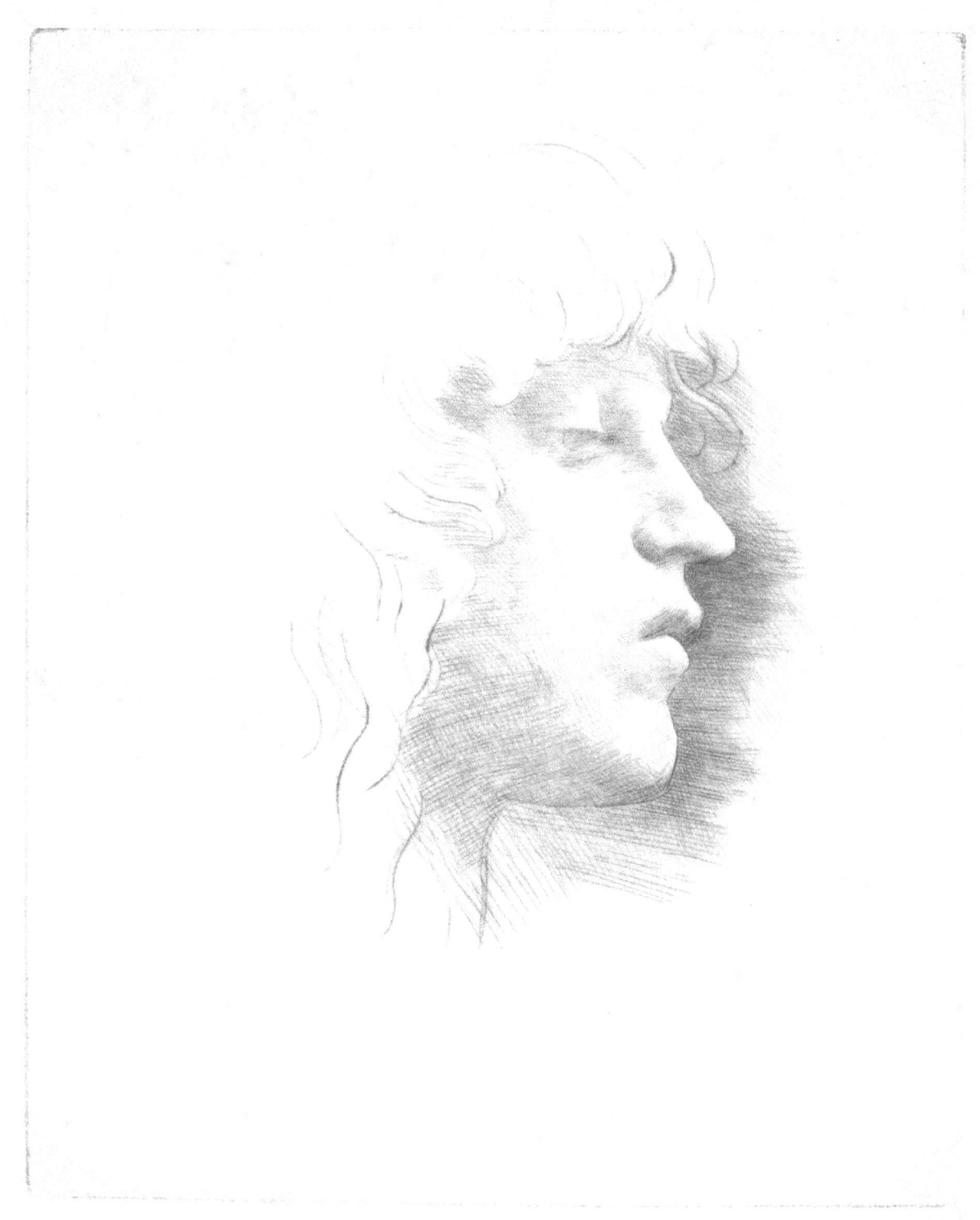

I am now in control

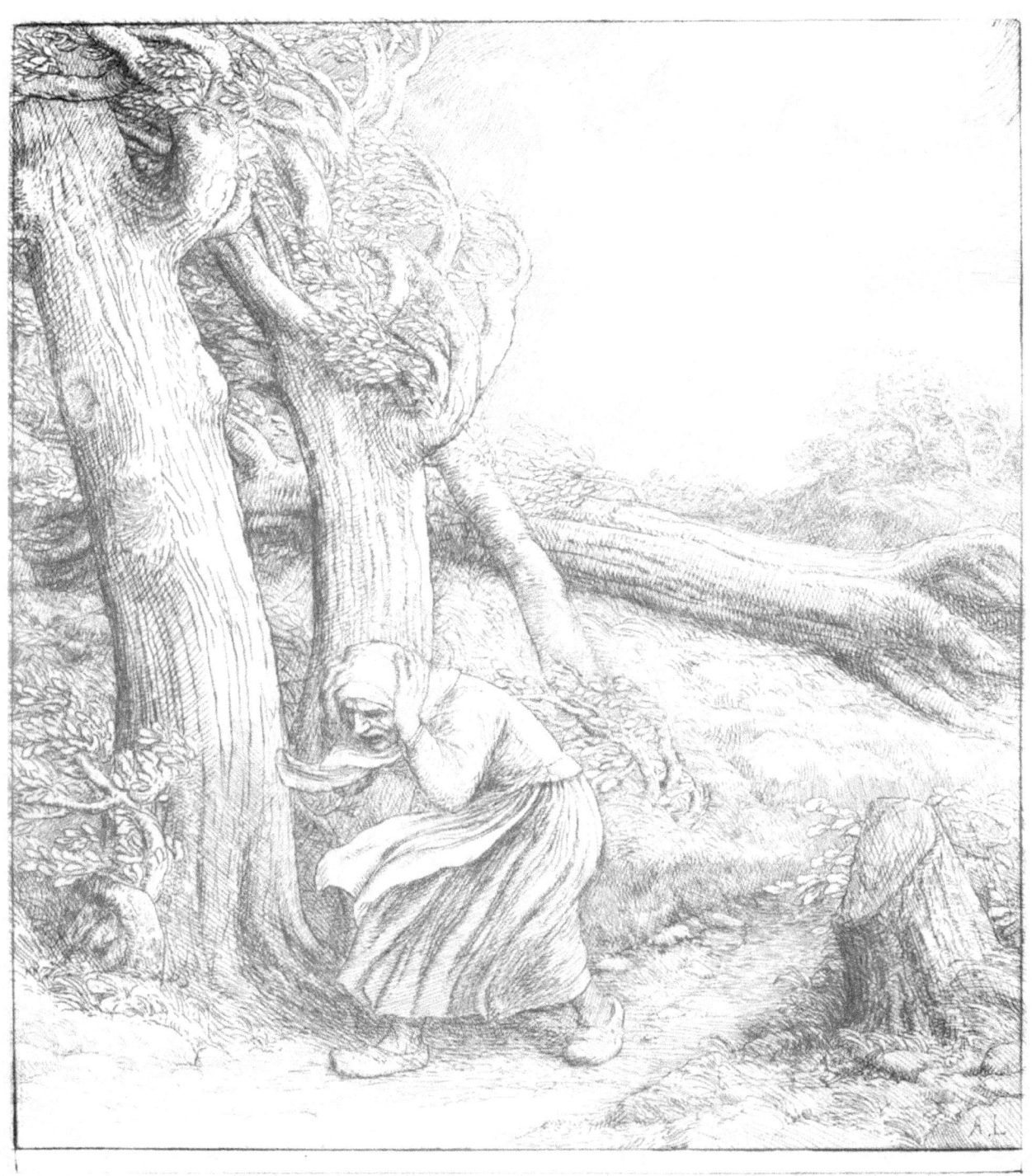

I can learn to trust myself

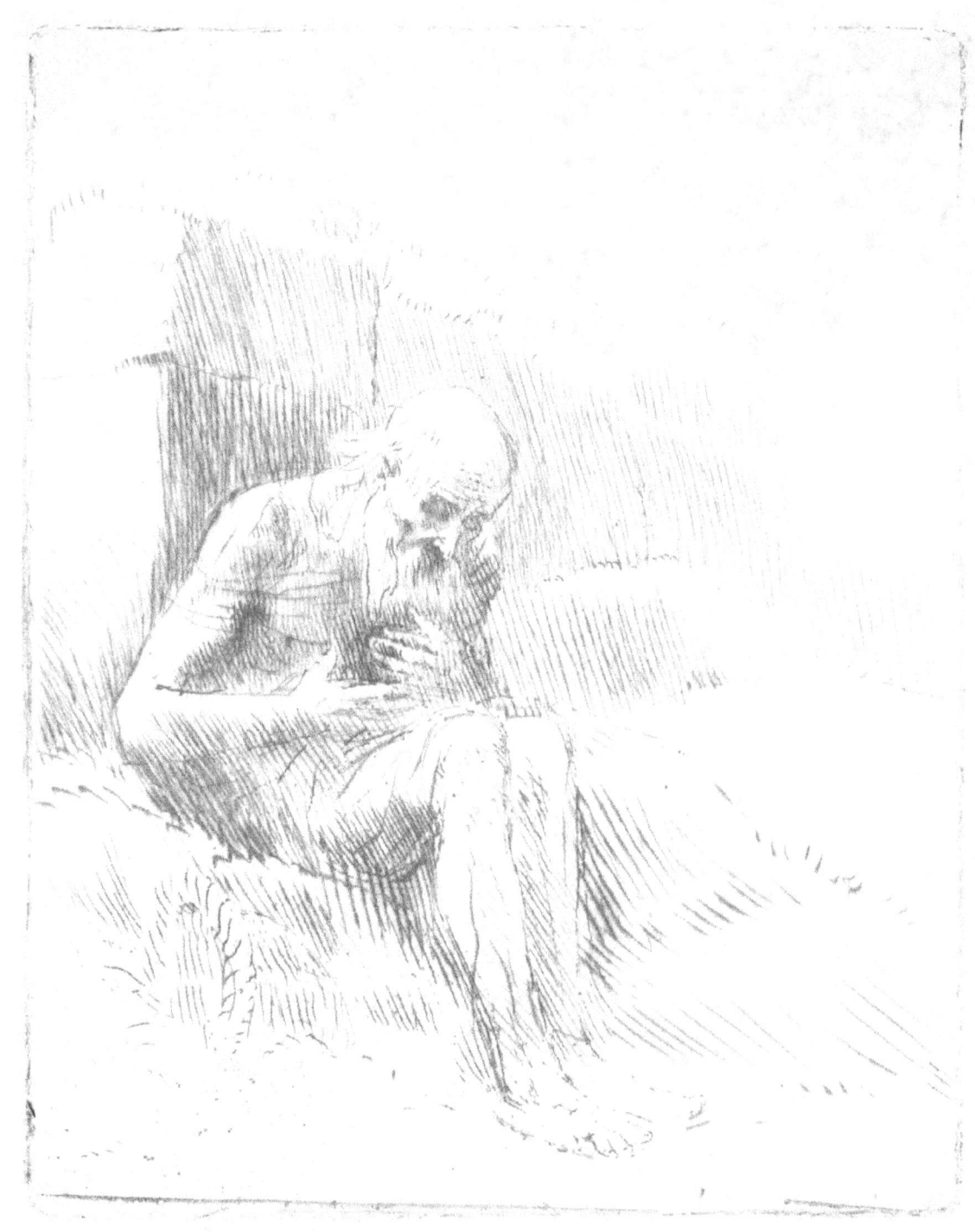

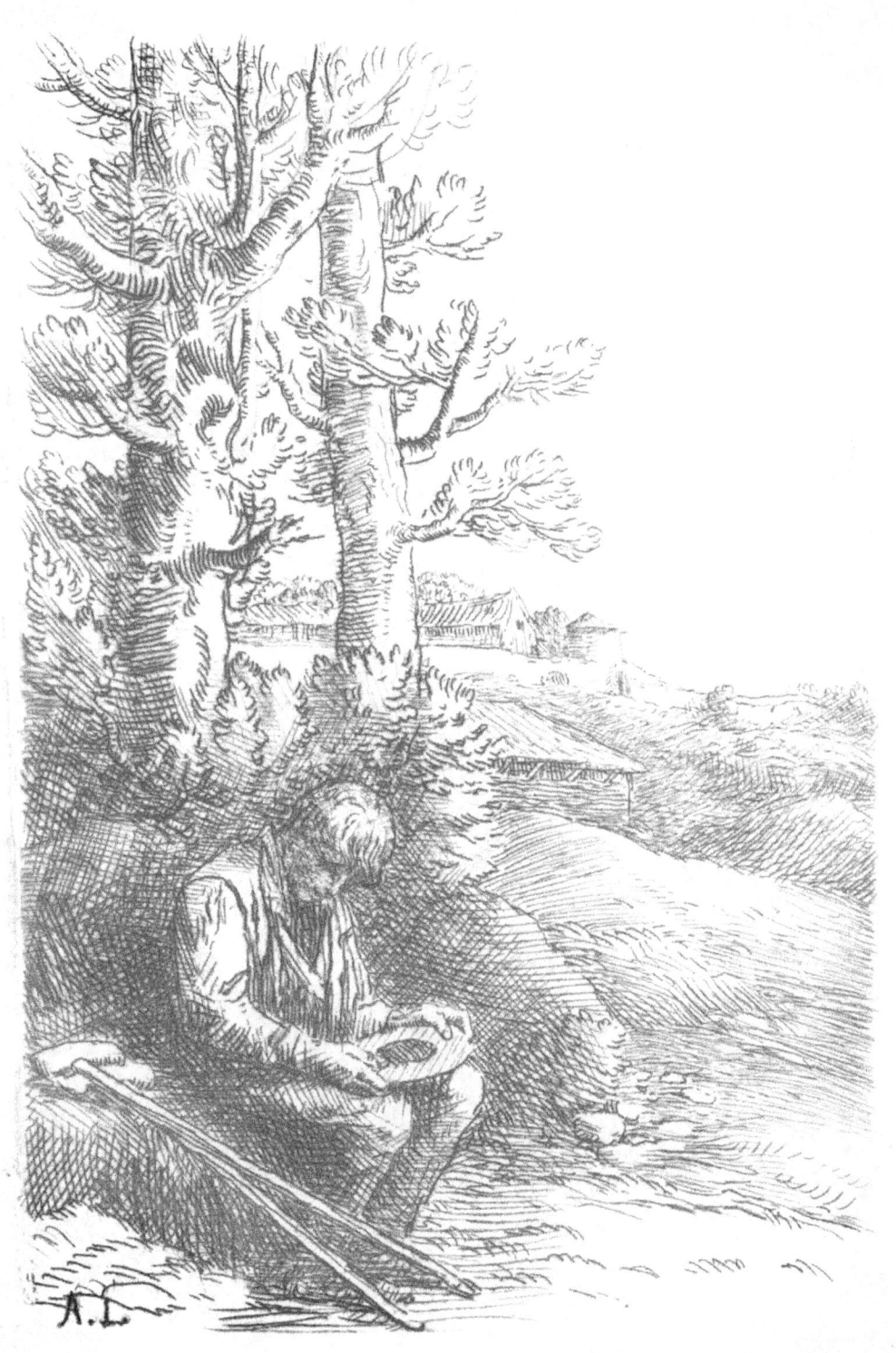

I deserve to live

I am not alone

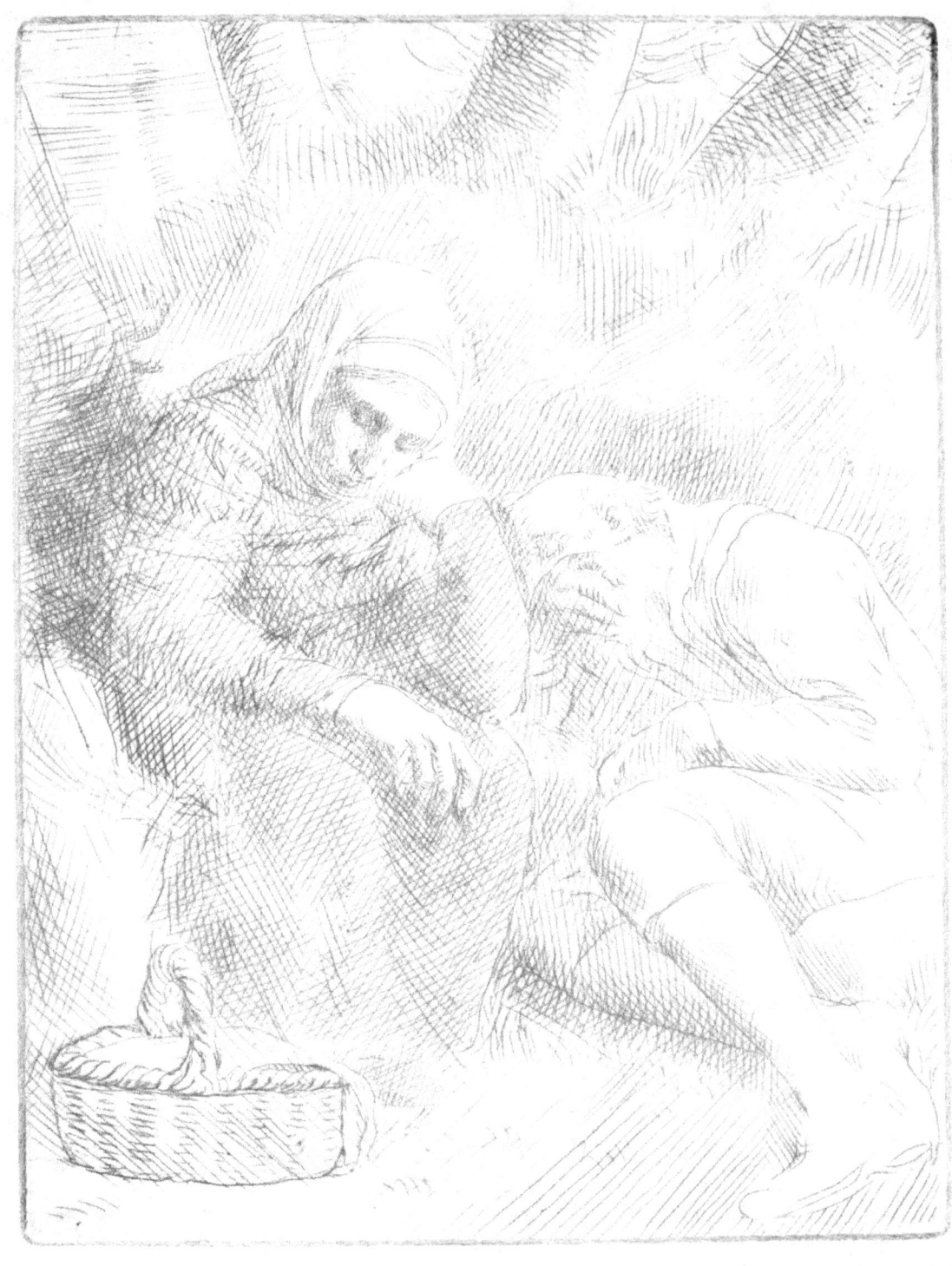

I am able to succeed

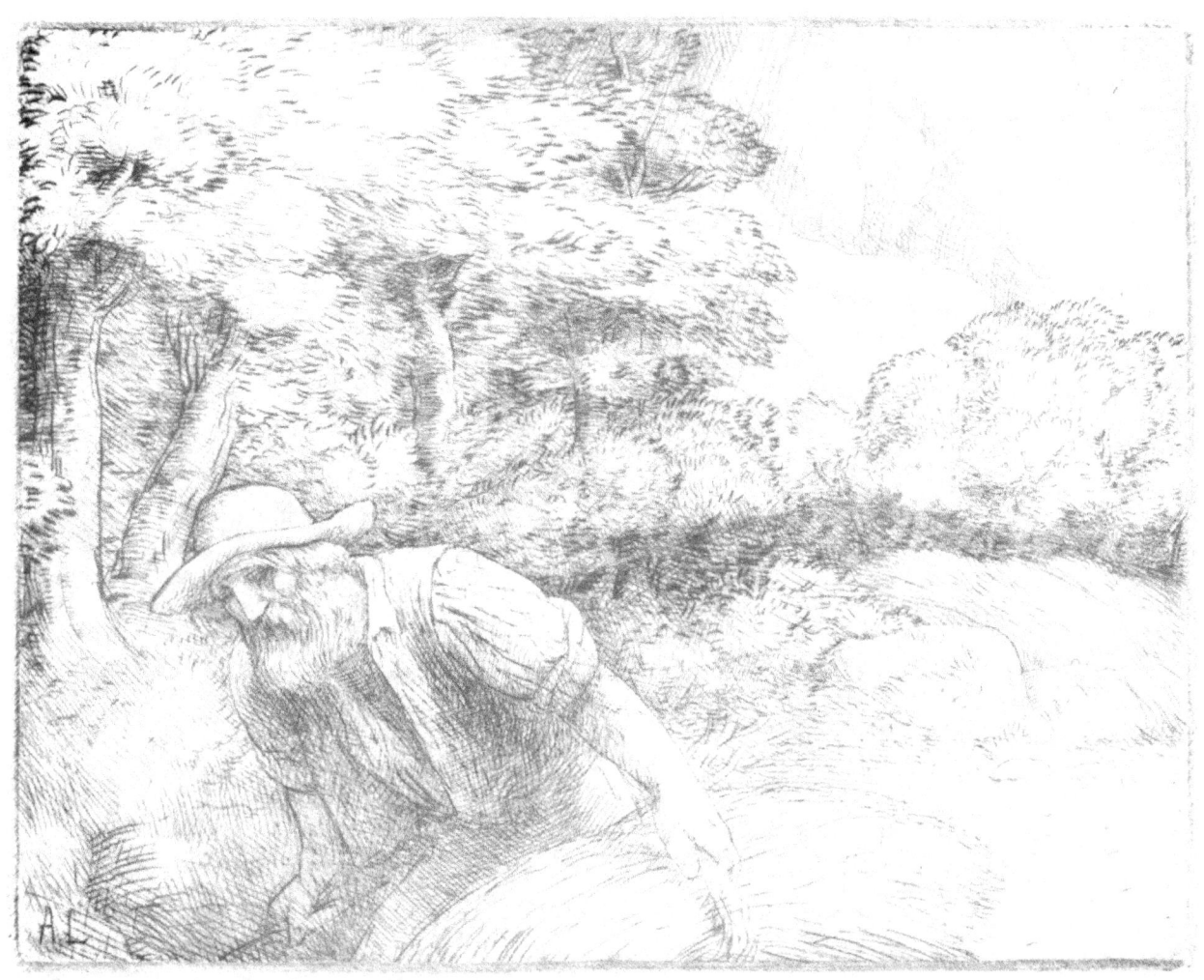

I am worthy of love

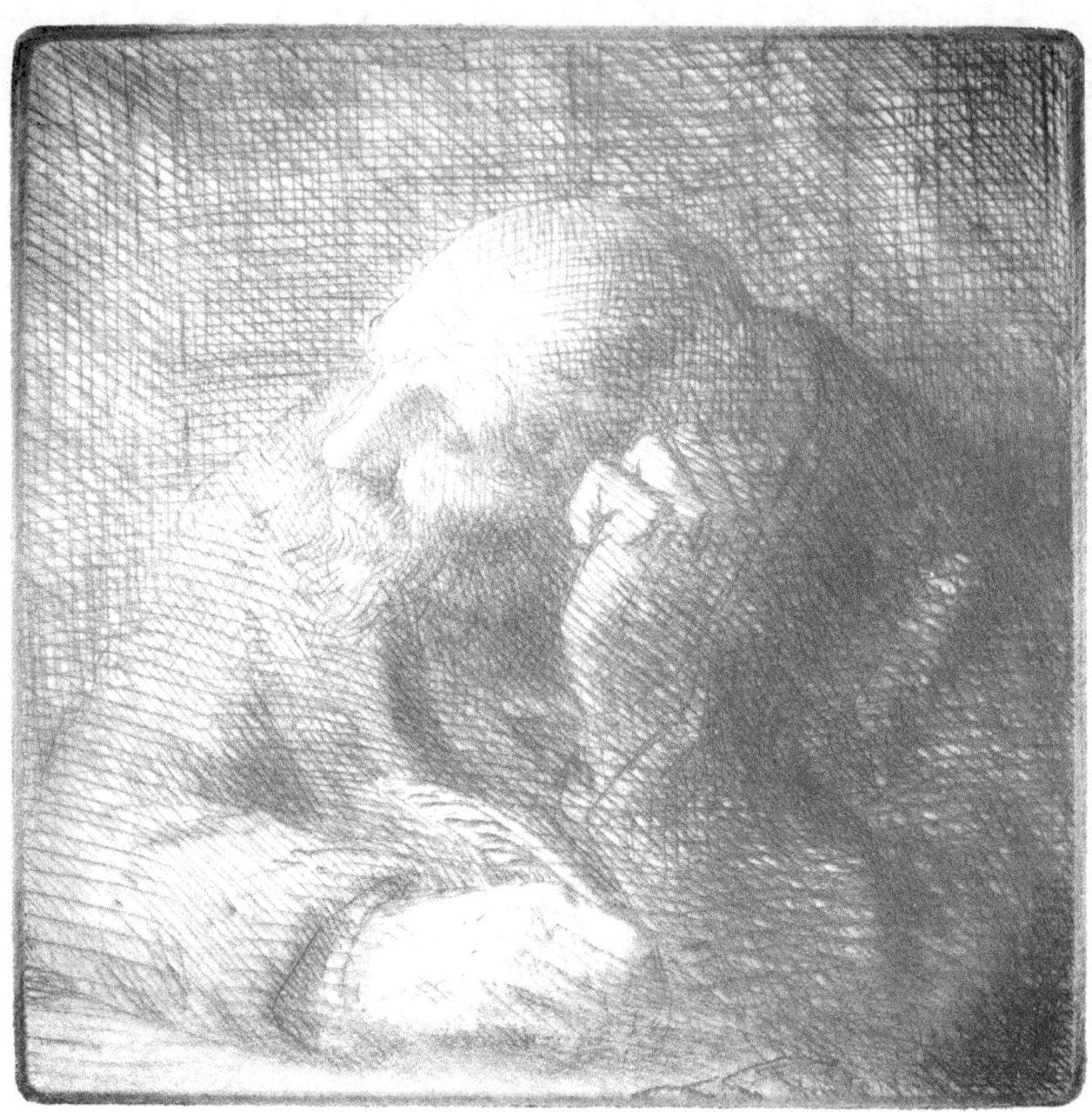

I can be trusted

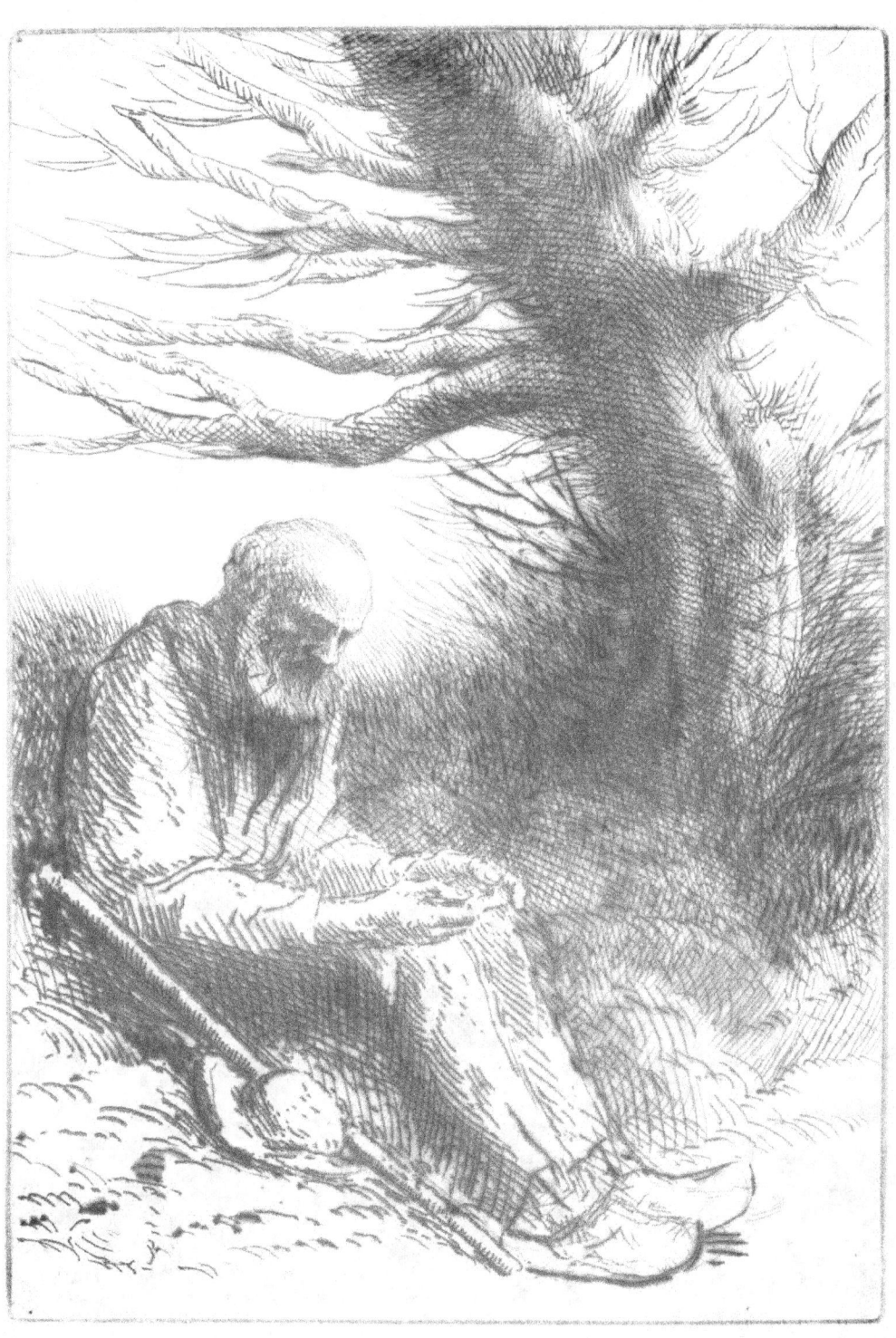

I am honorable

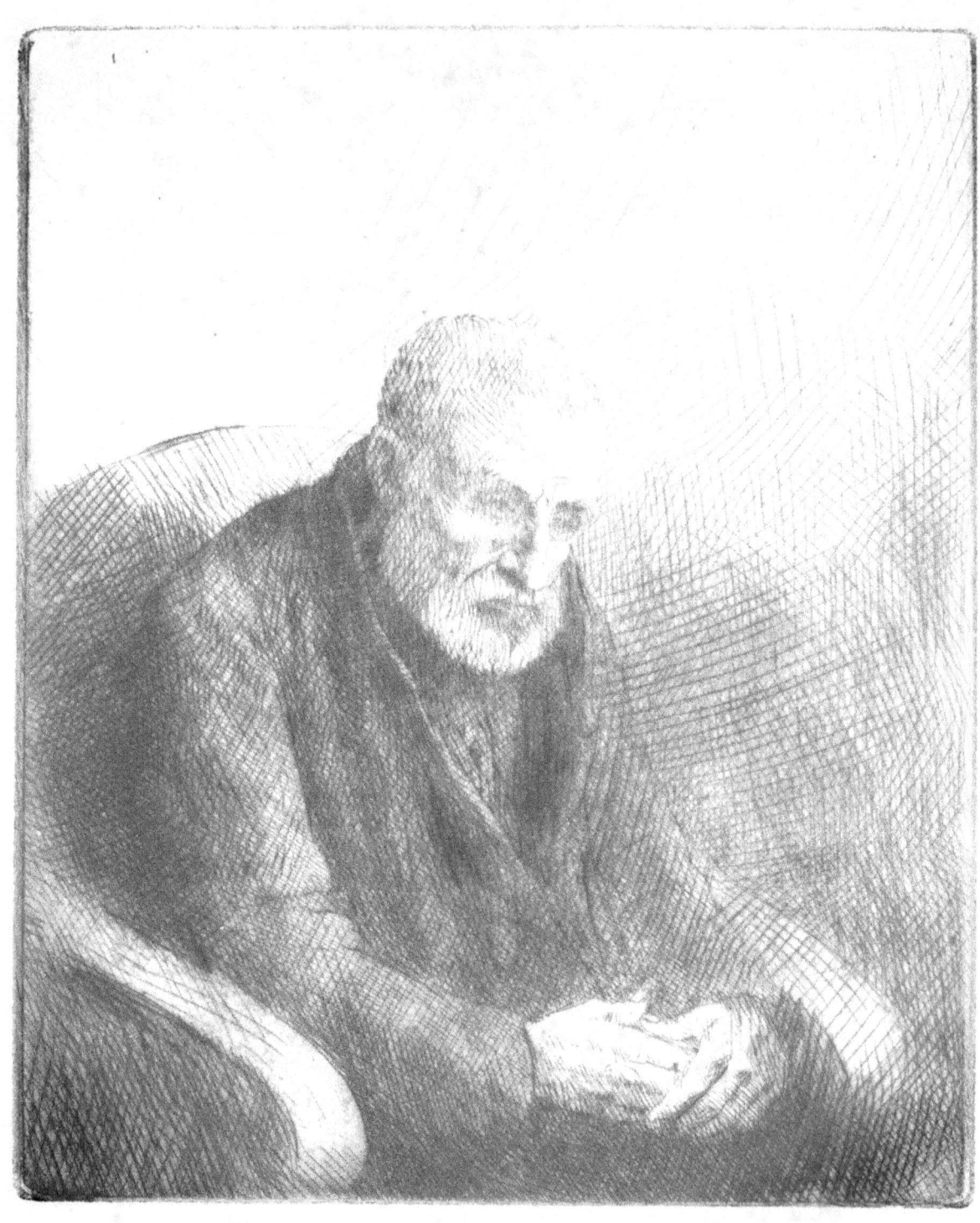

I have dignity

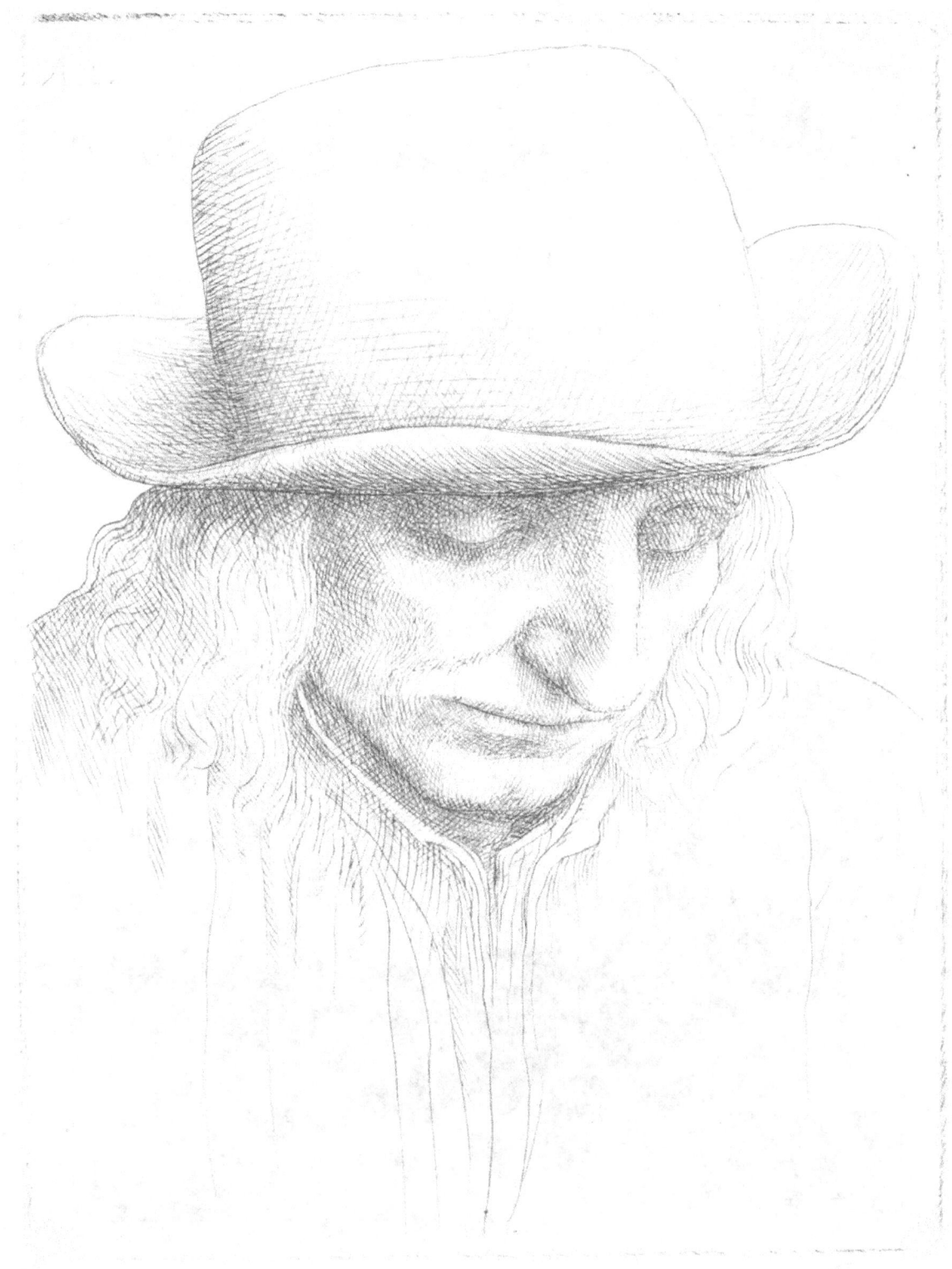

I am valuable

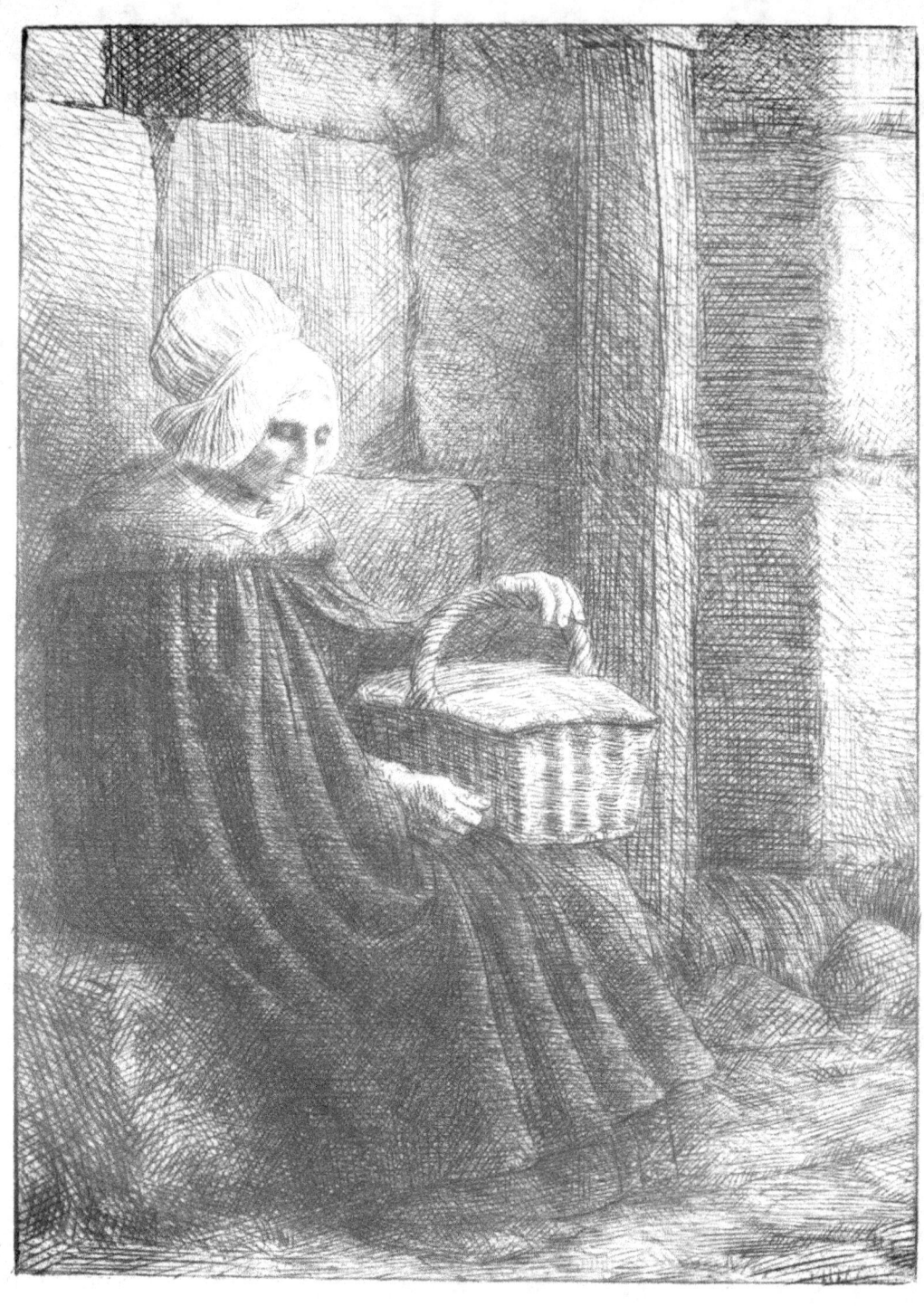

I am able to learn

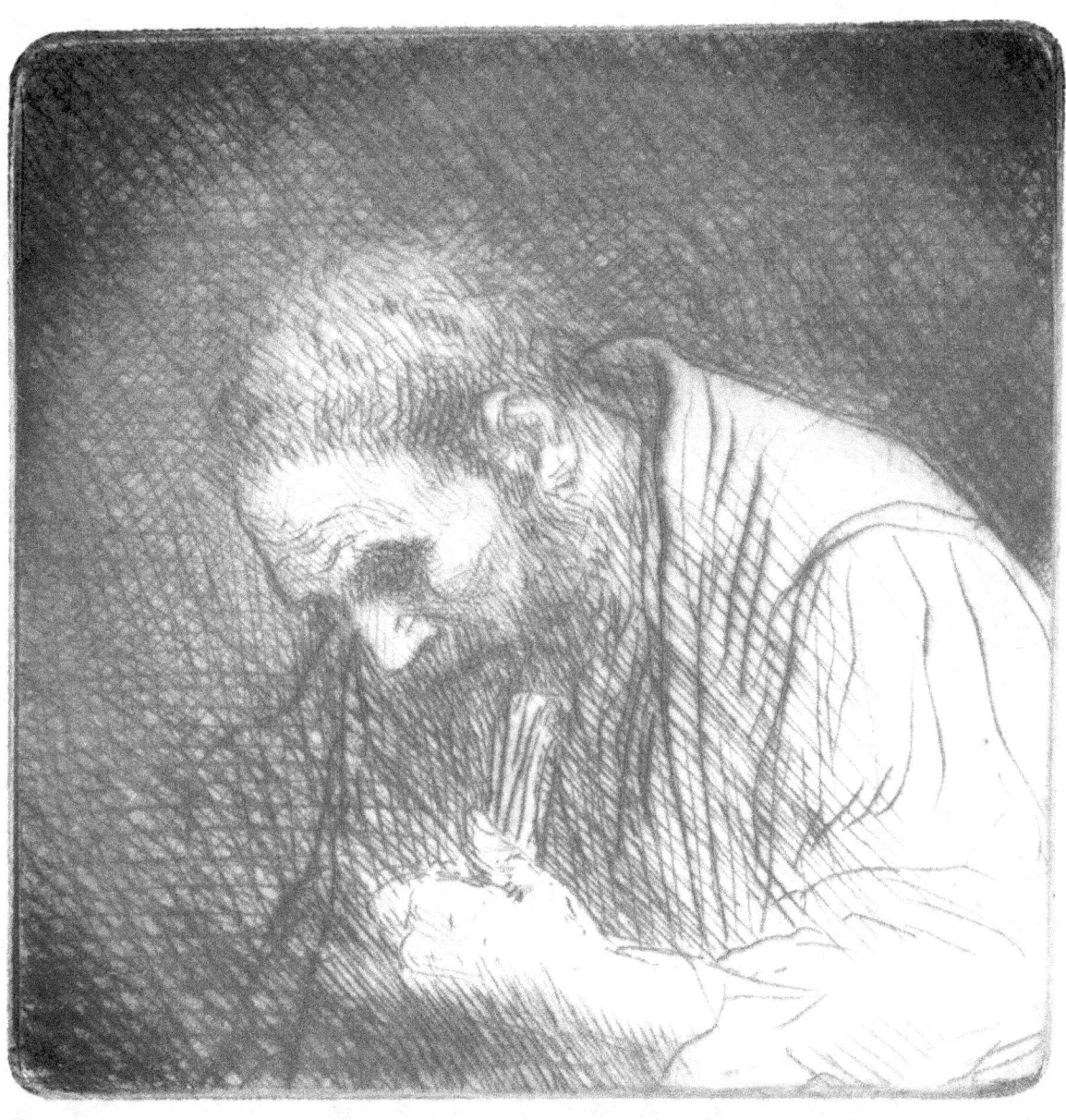

I am fine as I am

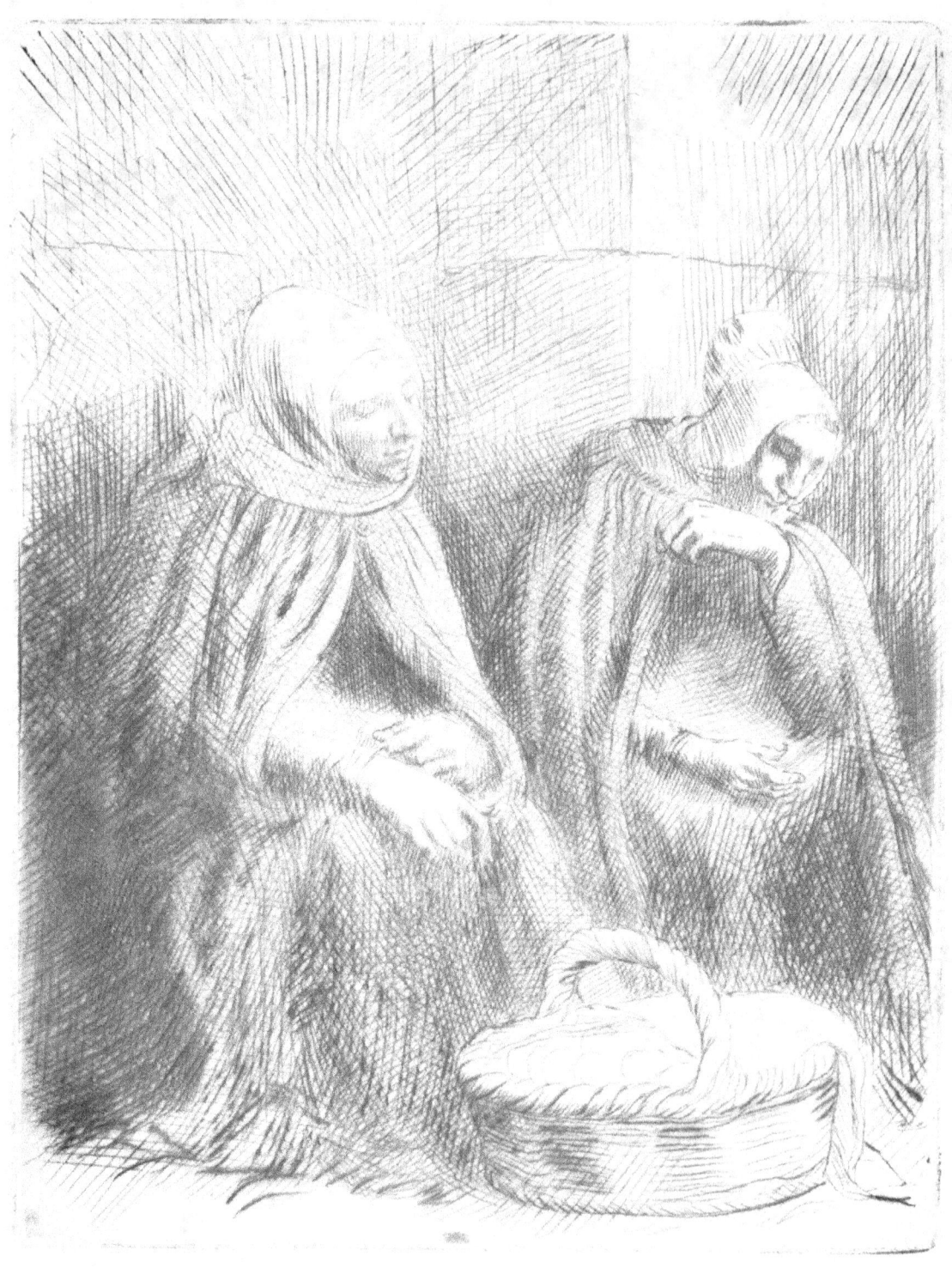

I am only human

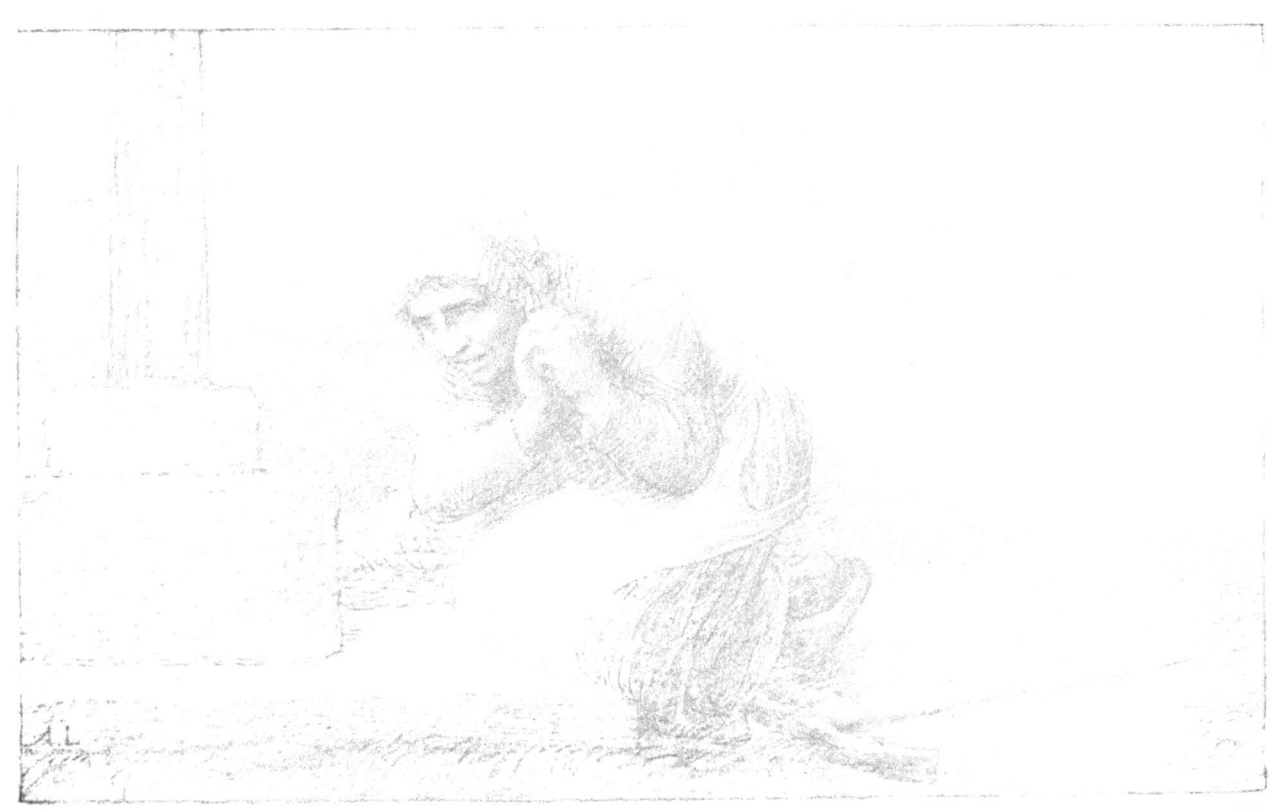

I am smart

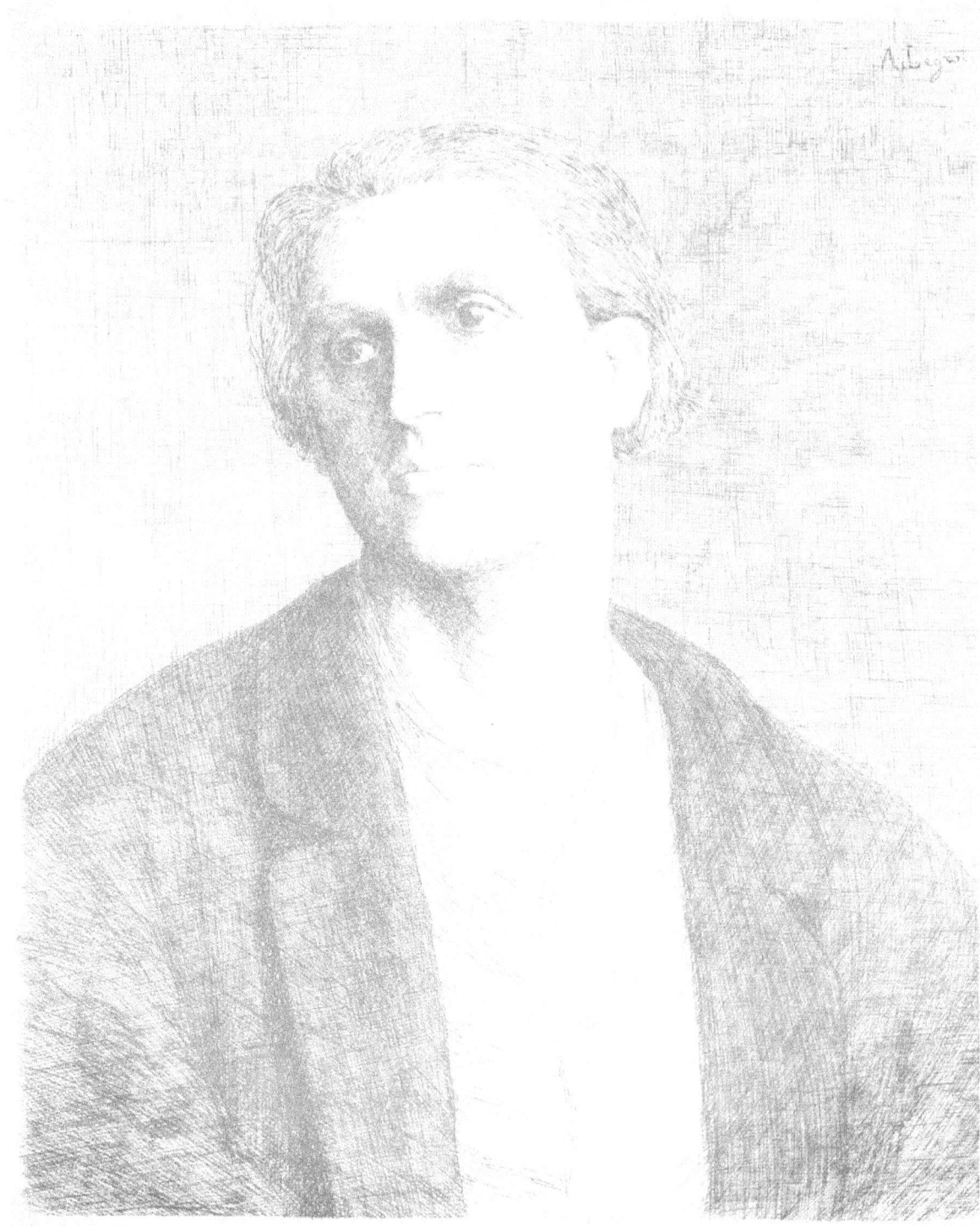

I am whole

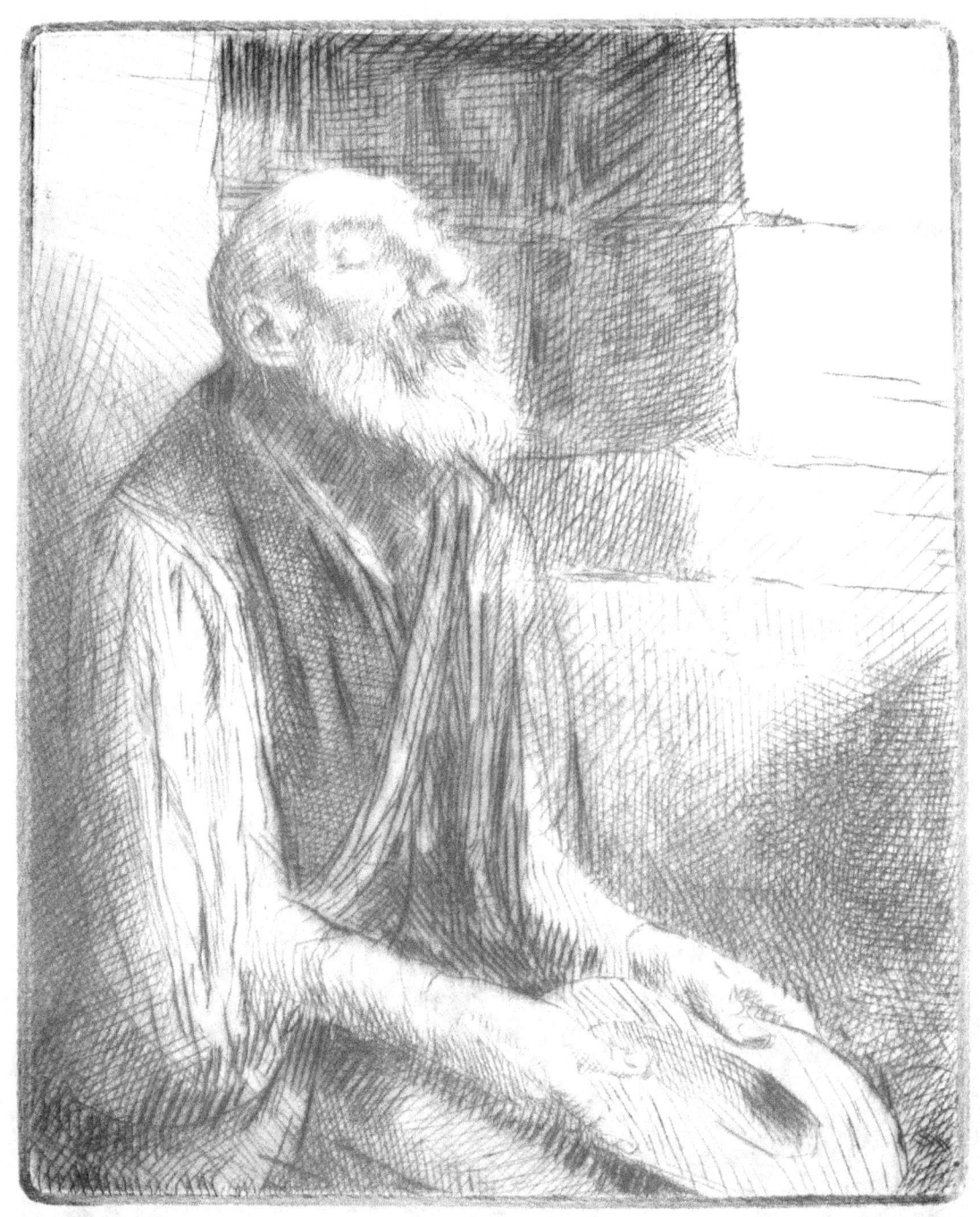

I can handle it

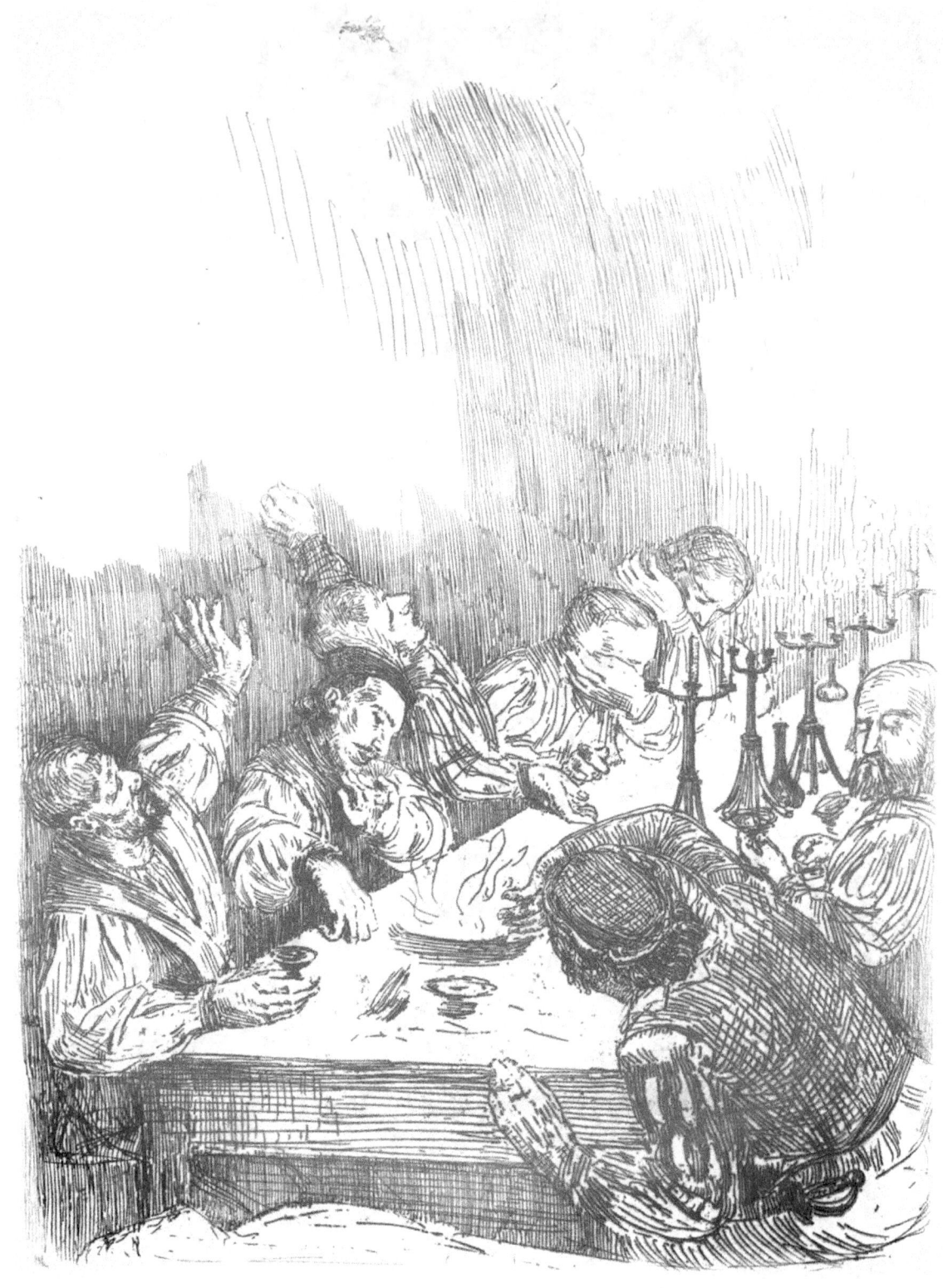

I am enough

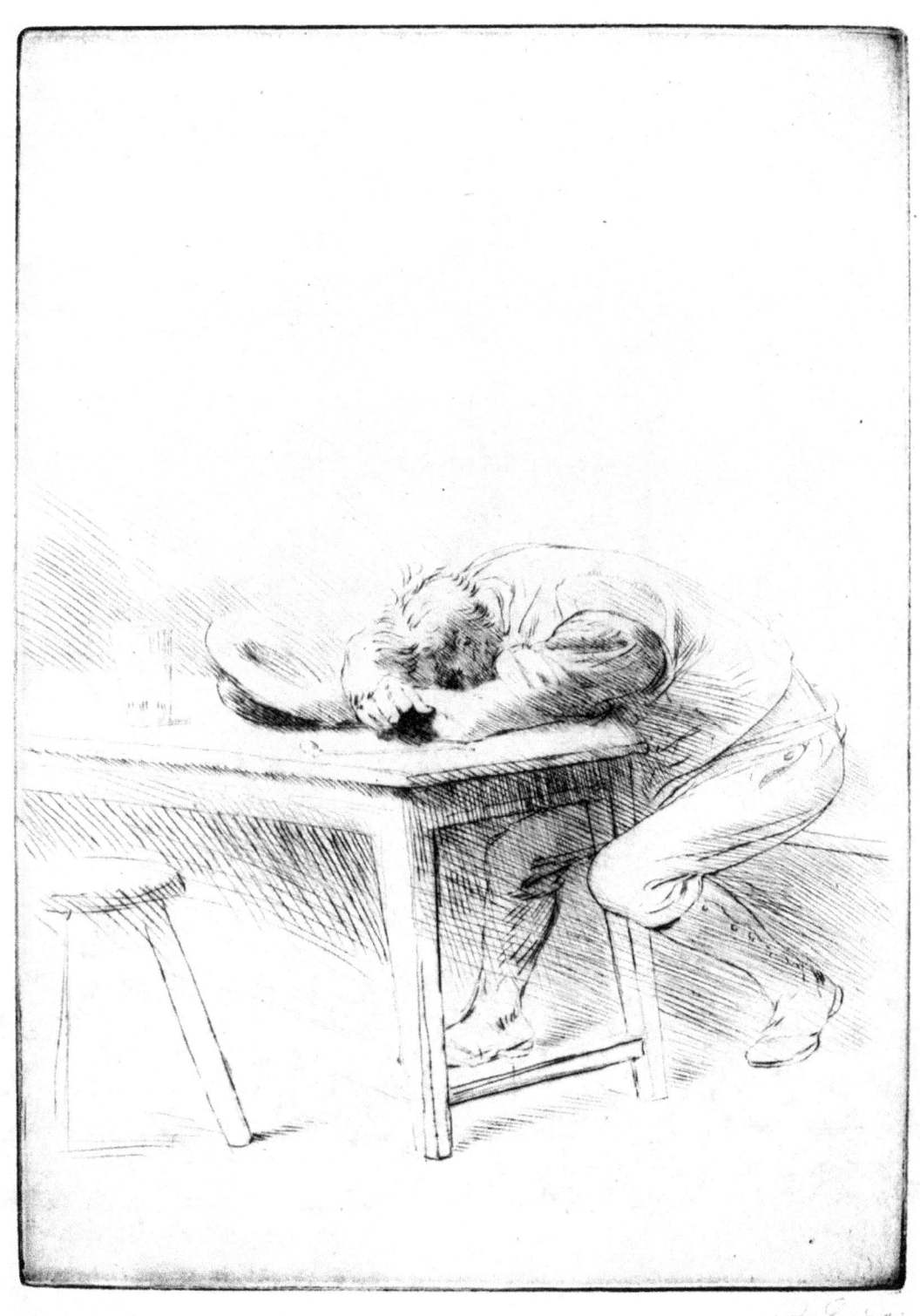

I can be myself

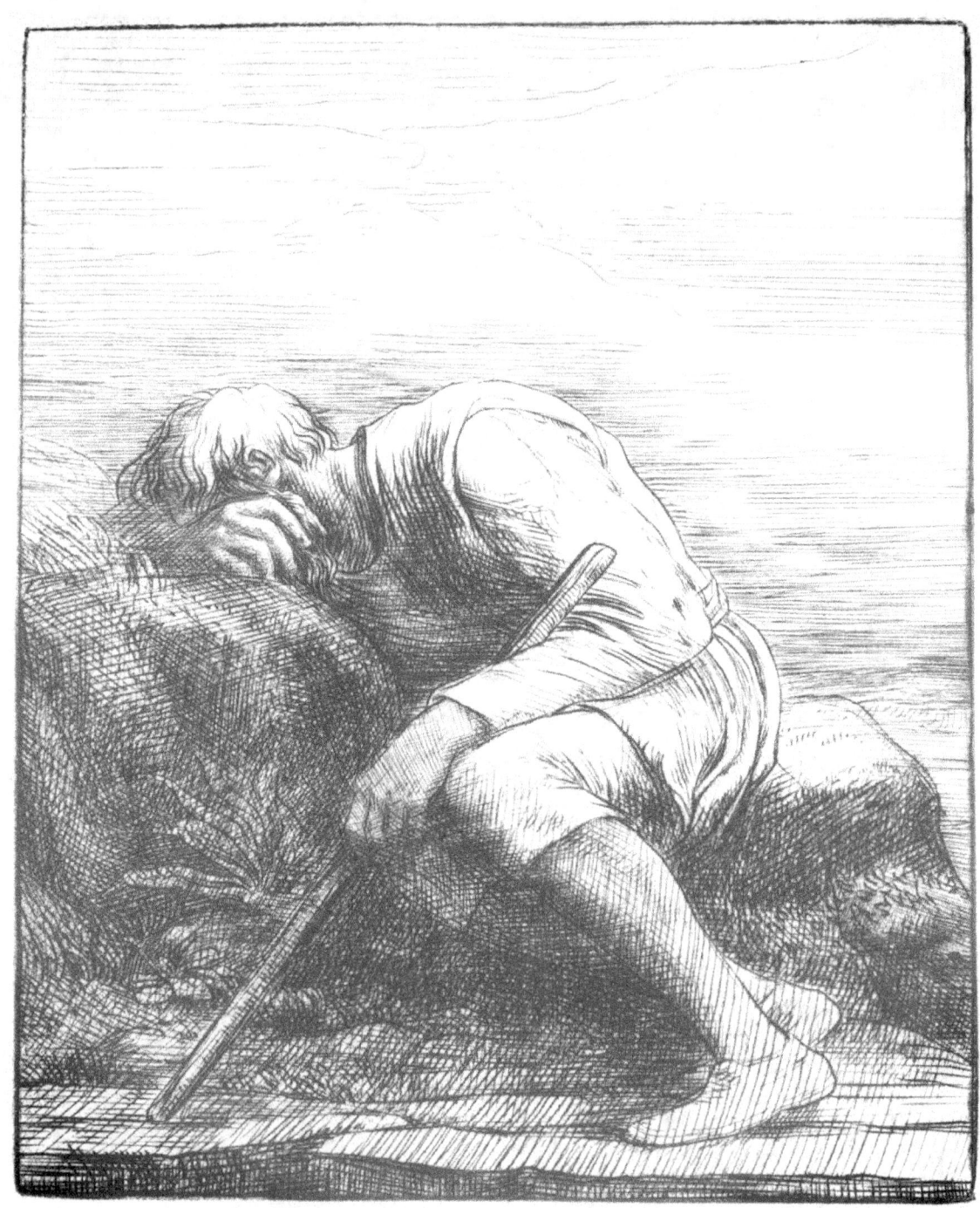

I can make mistakes

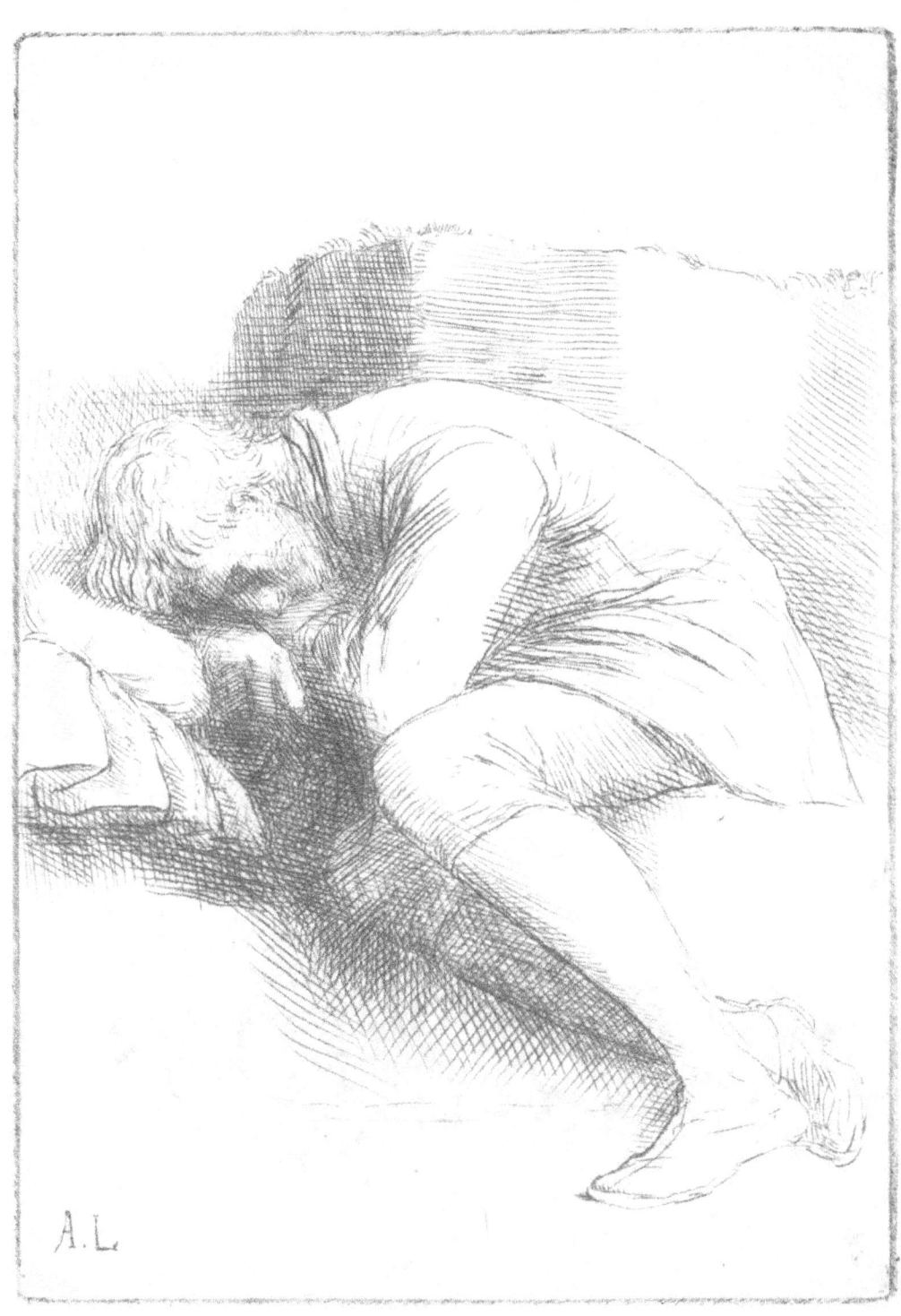

I am intelligent

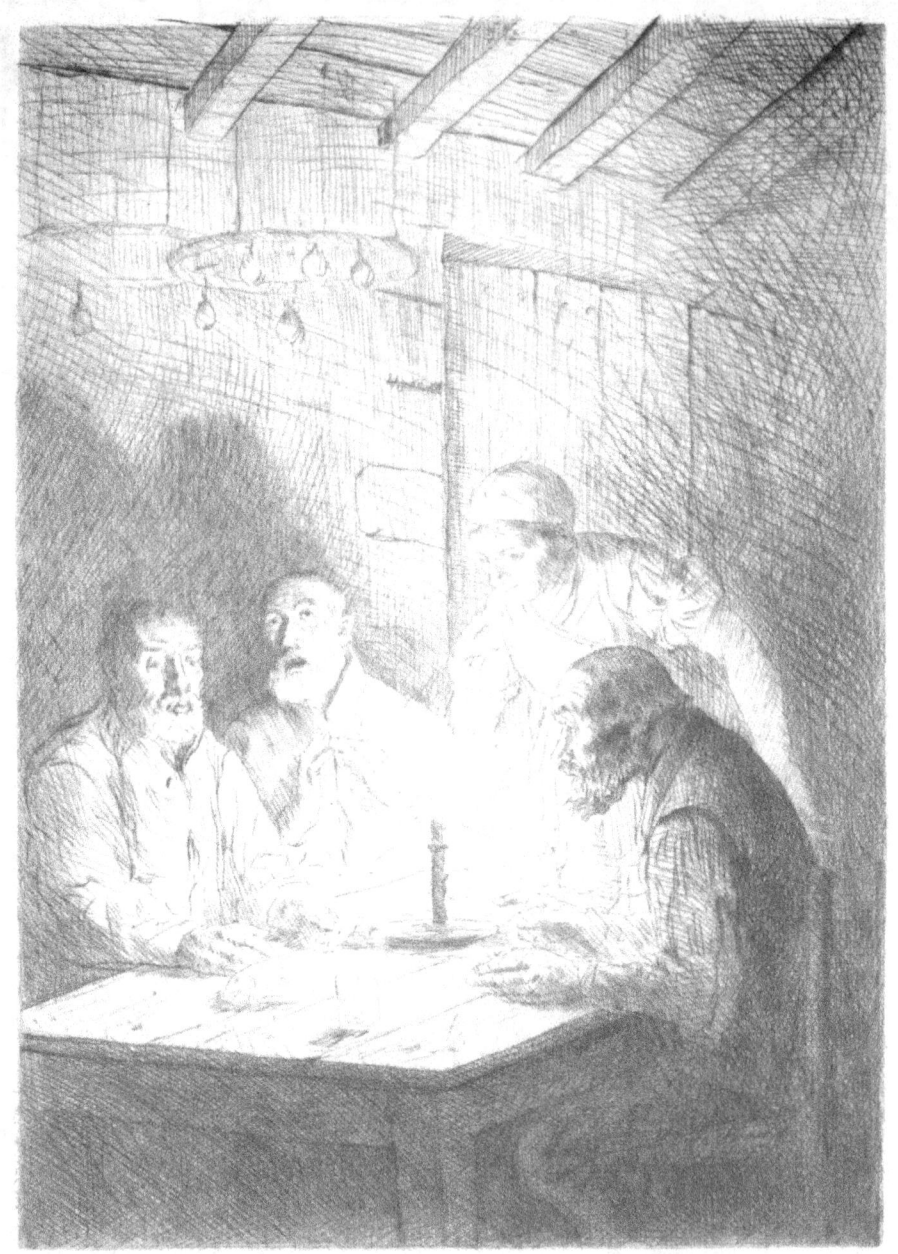

I am strong now

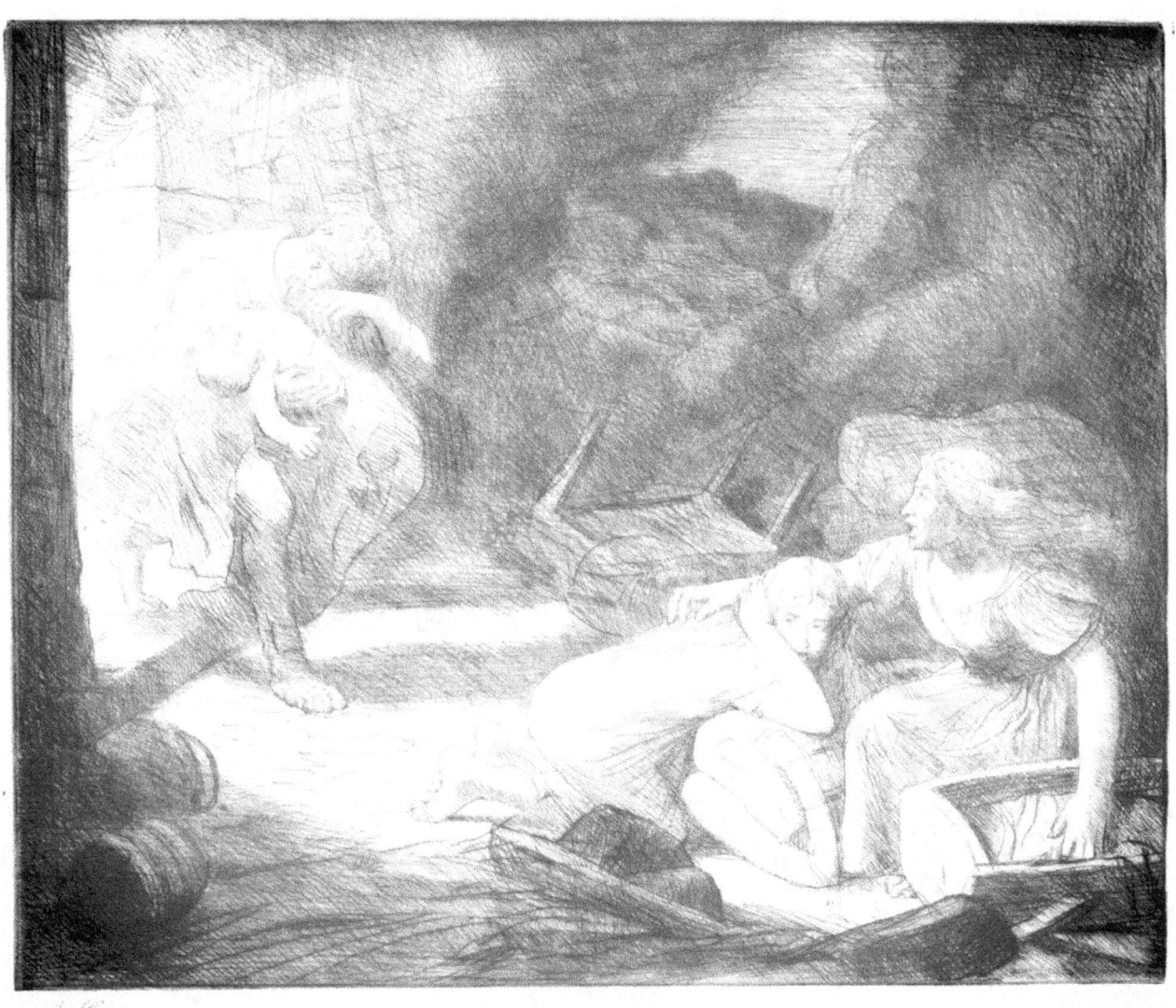

I can be healthy

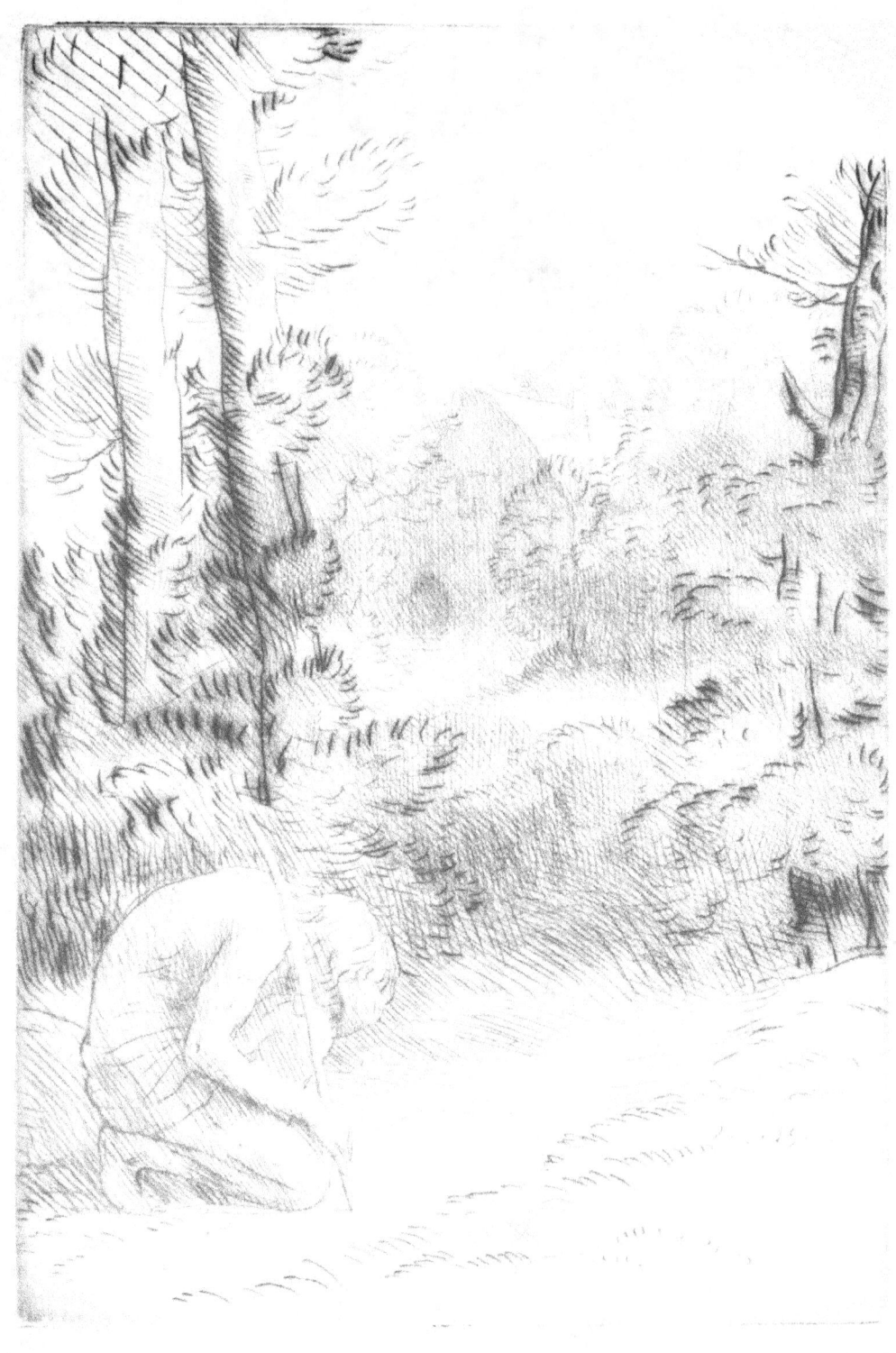

I am a work in progress

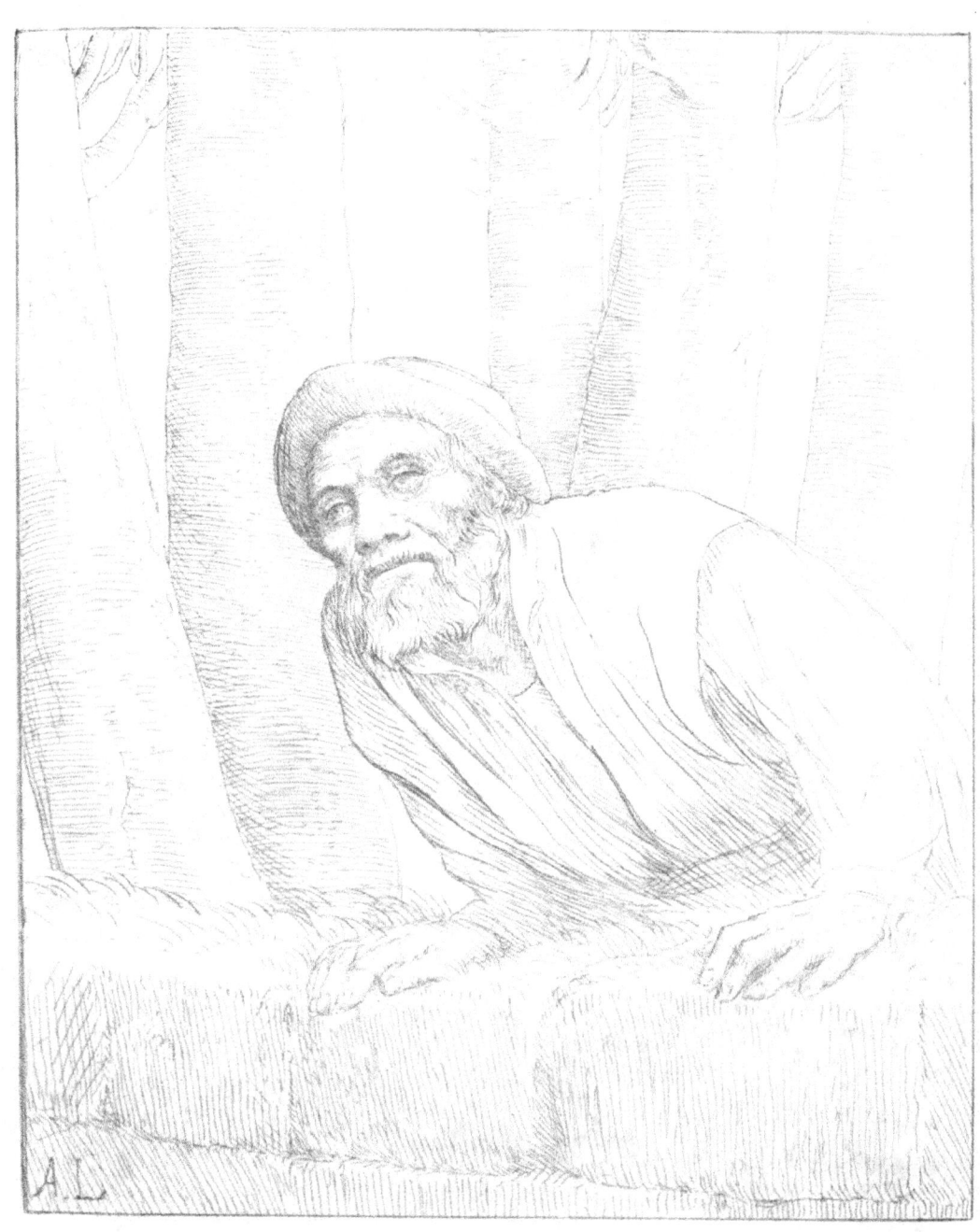

I do the best I can

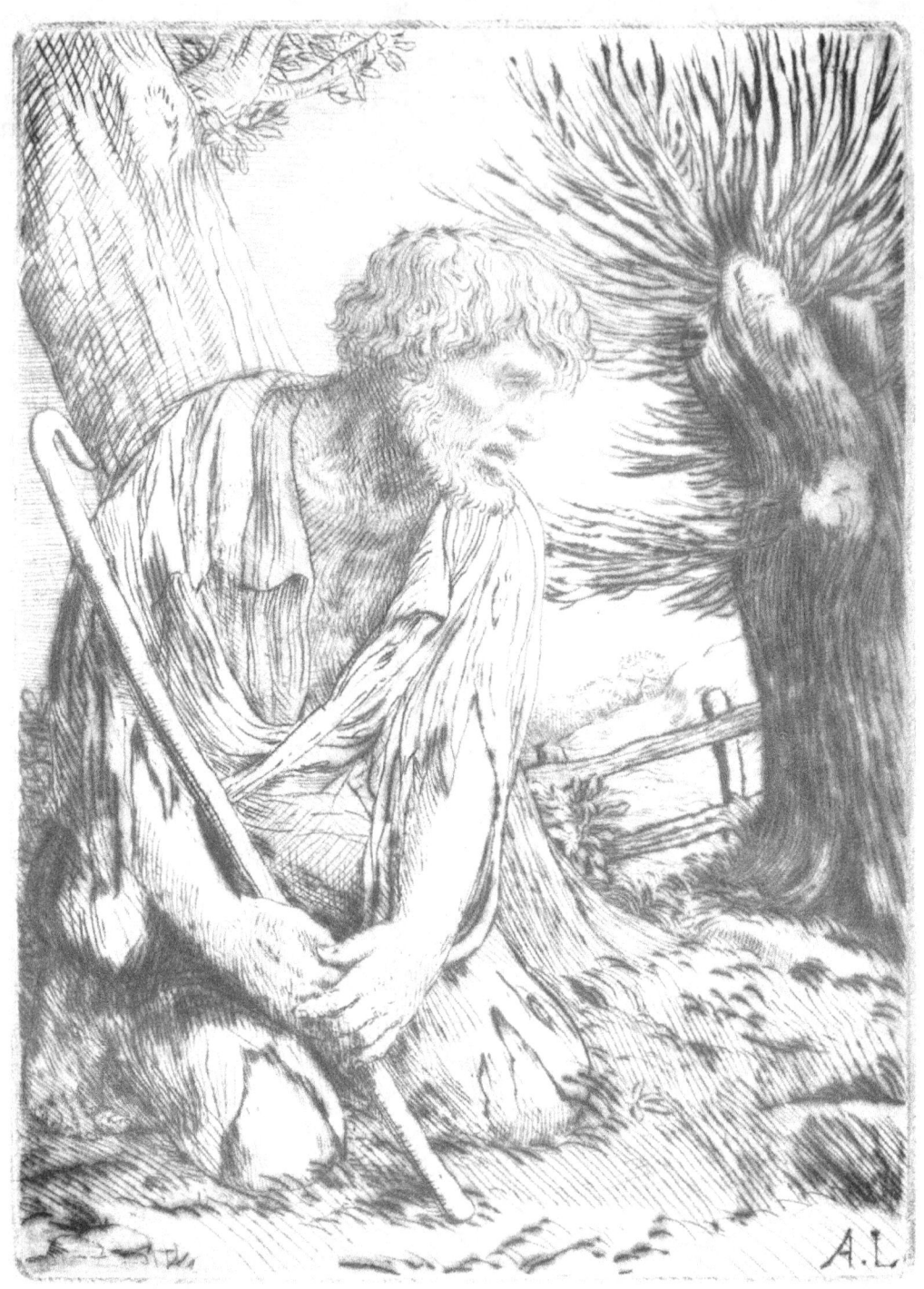

I am a good person

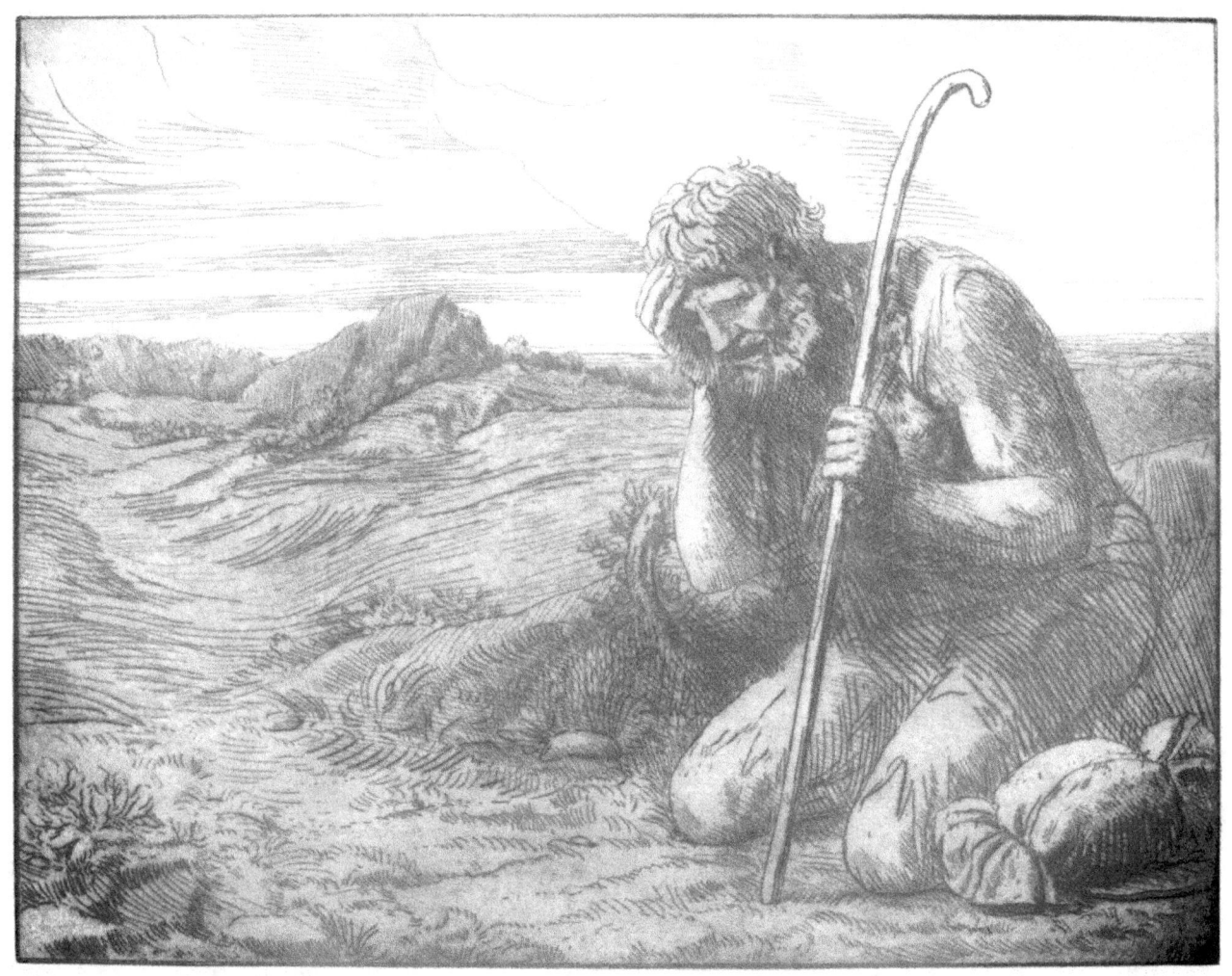

I am okay just the way I am

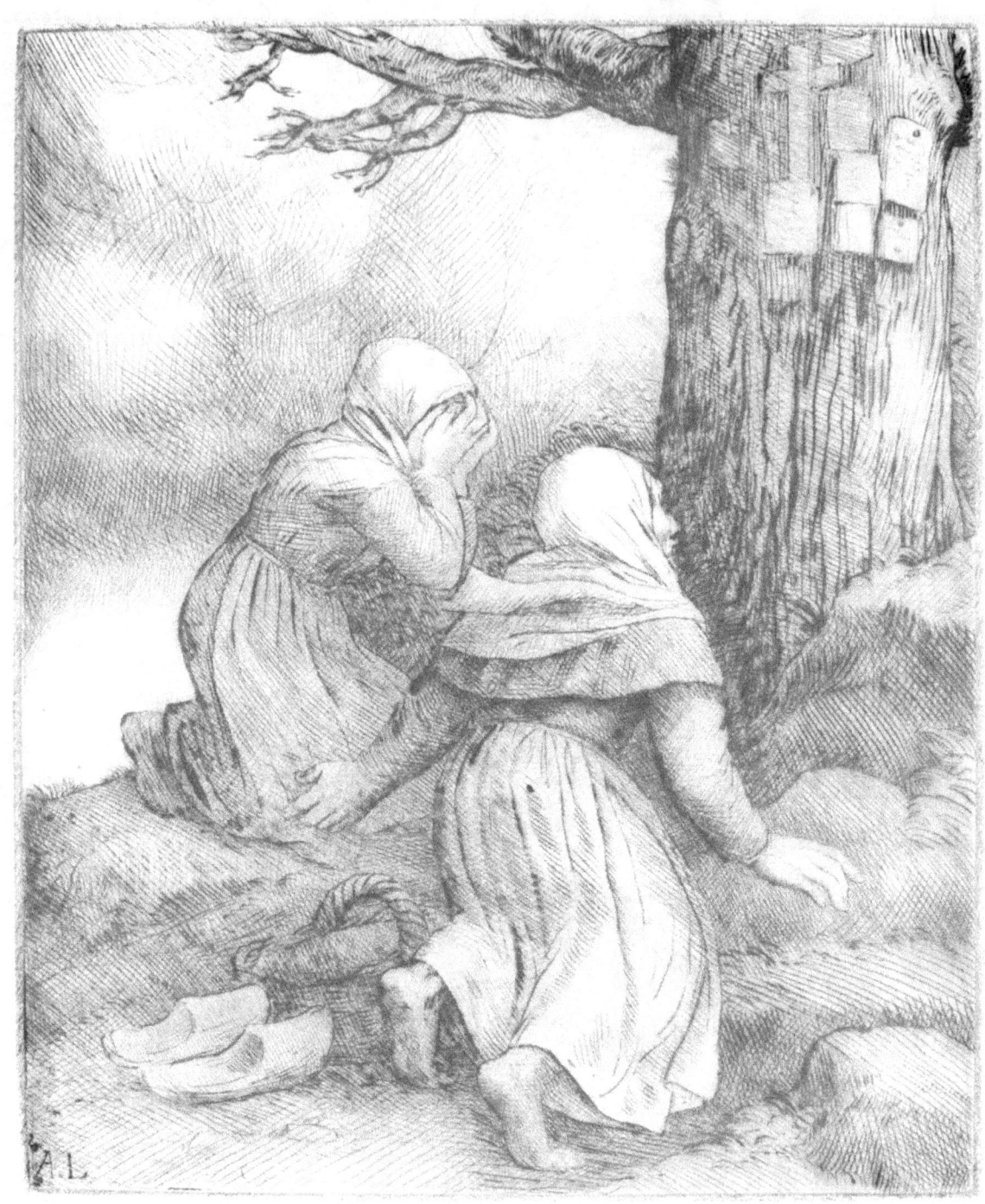

I am strong

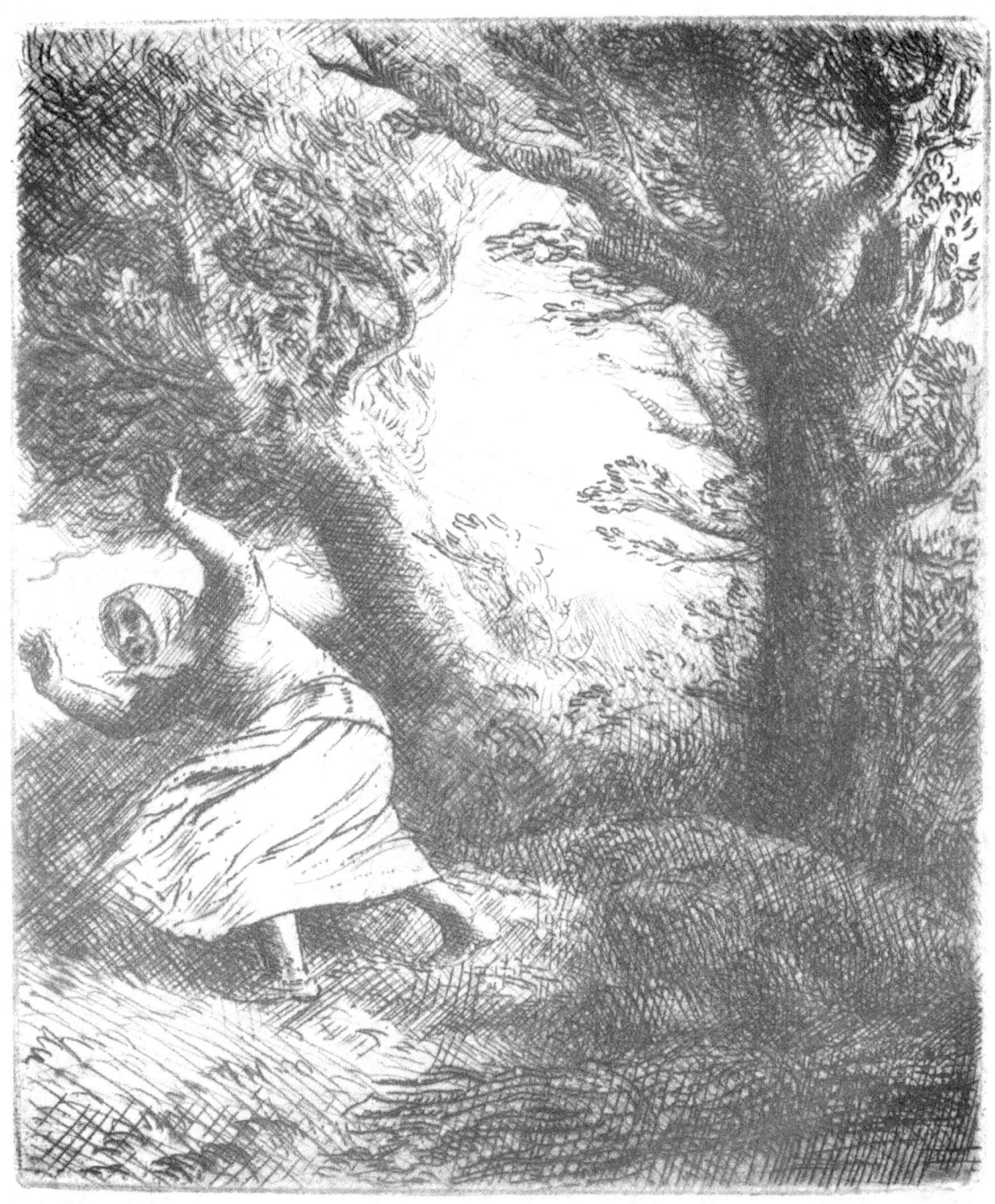

I can do it

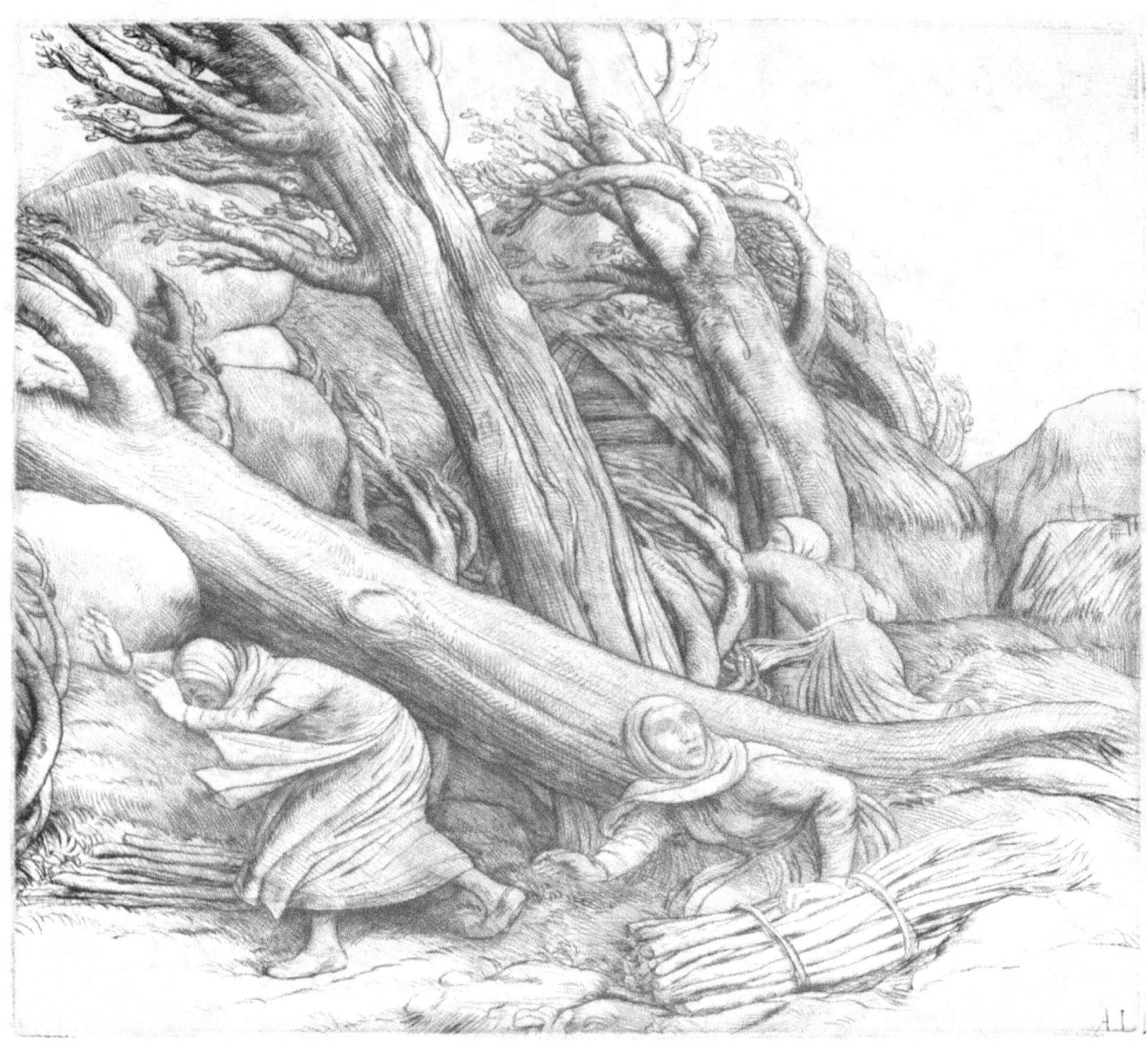

I am forgiven

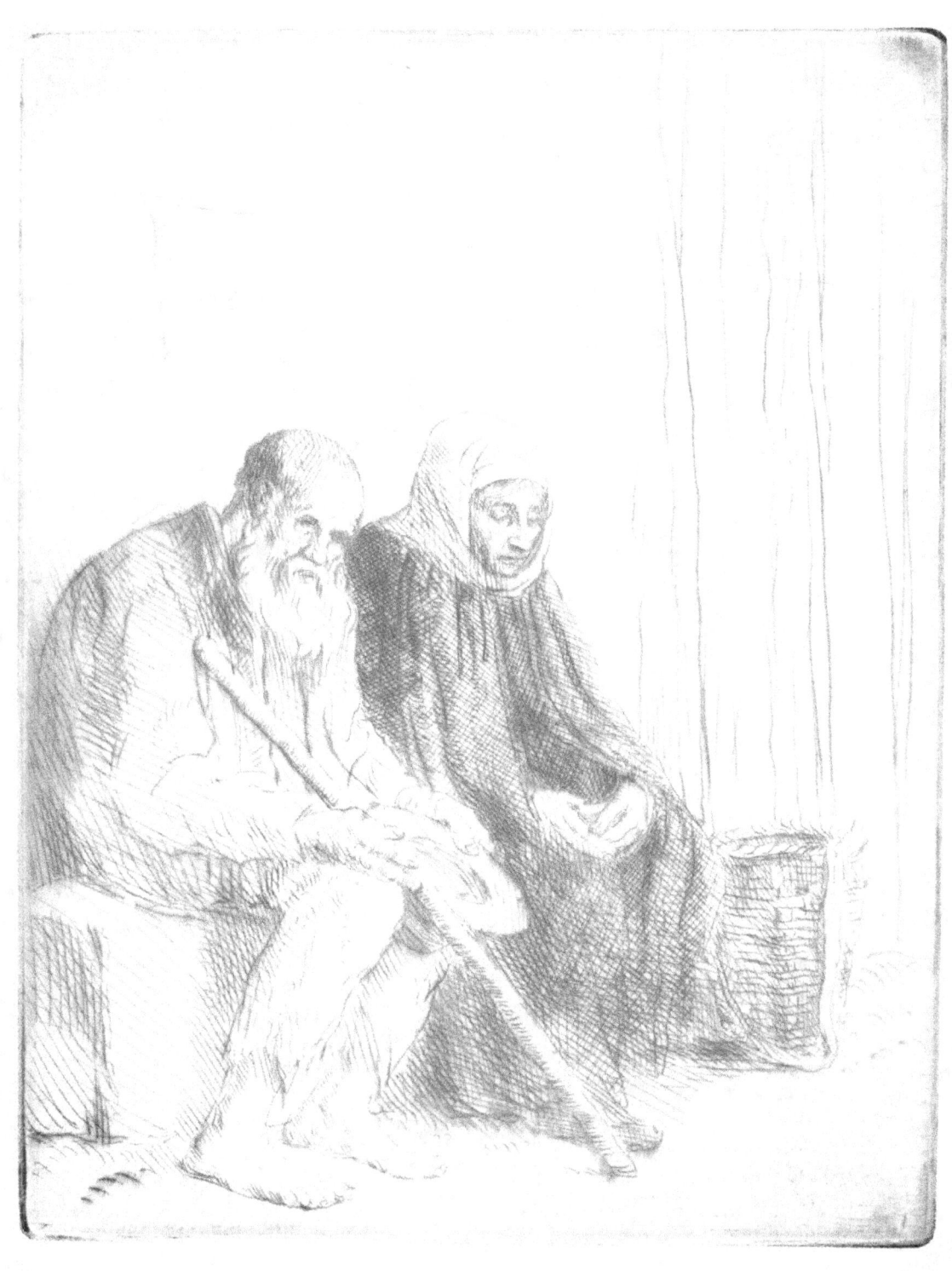

I have what it takes

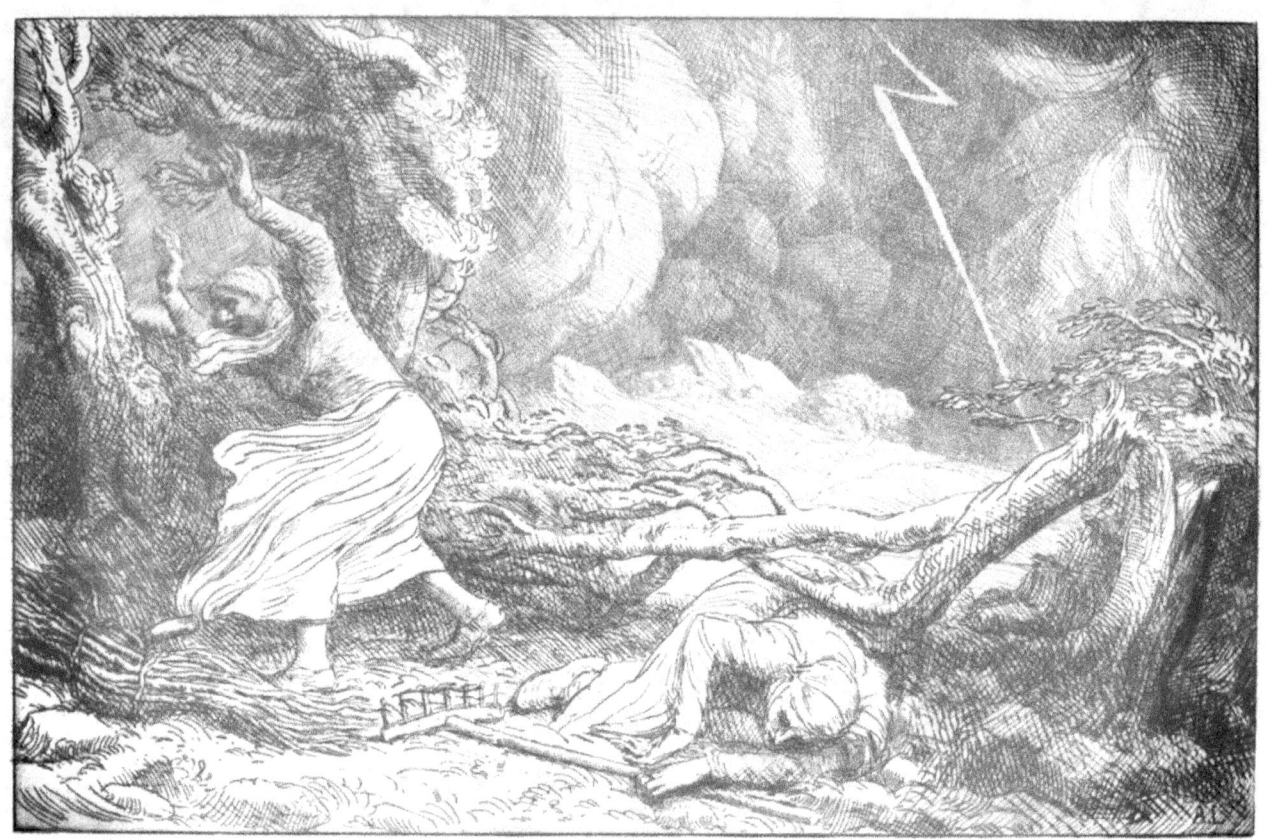

I am okay as I am

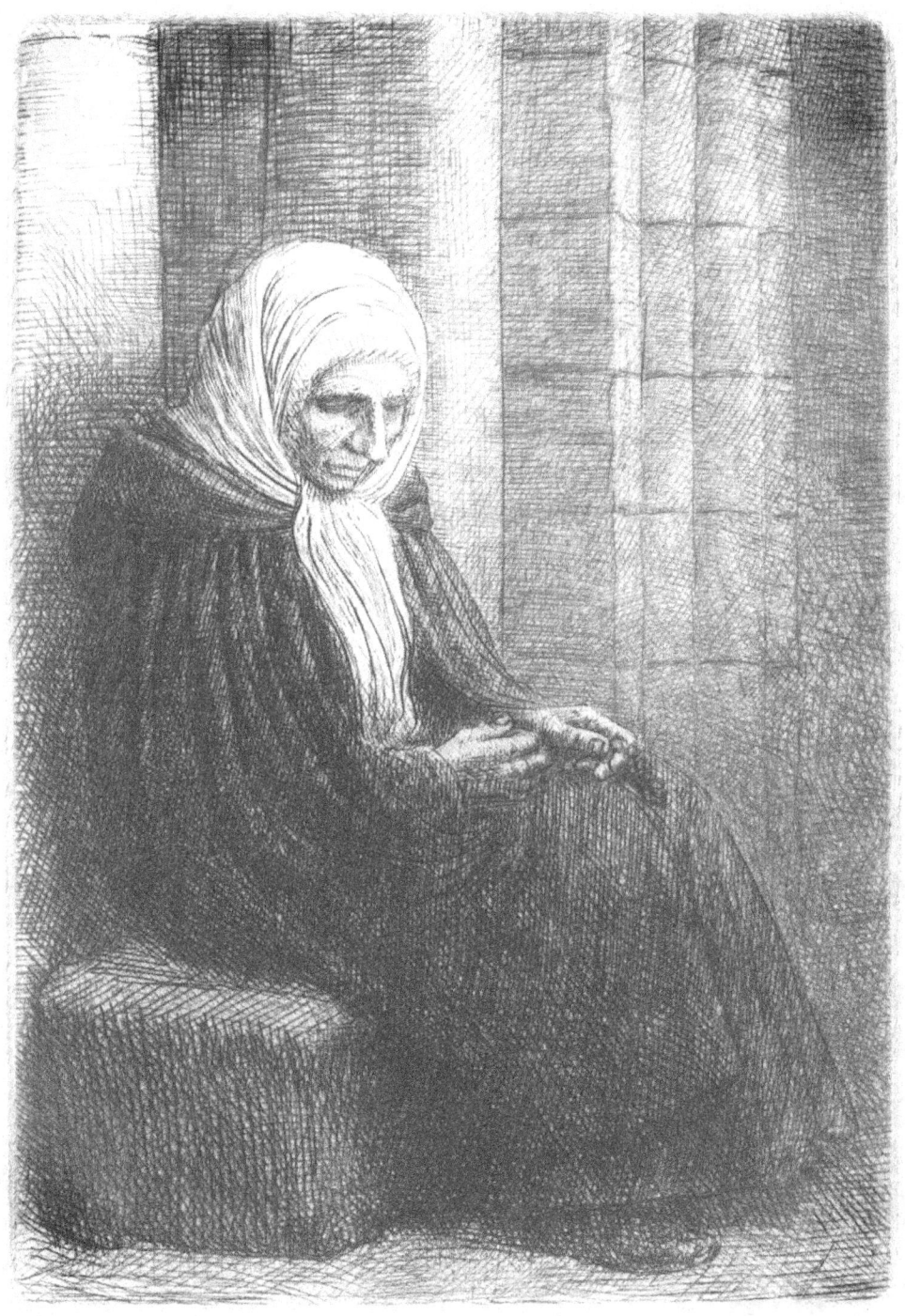

It is okay to be me

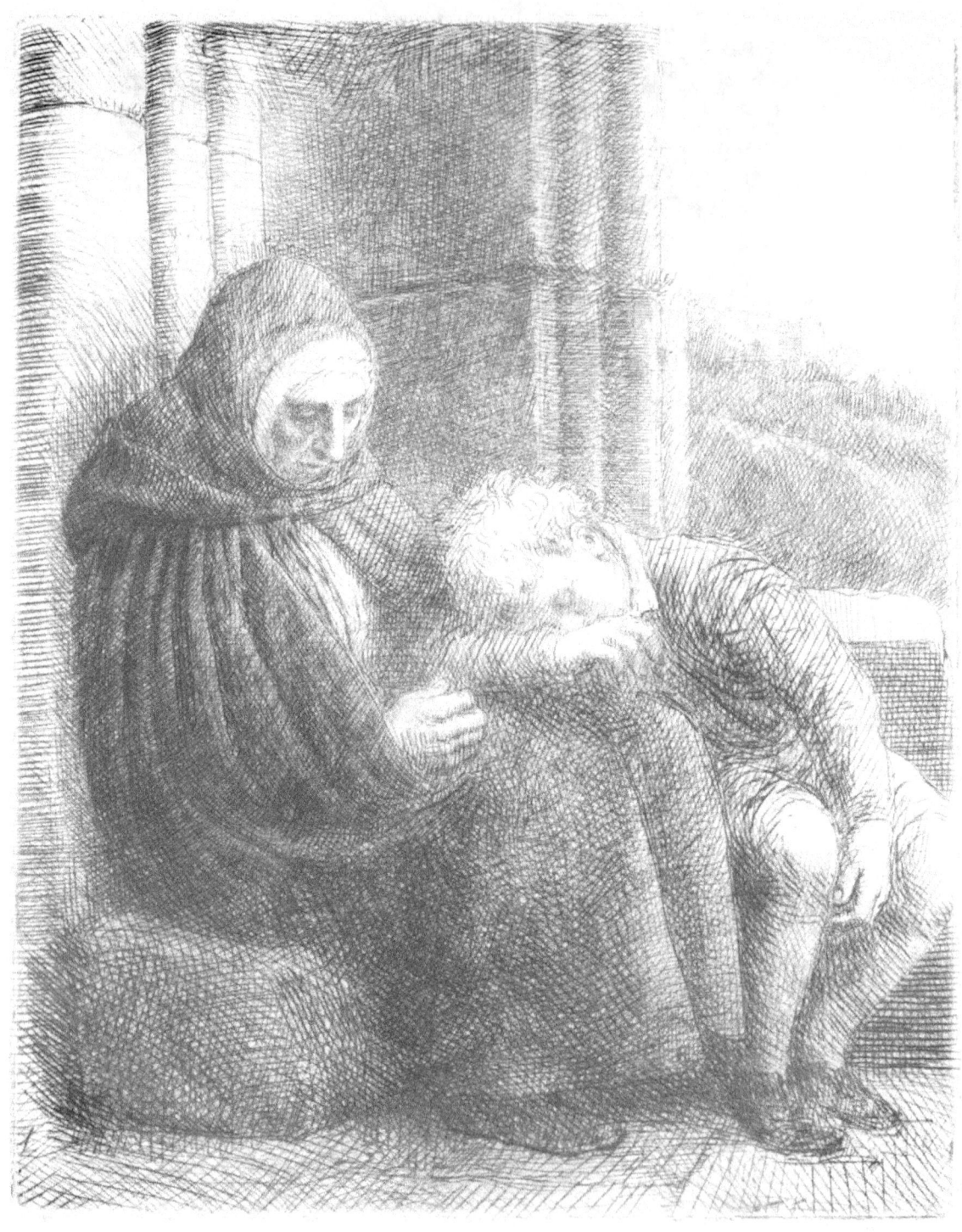

I can accomplish my goals

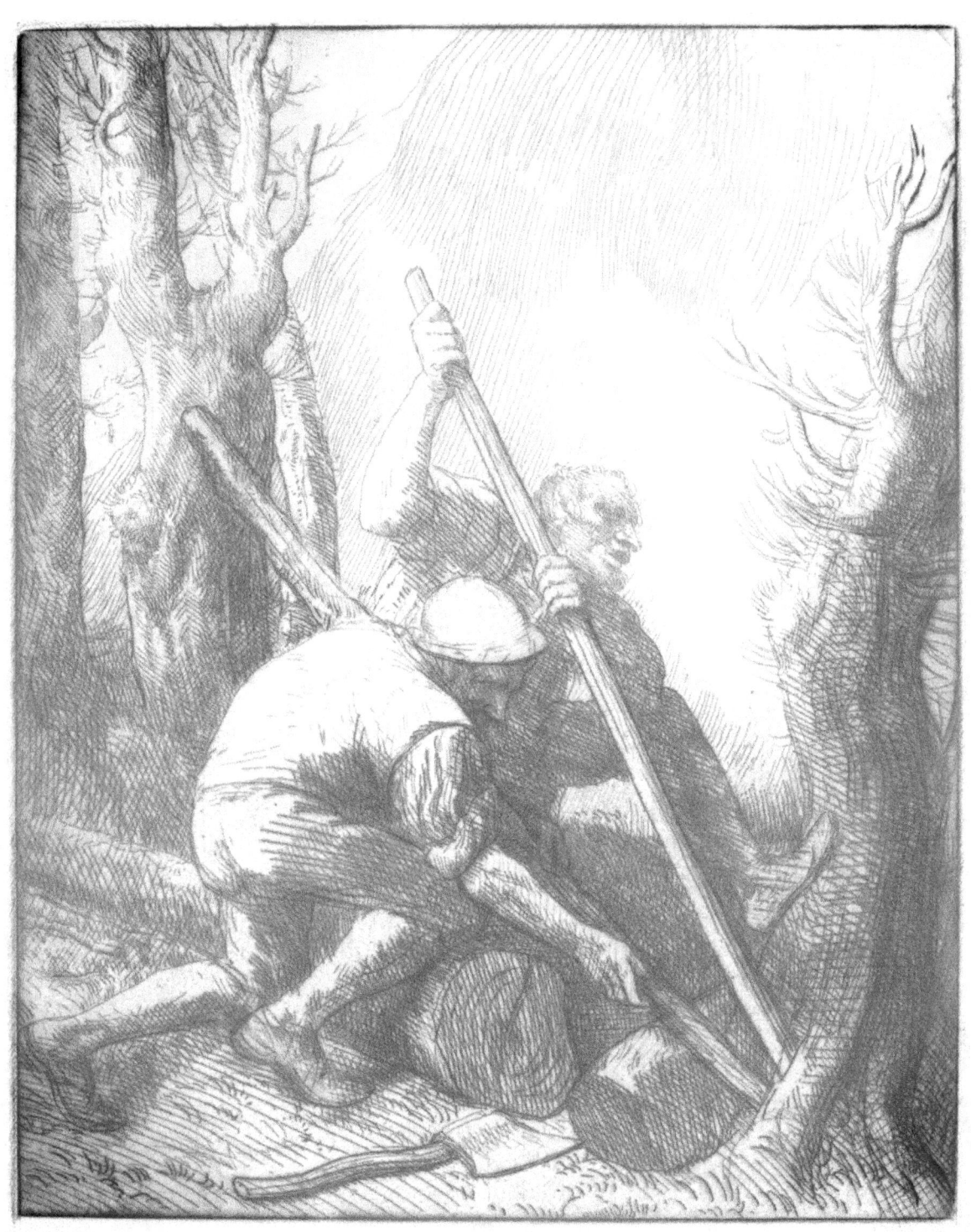

I am unforgettable

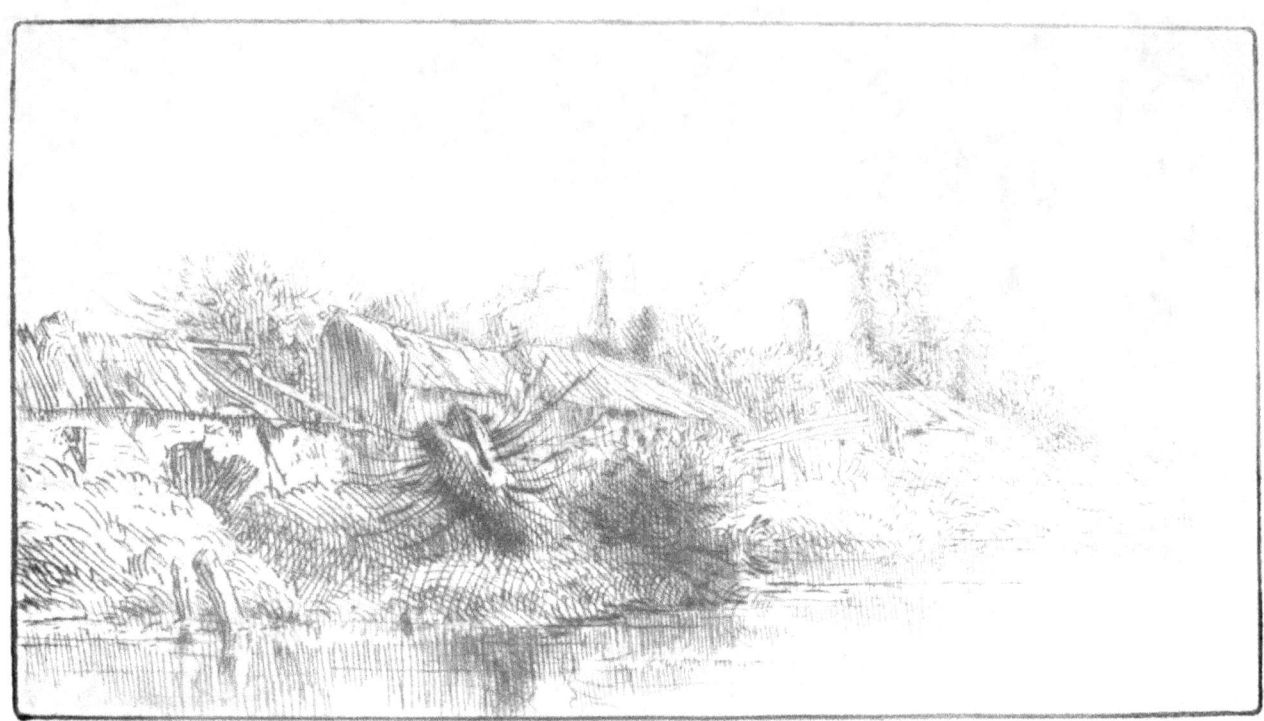

I am worthy of joy

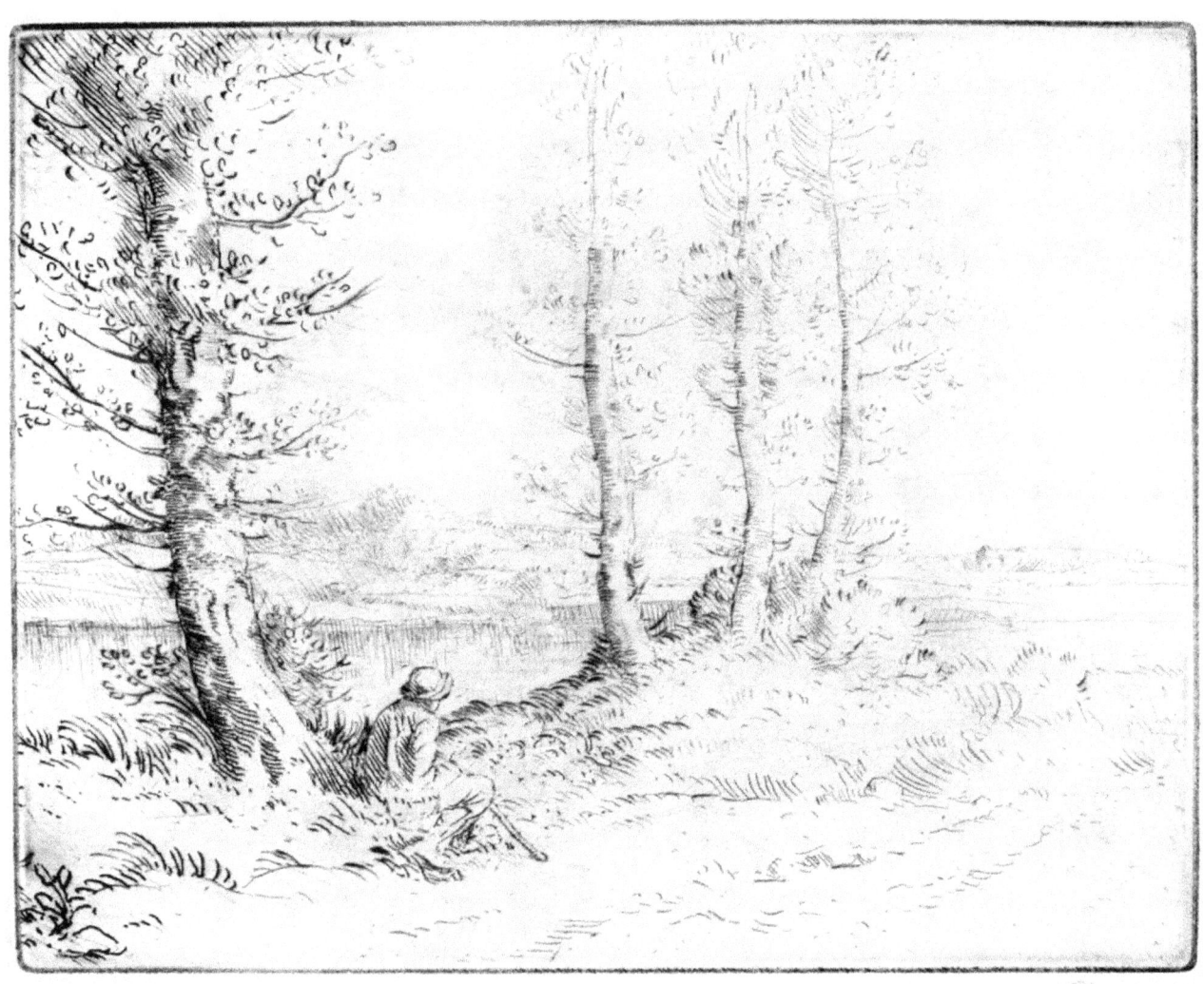

I have mastery

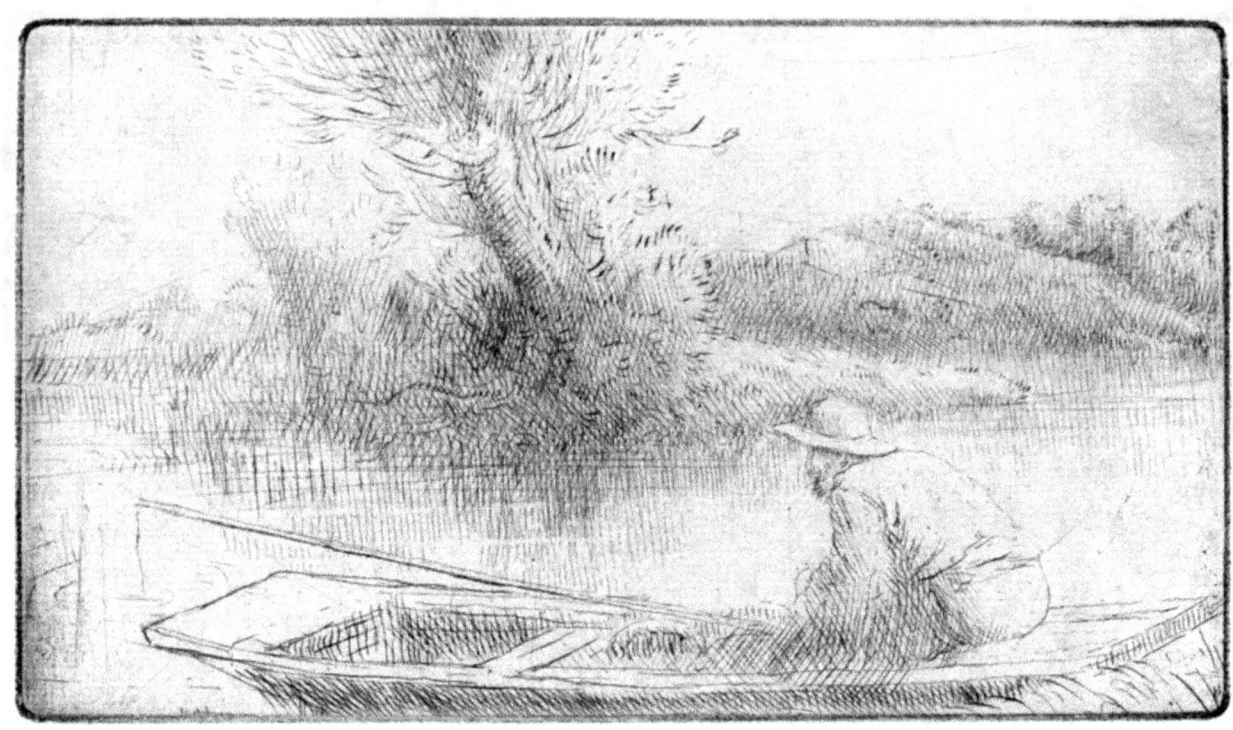

I did enough

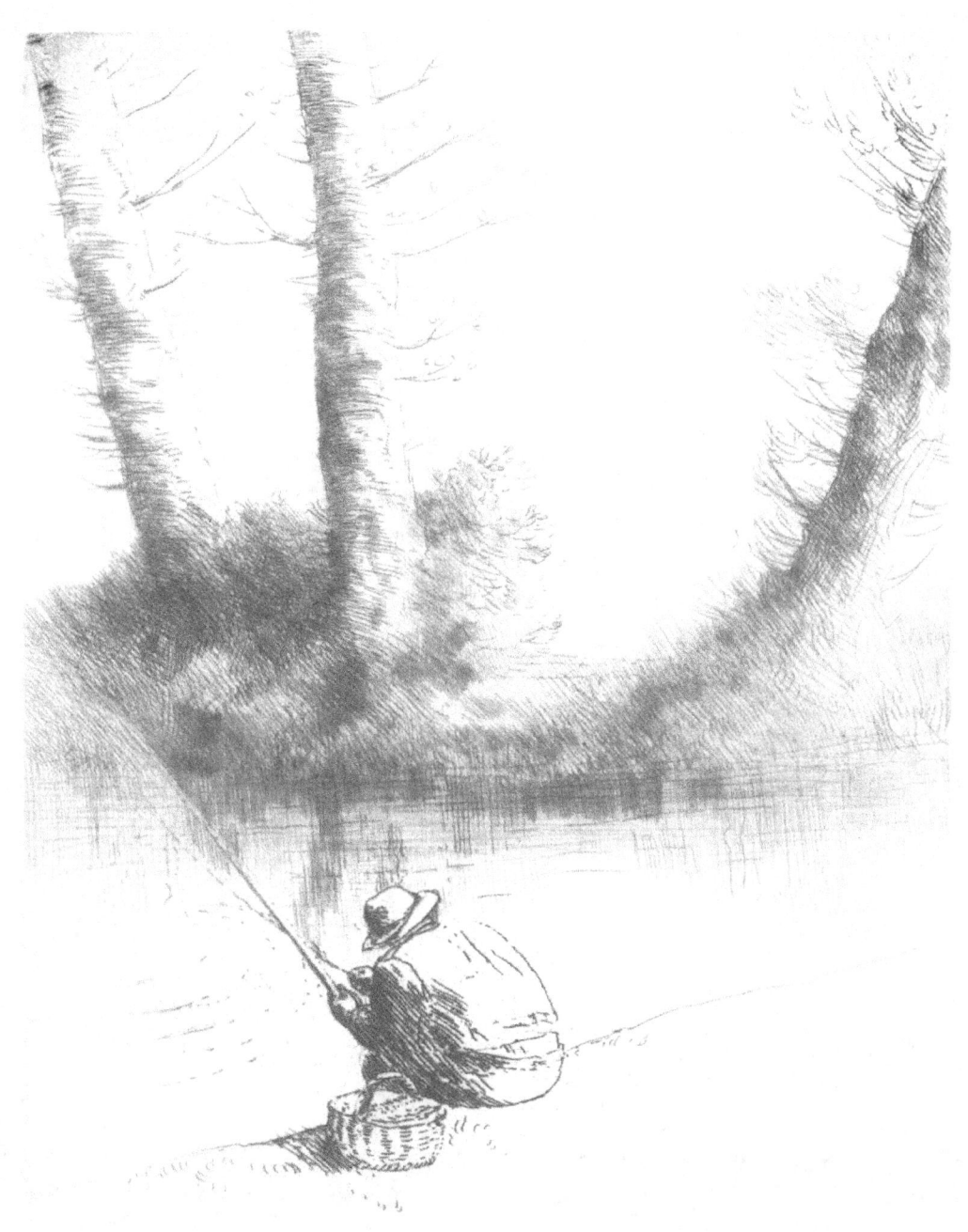

I can be free

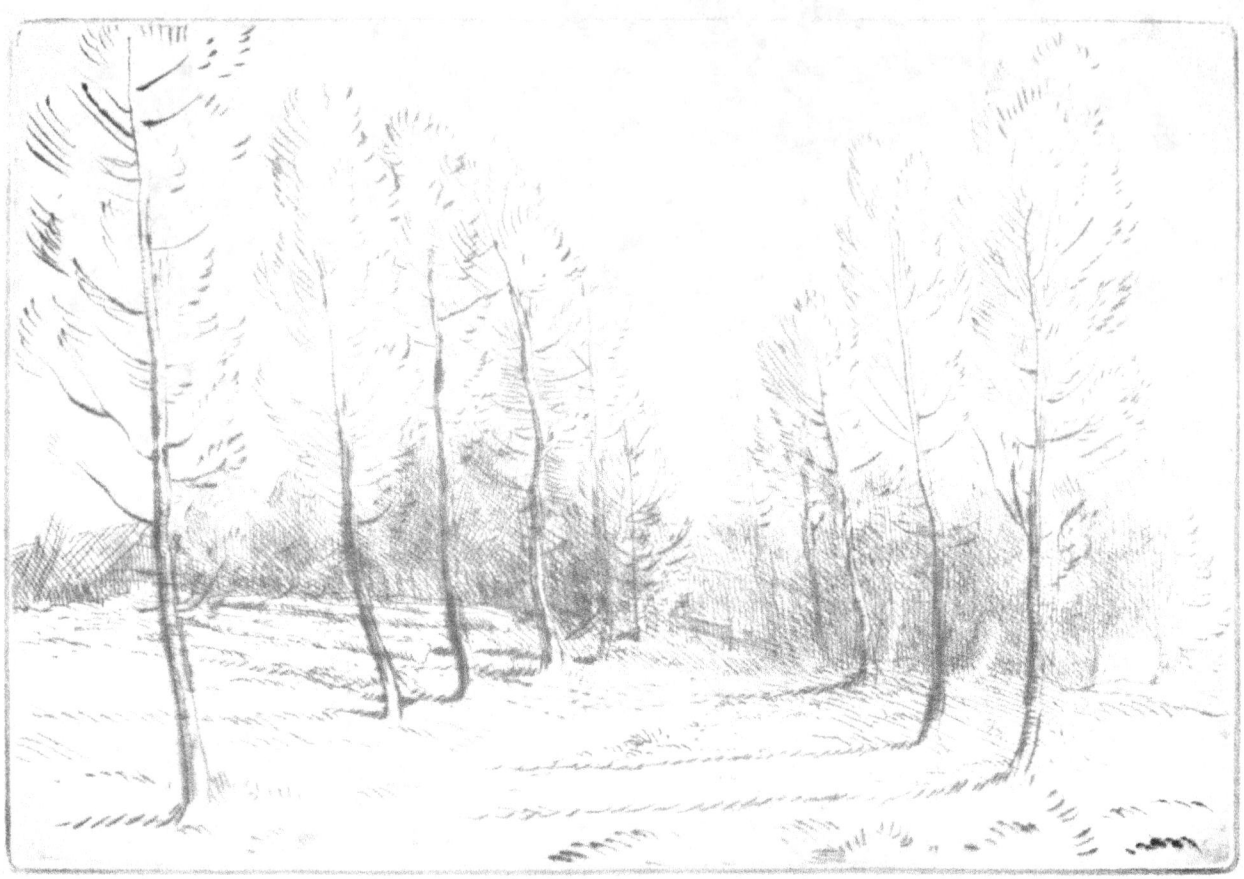

I can make good decisions

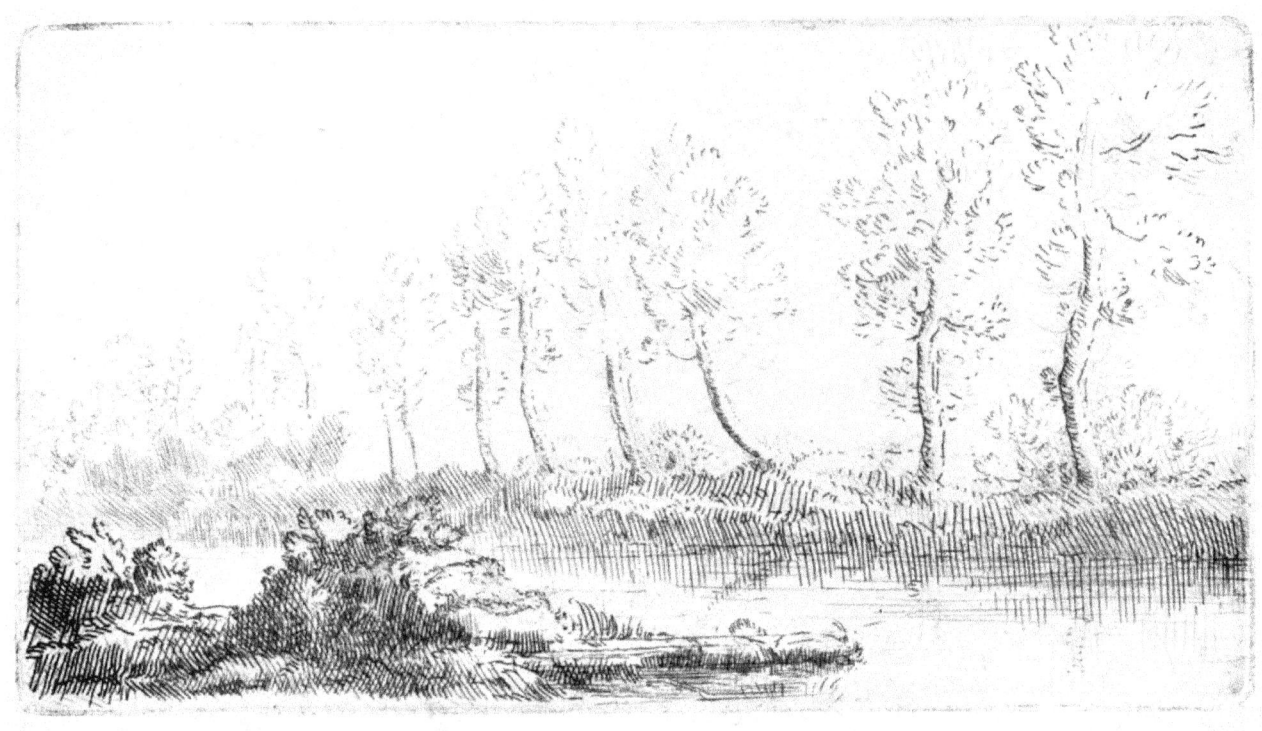

I am alright

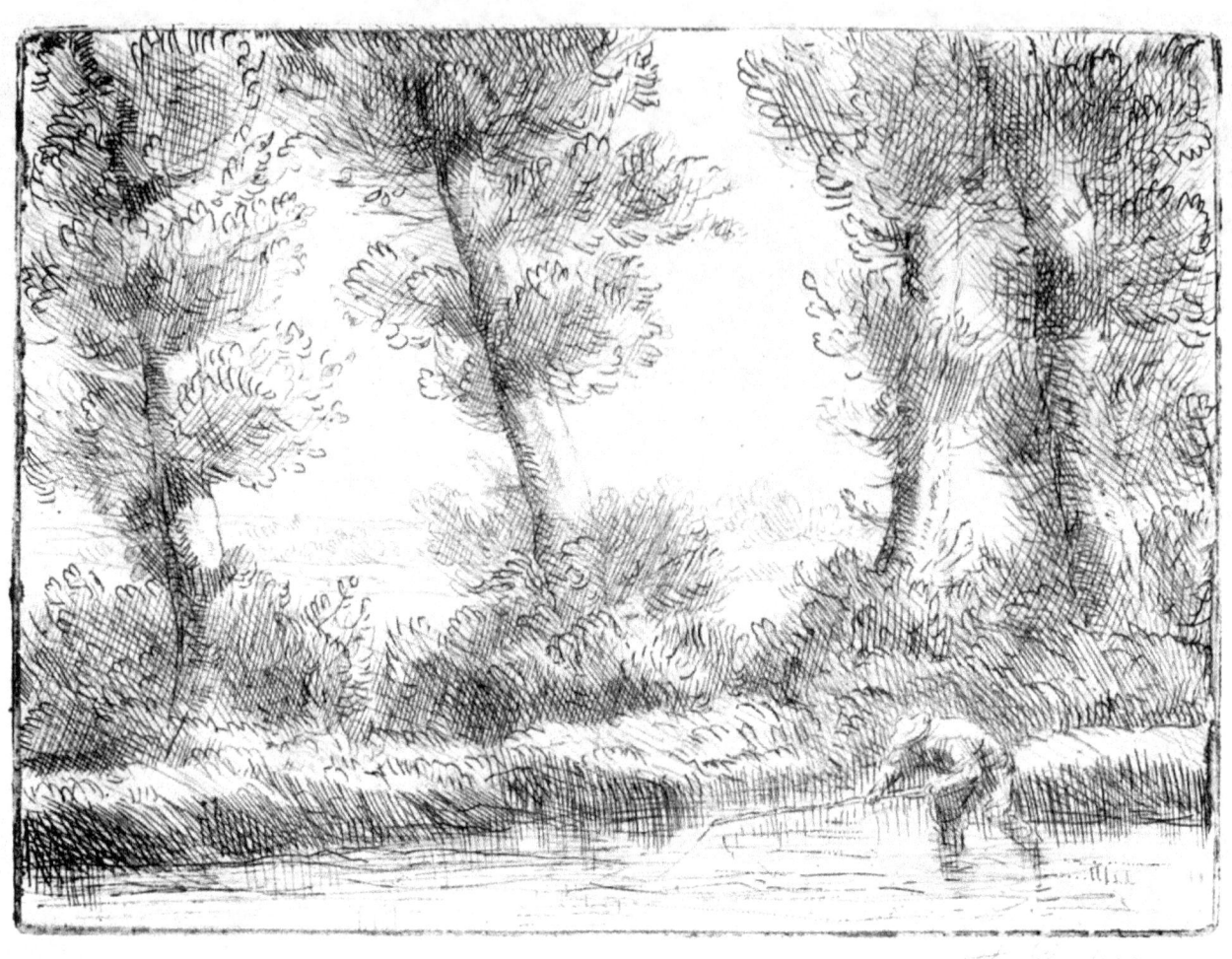

I am lovely

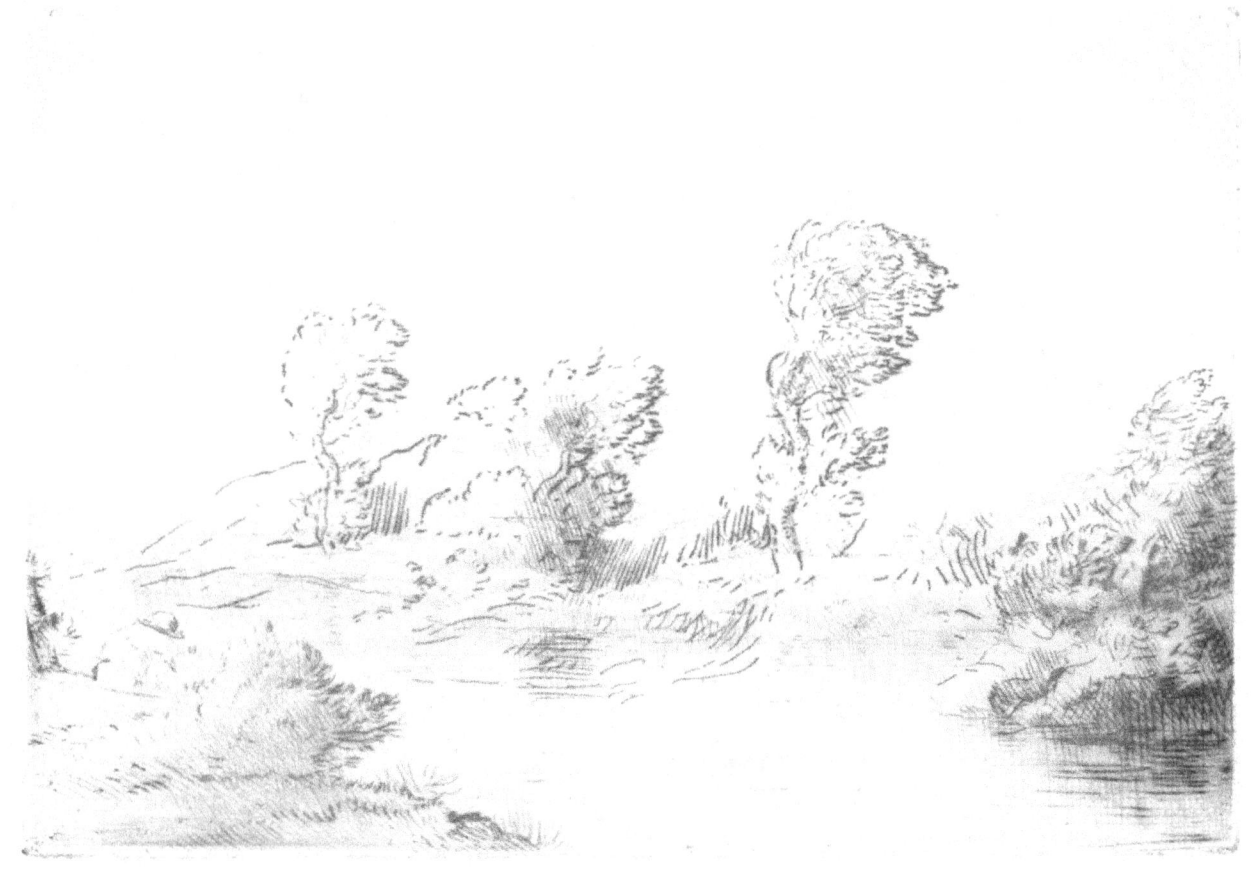

I am remarkable

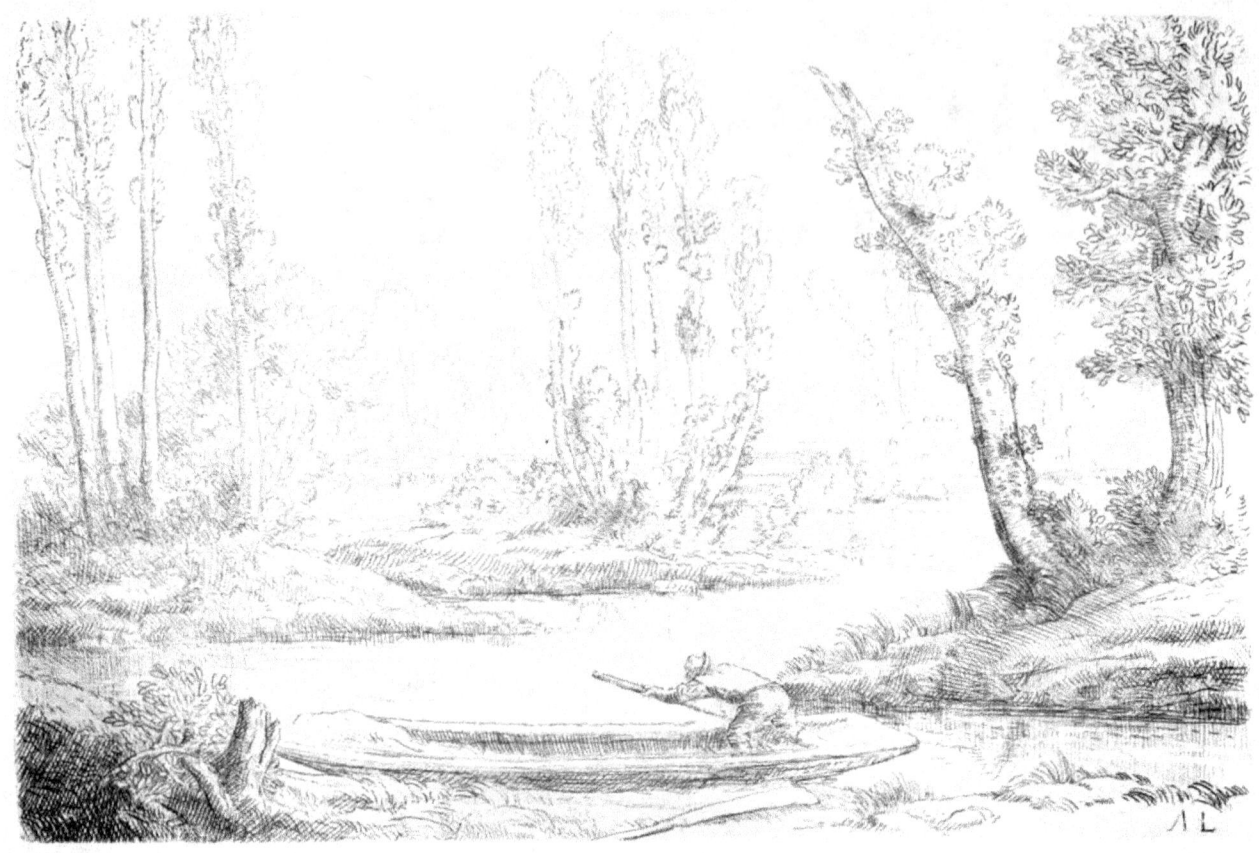

I was just a kid

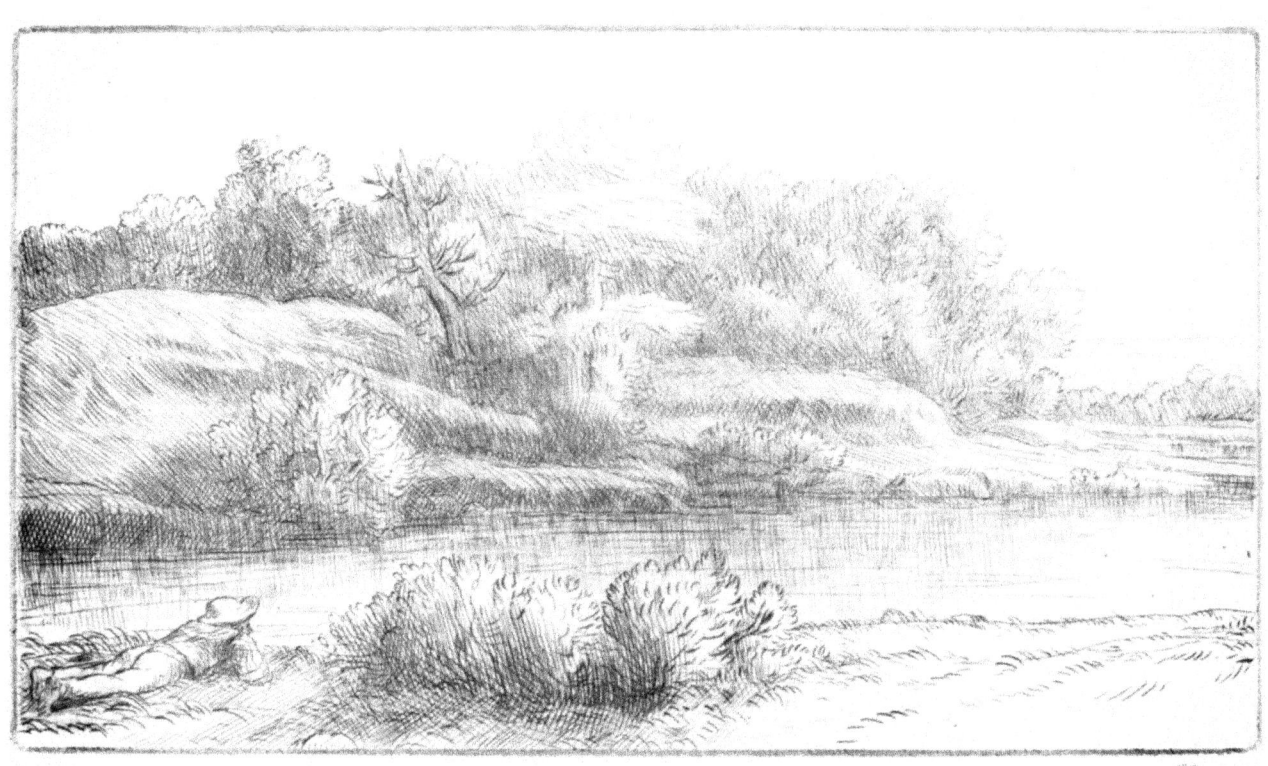

I am excellent

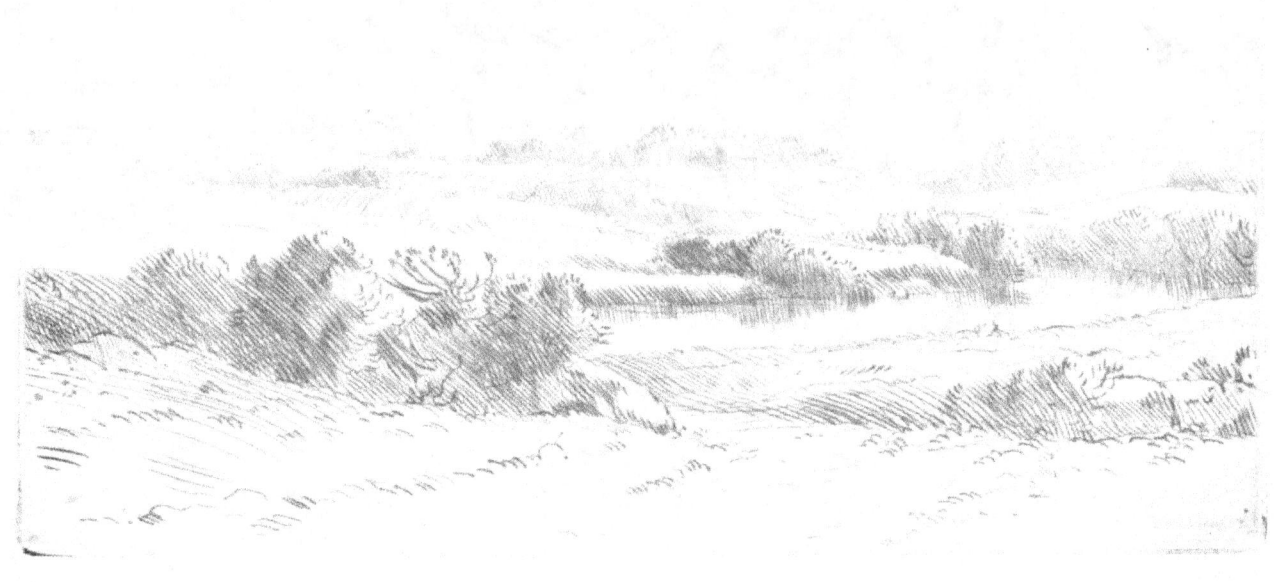

I can move on

I am able

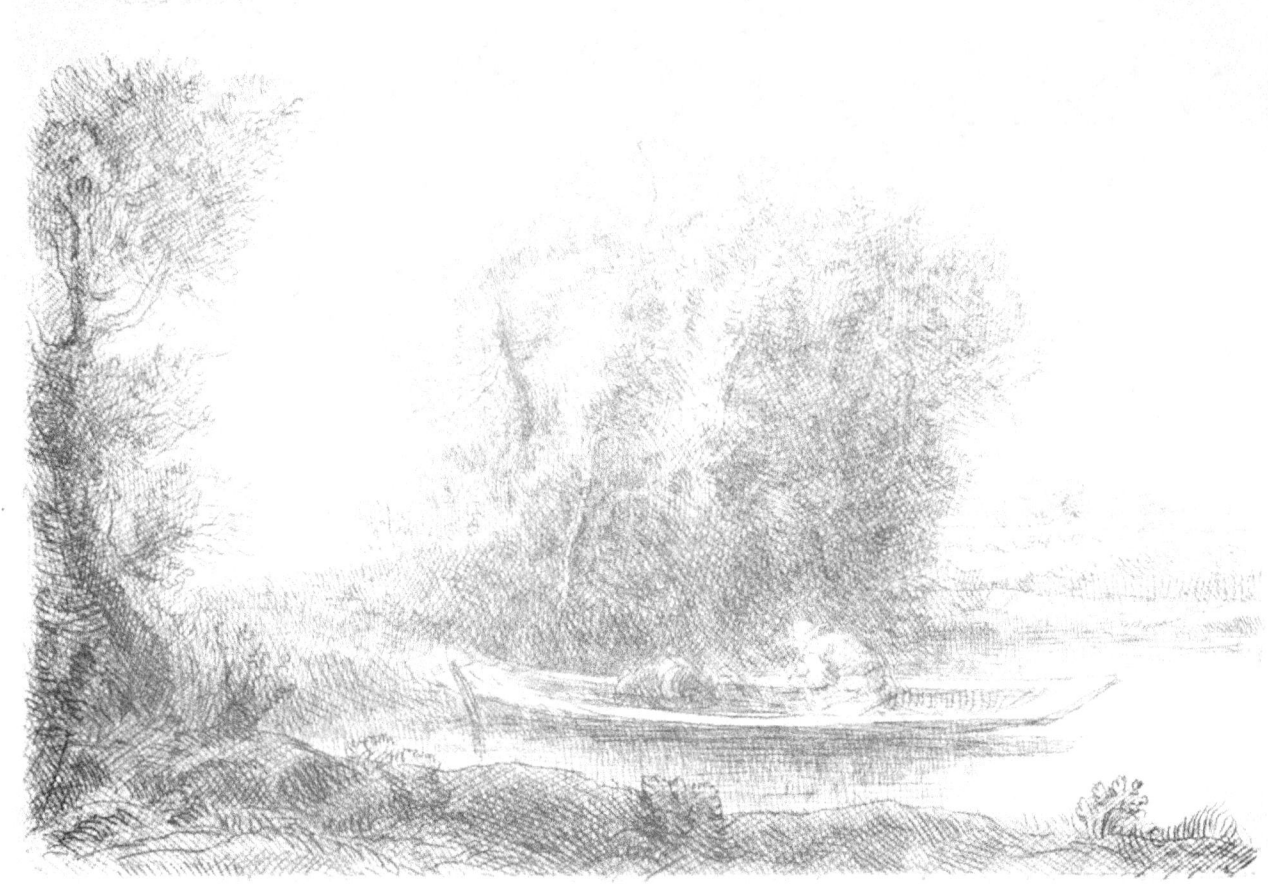

I can conquer my fears

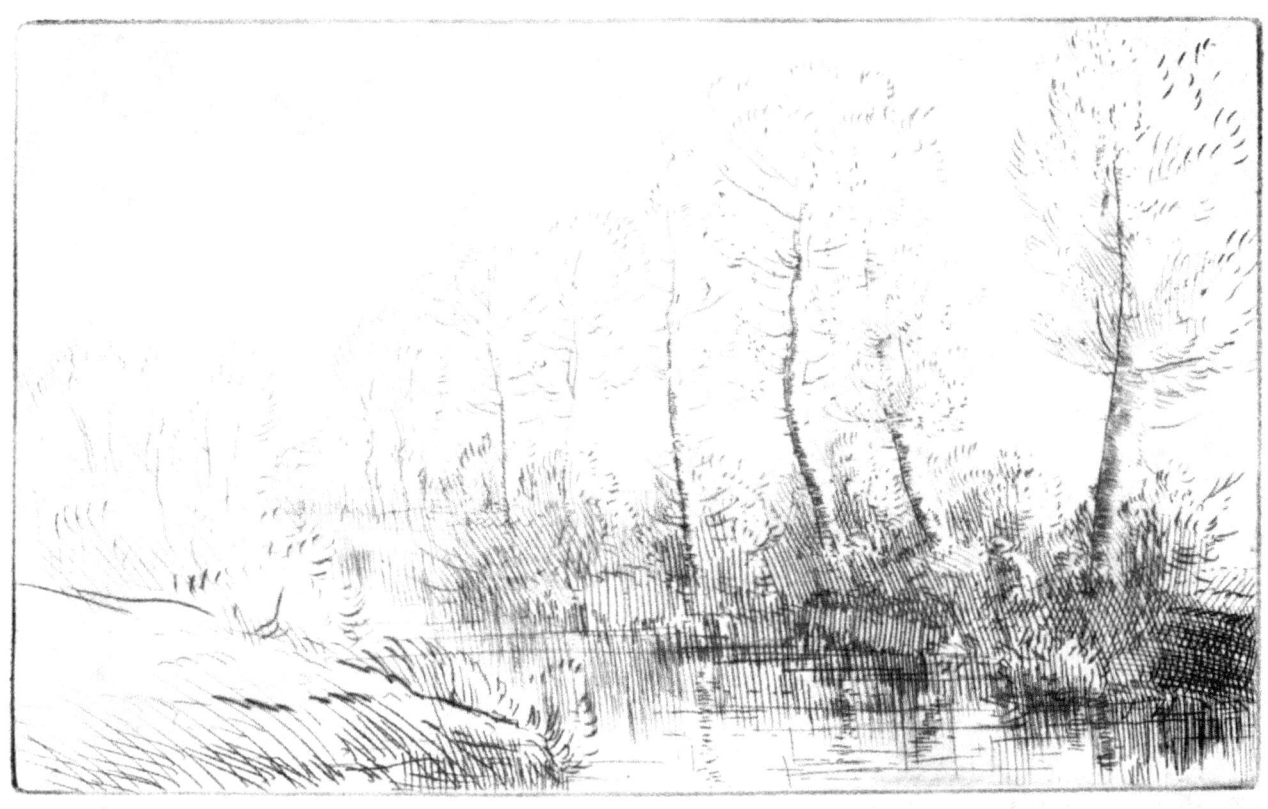

I am a masterpiece

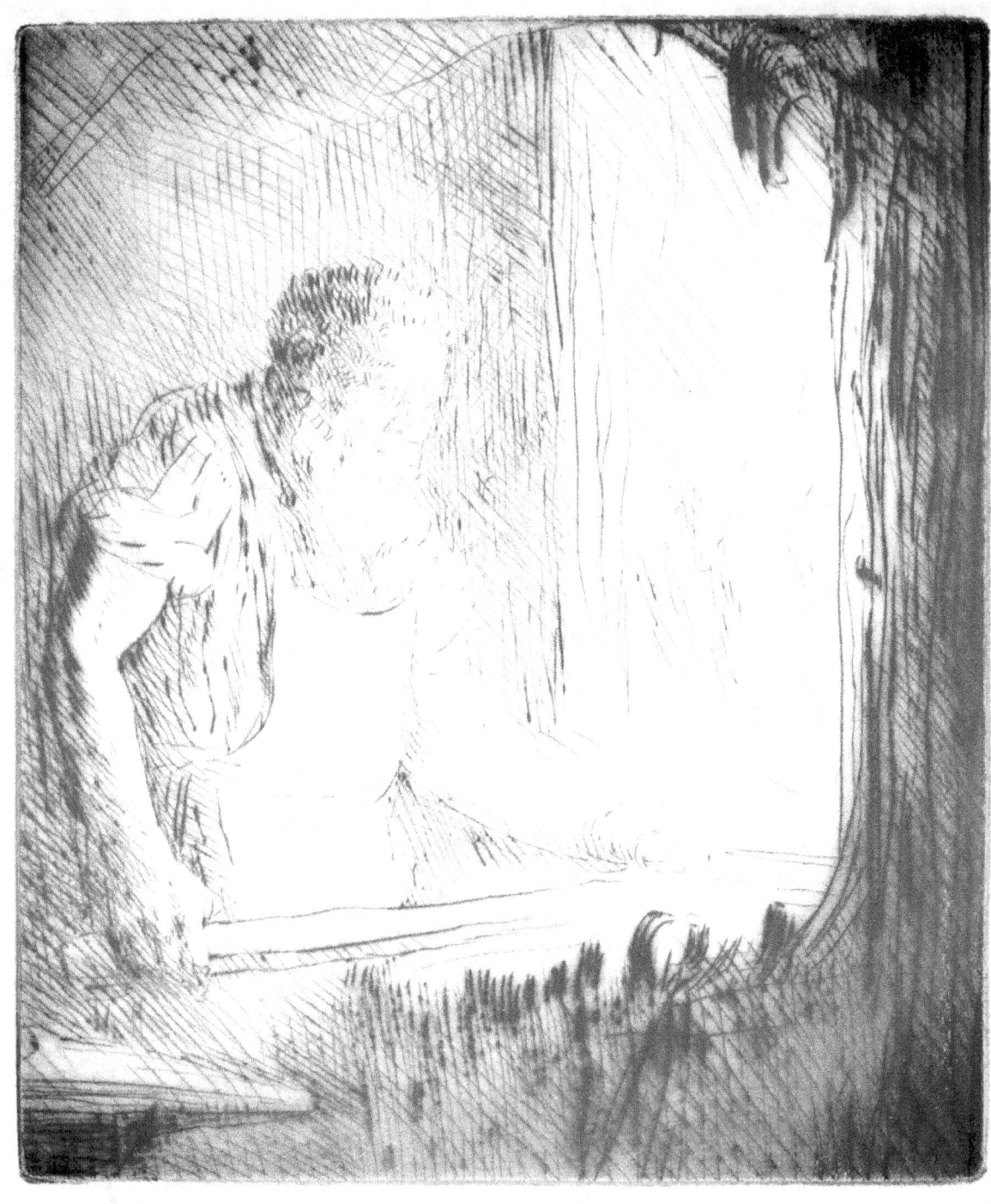

I am a person of integrity

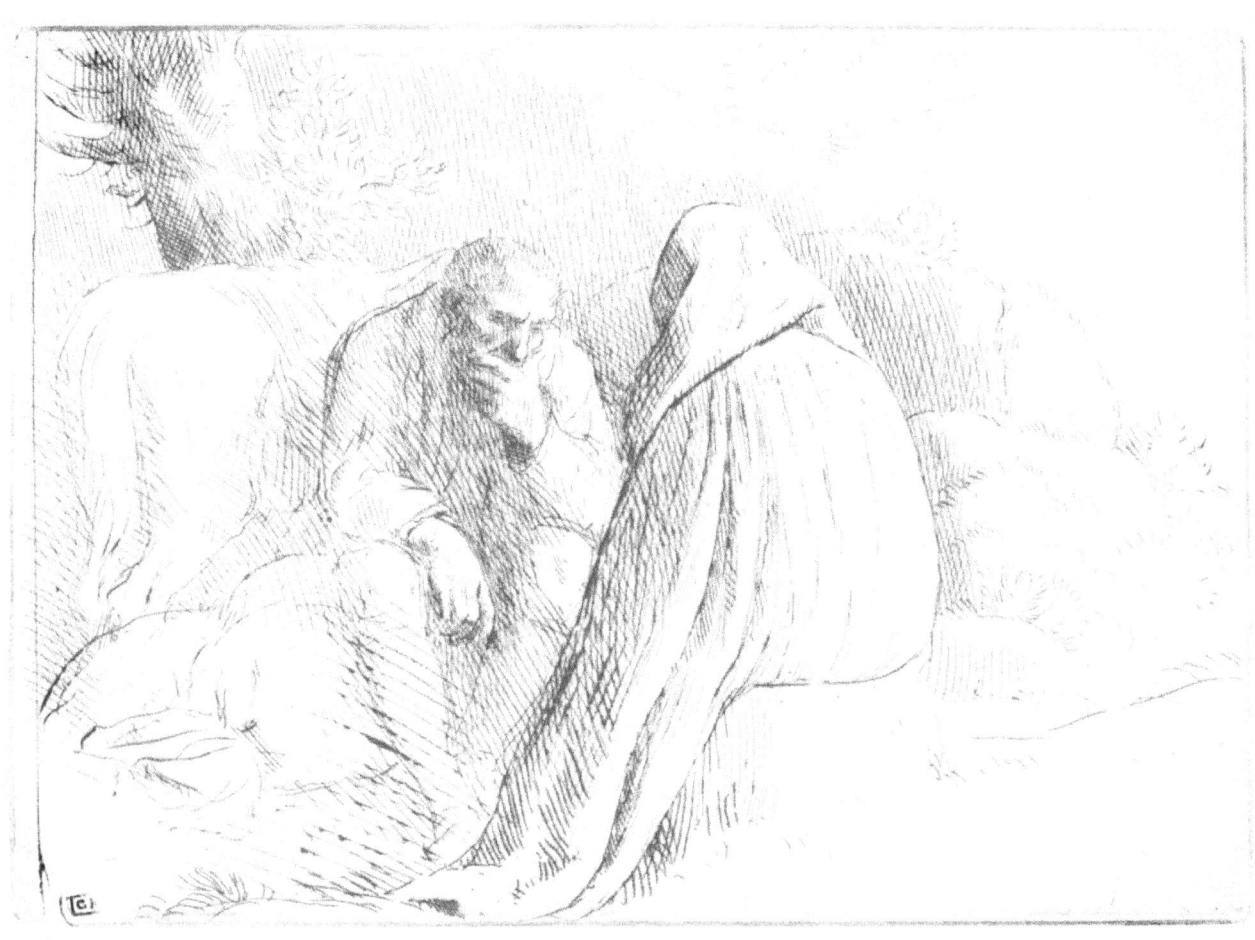

I am priceless

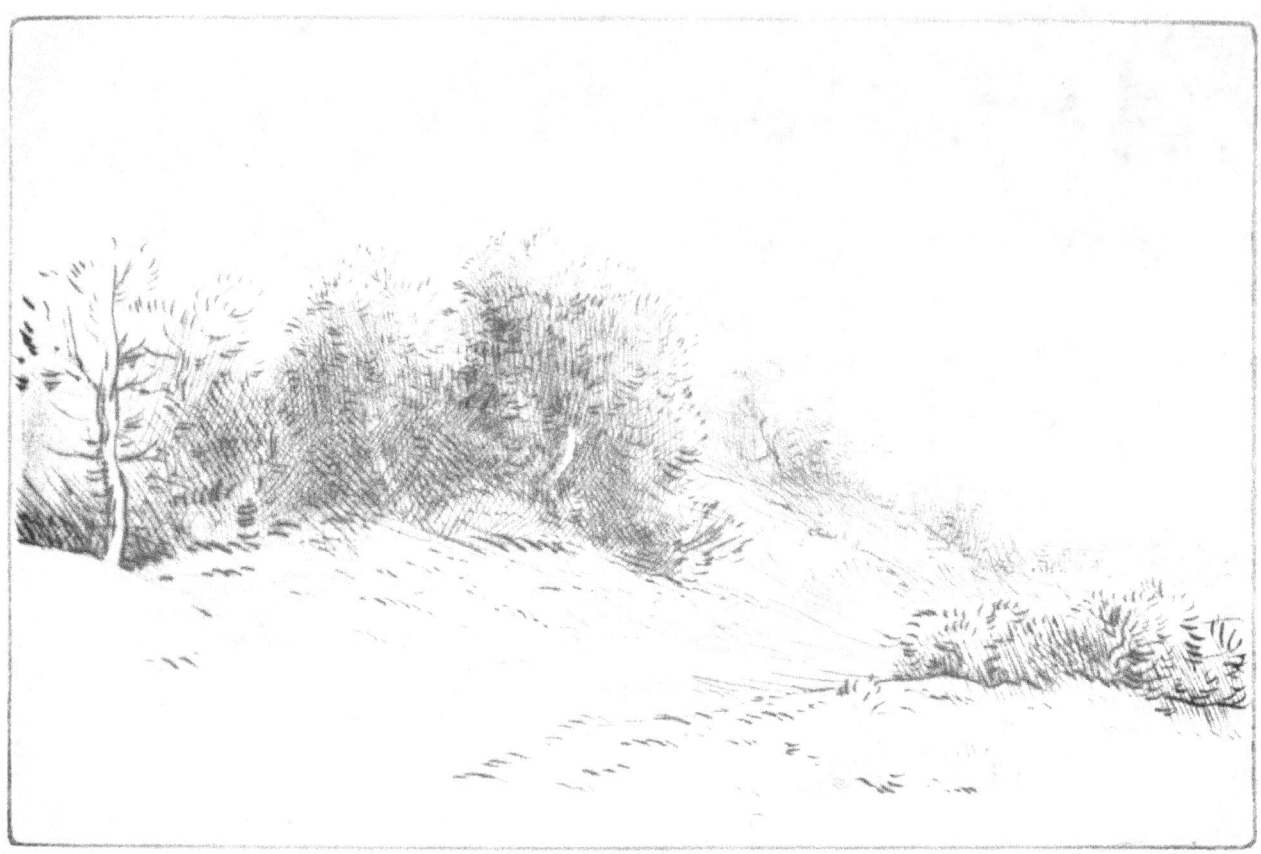

I am respectable

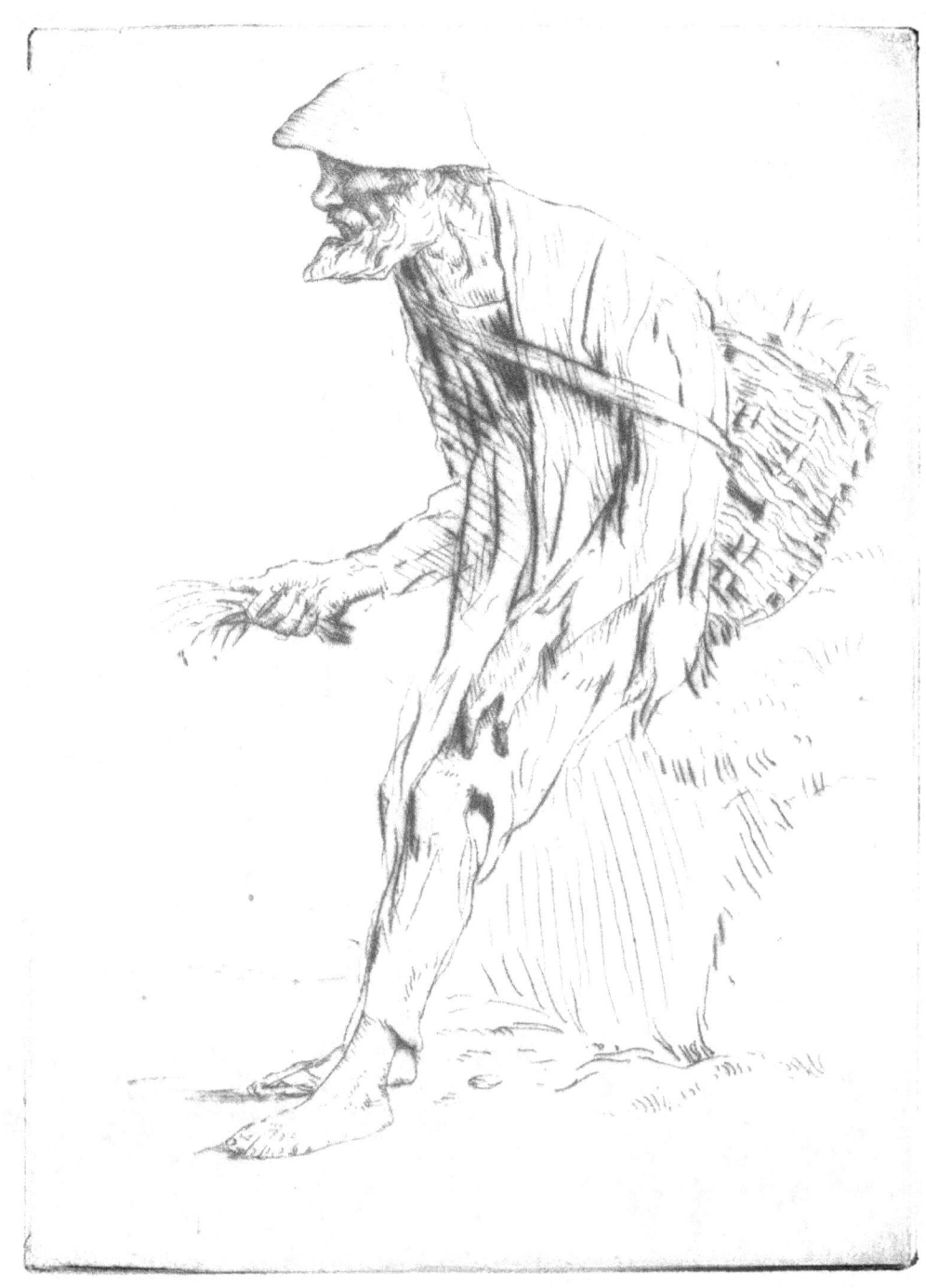

I am a work of art

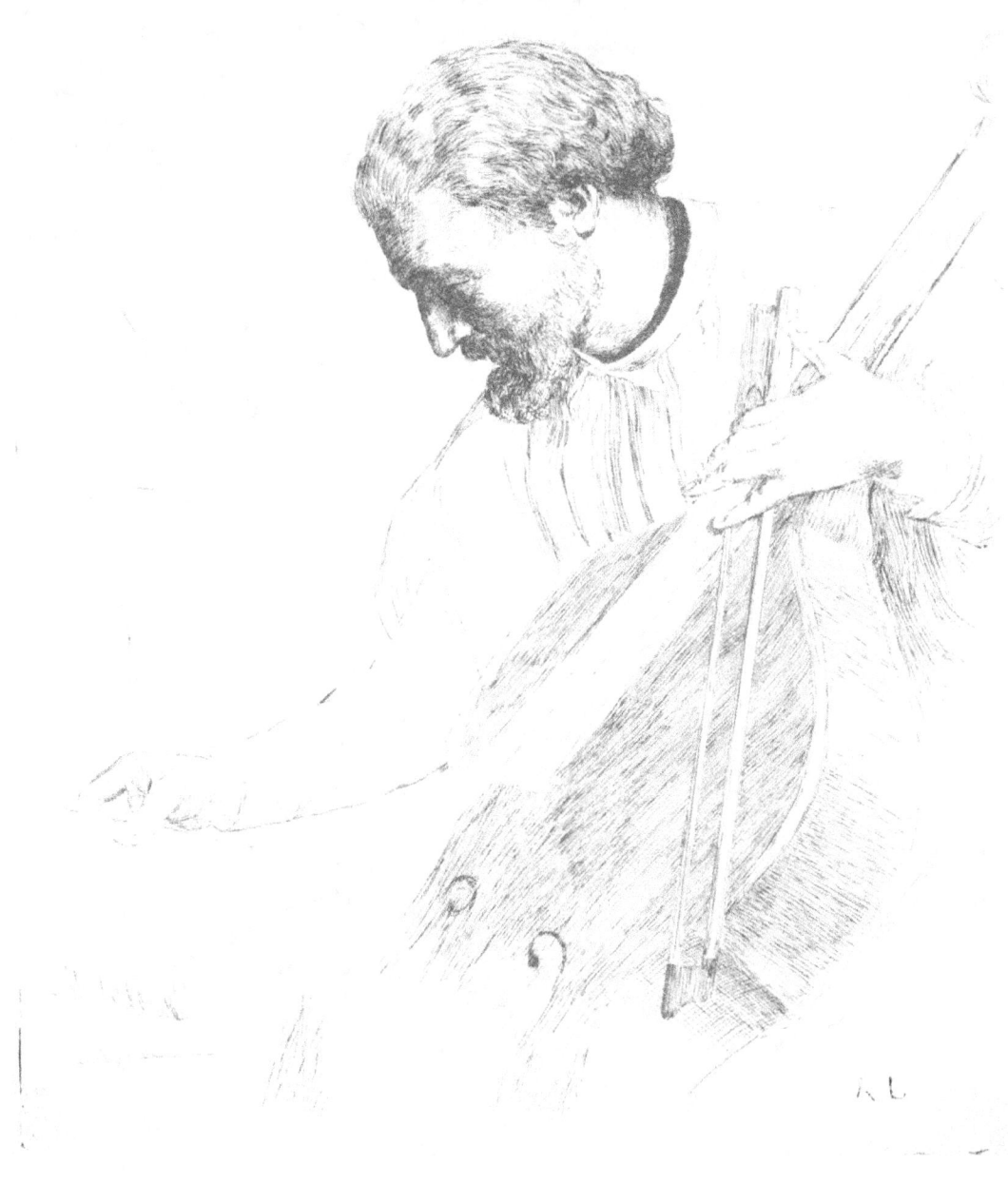

I deserve to thrive

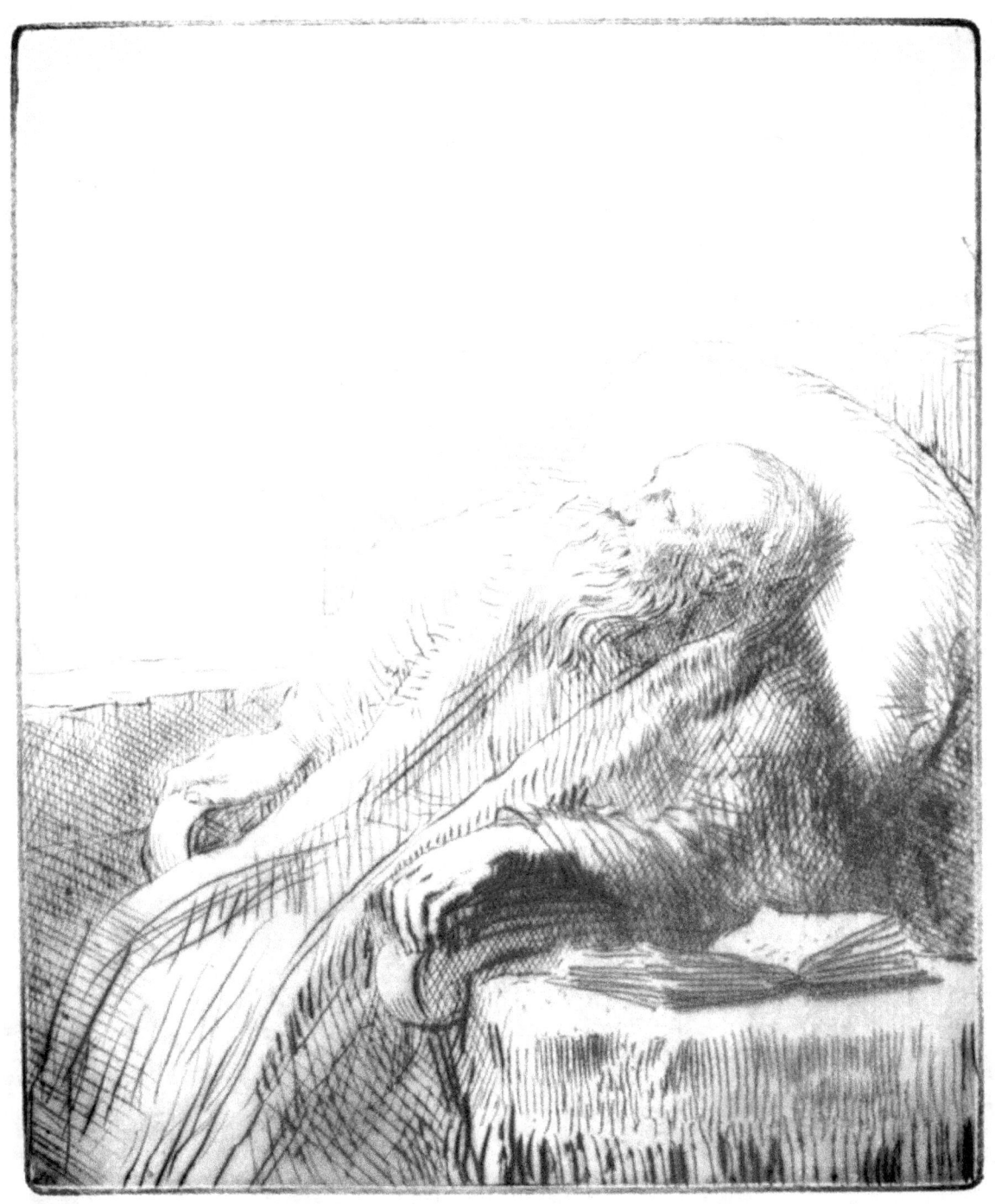

I am desirable

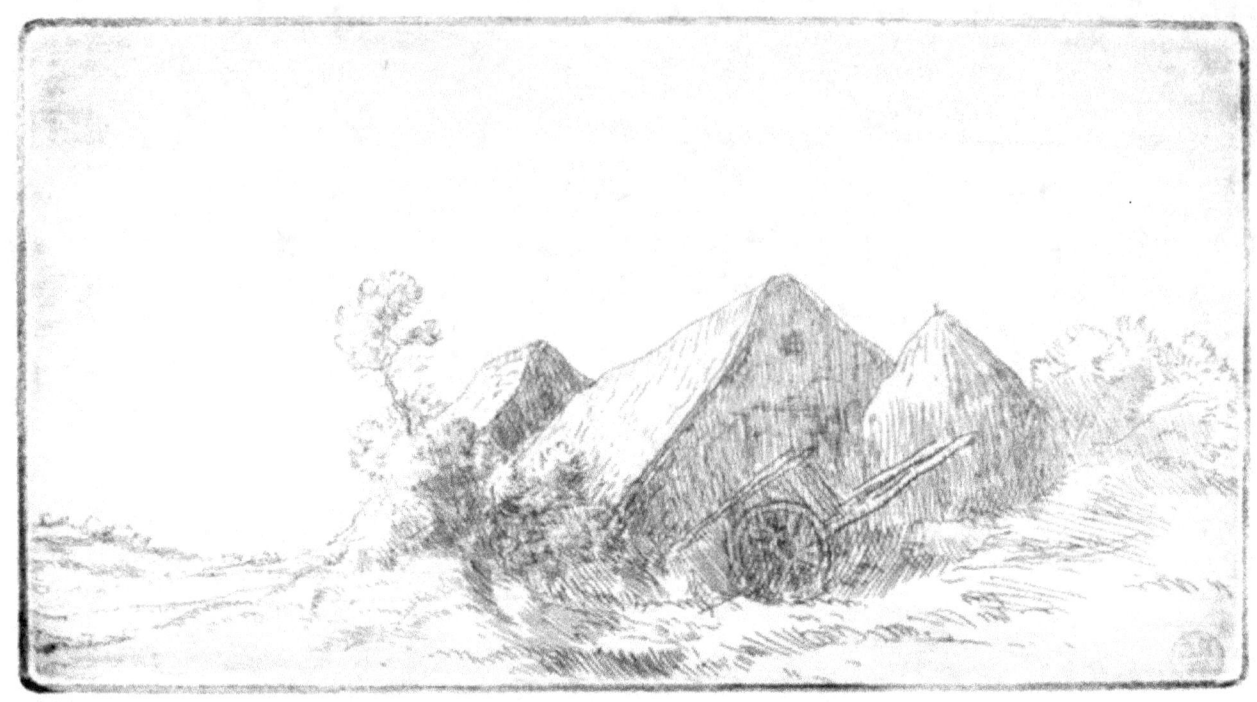

I am okay in my imperfection

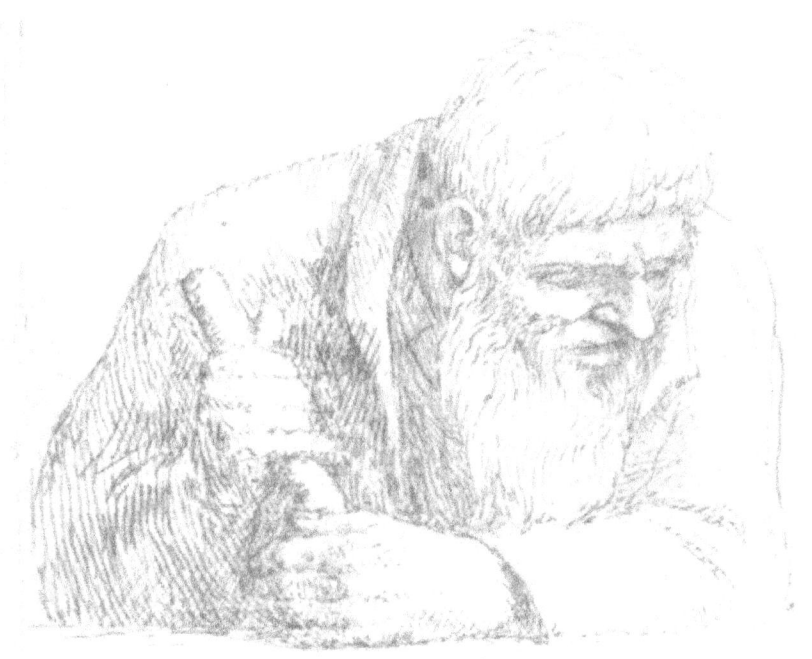

I am tough

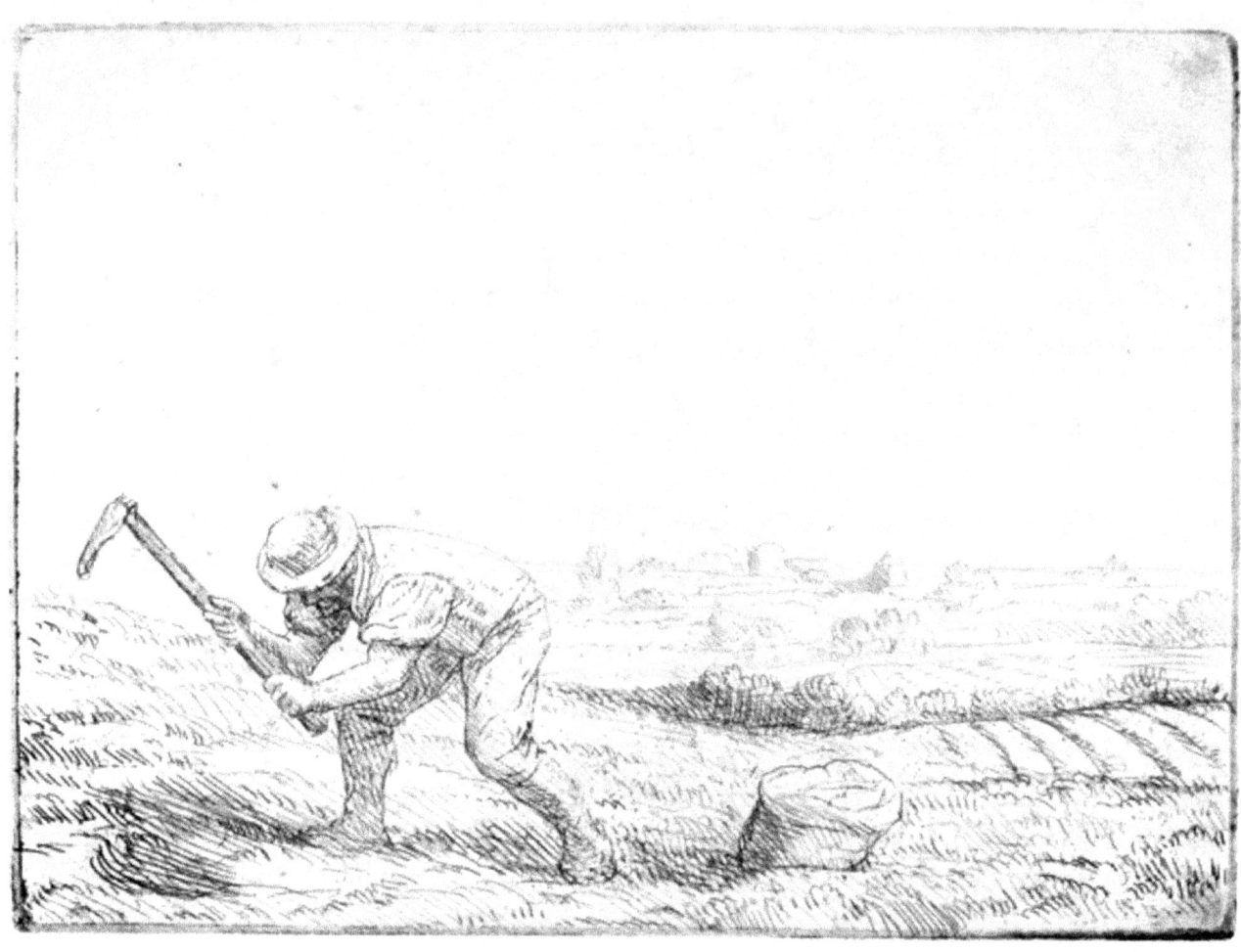

I am secure

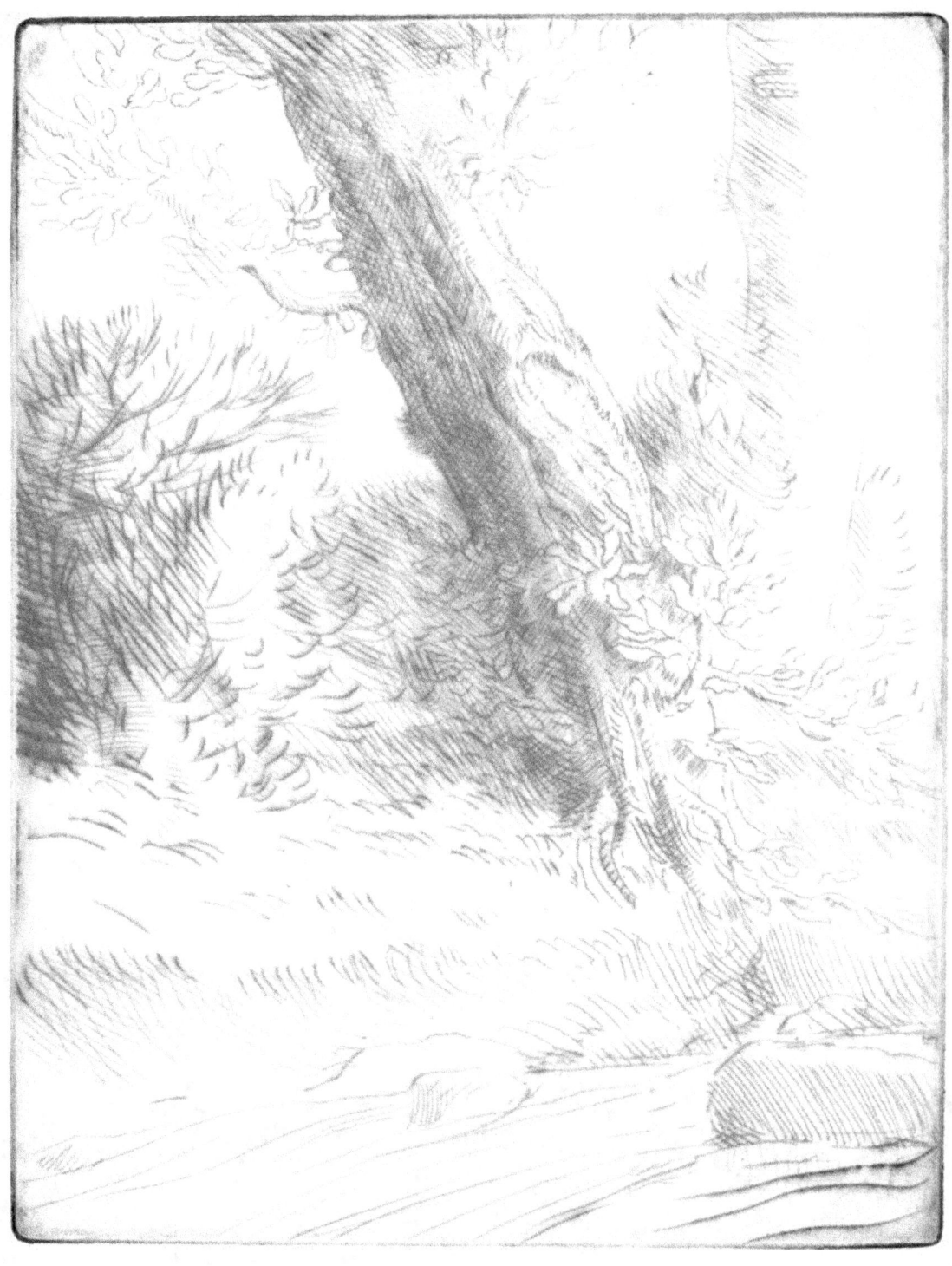

I can manage it

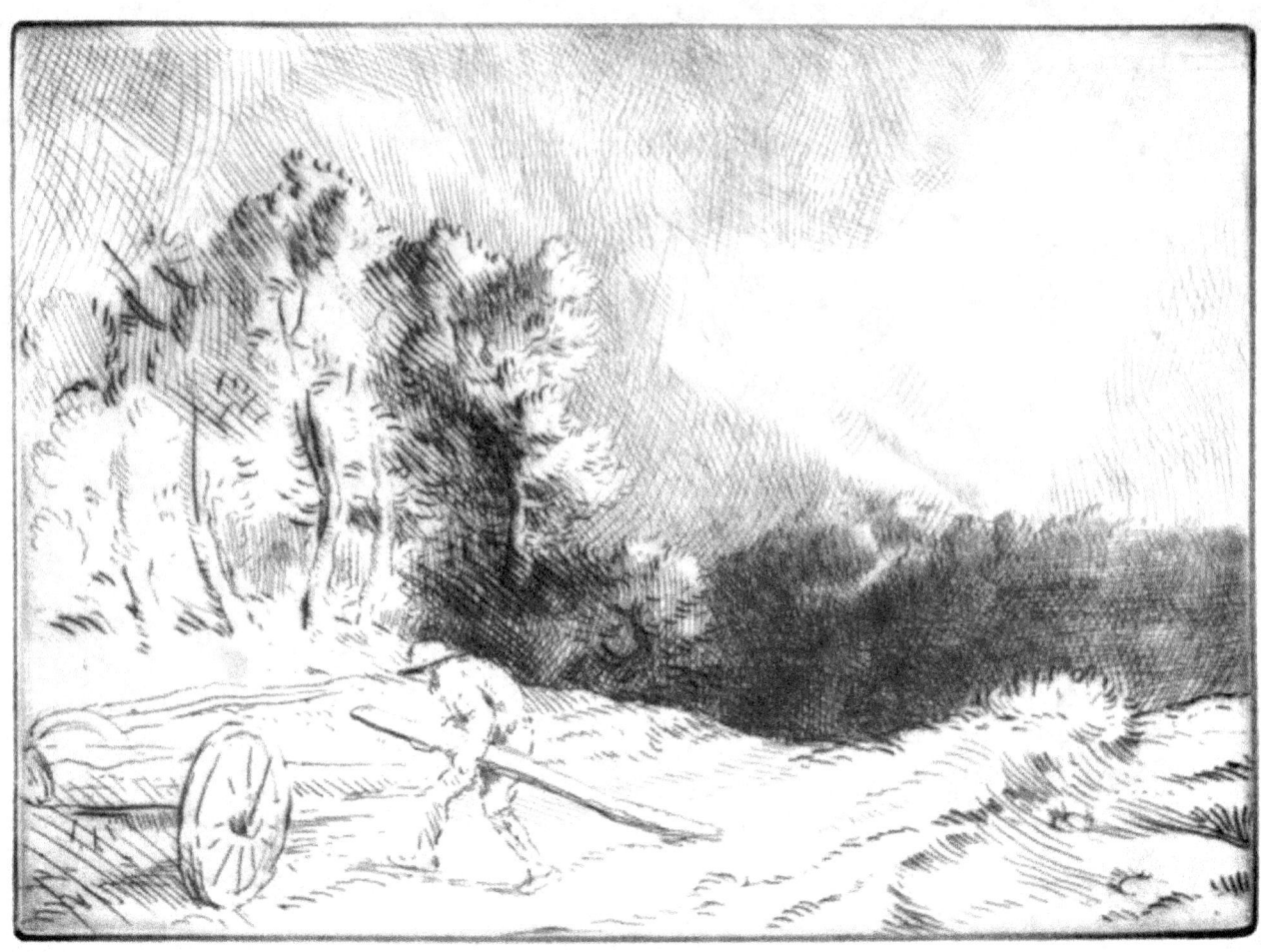

I am praiseworthy

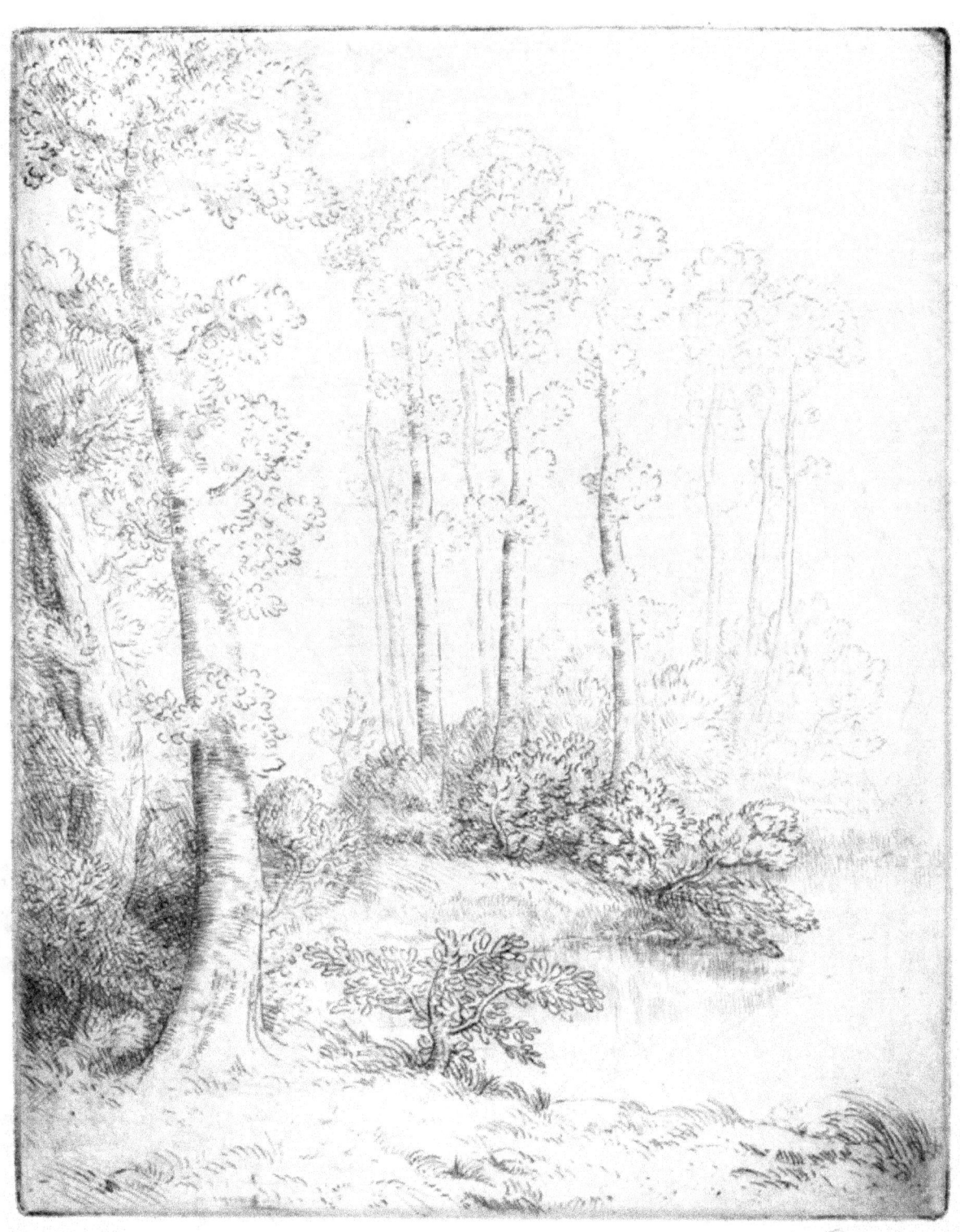

I am bright

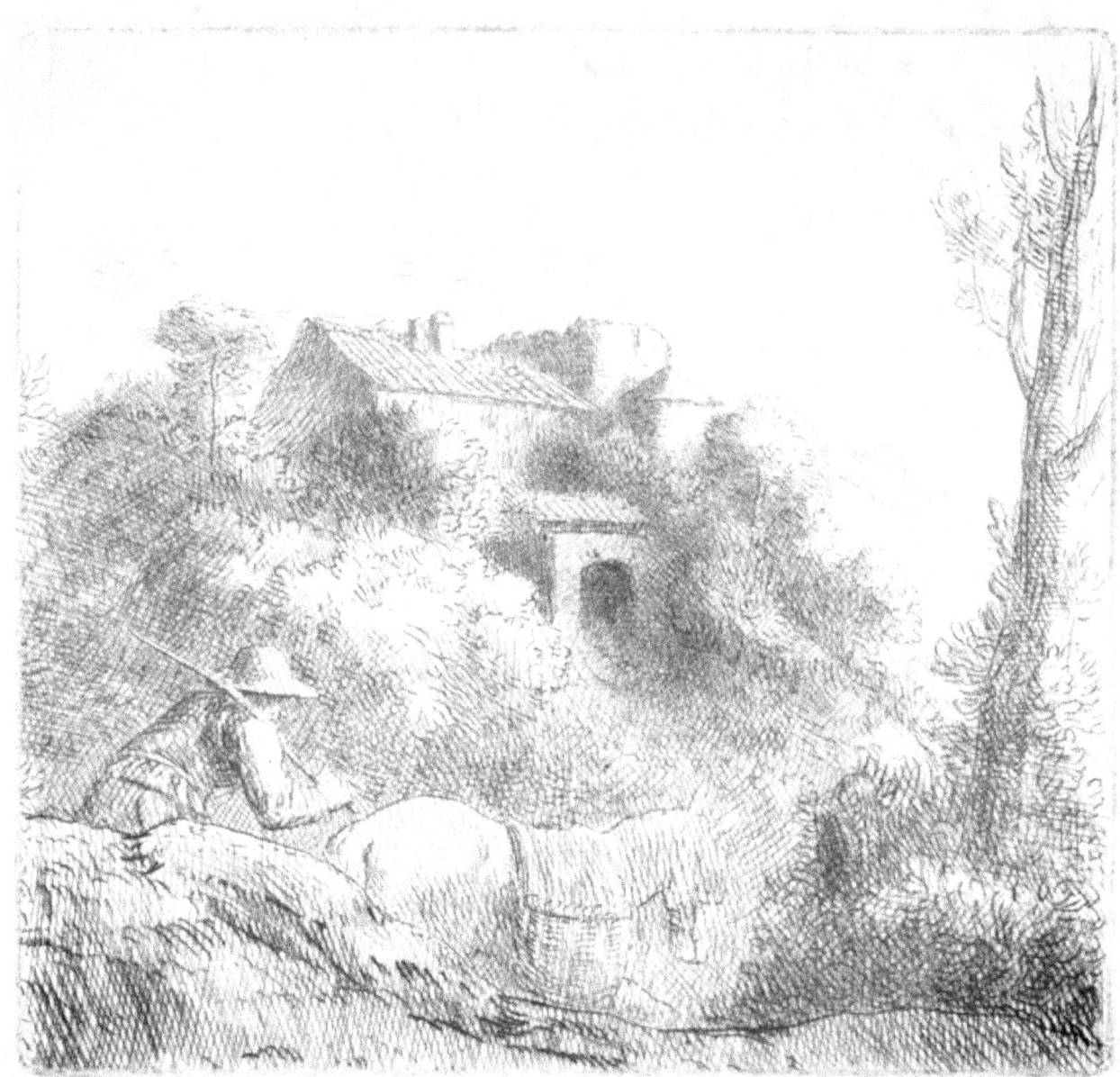

I am faithful

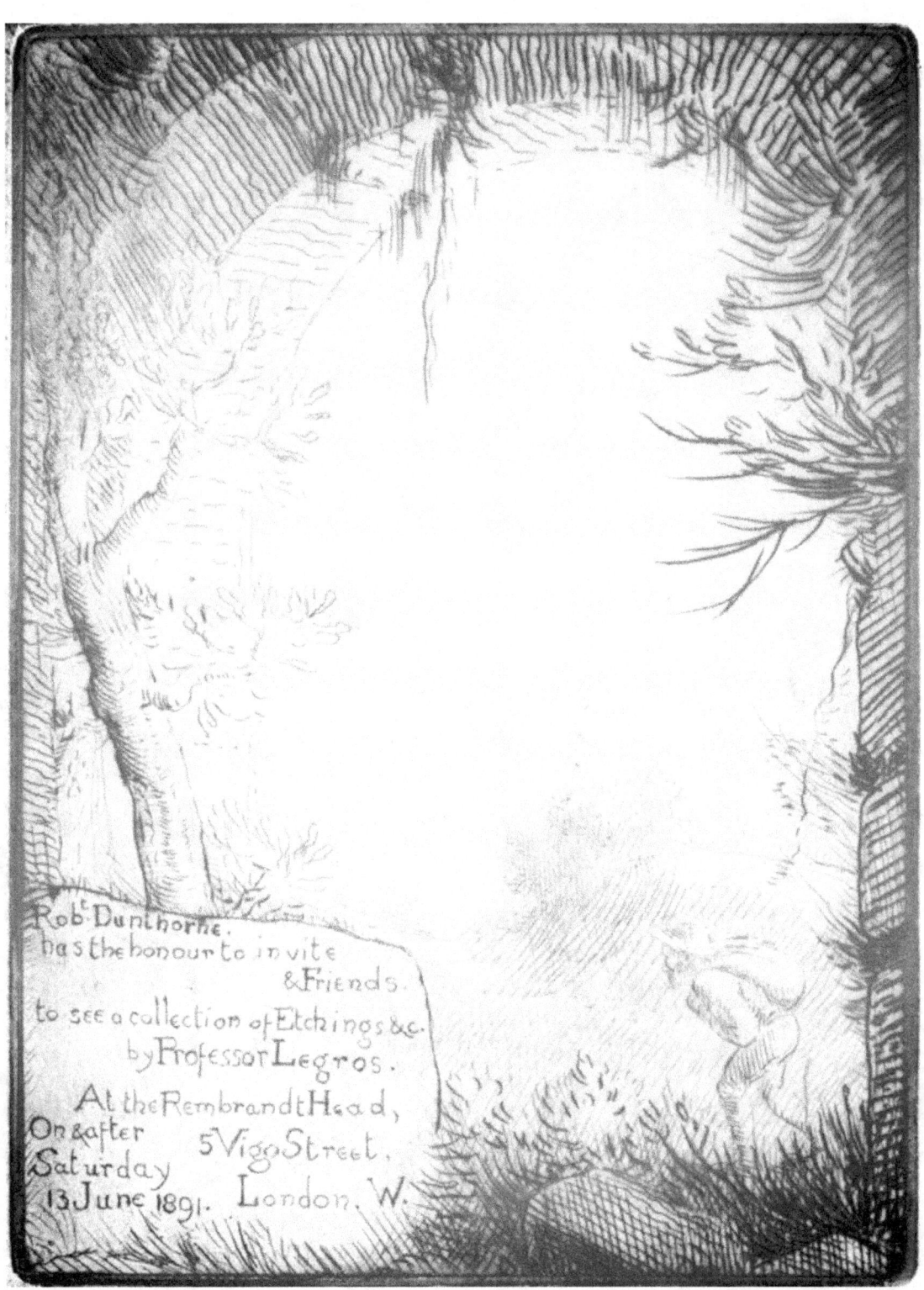

I am justified

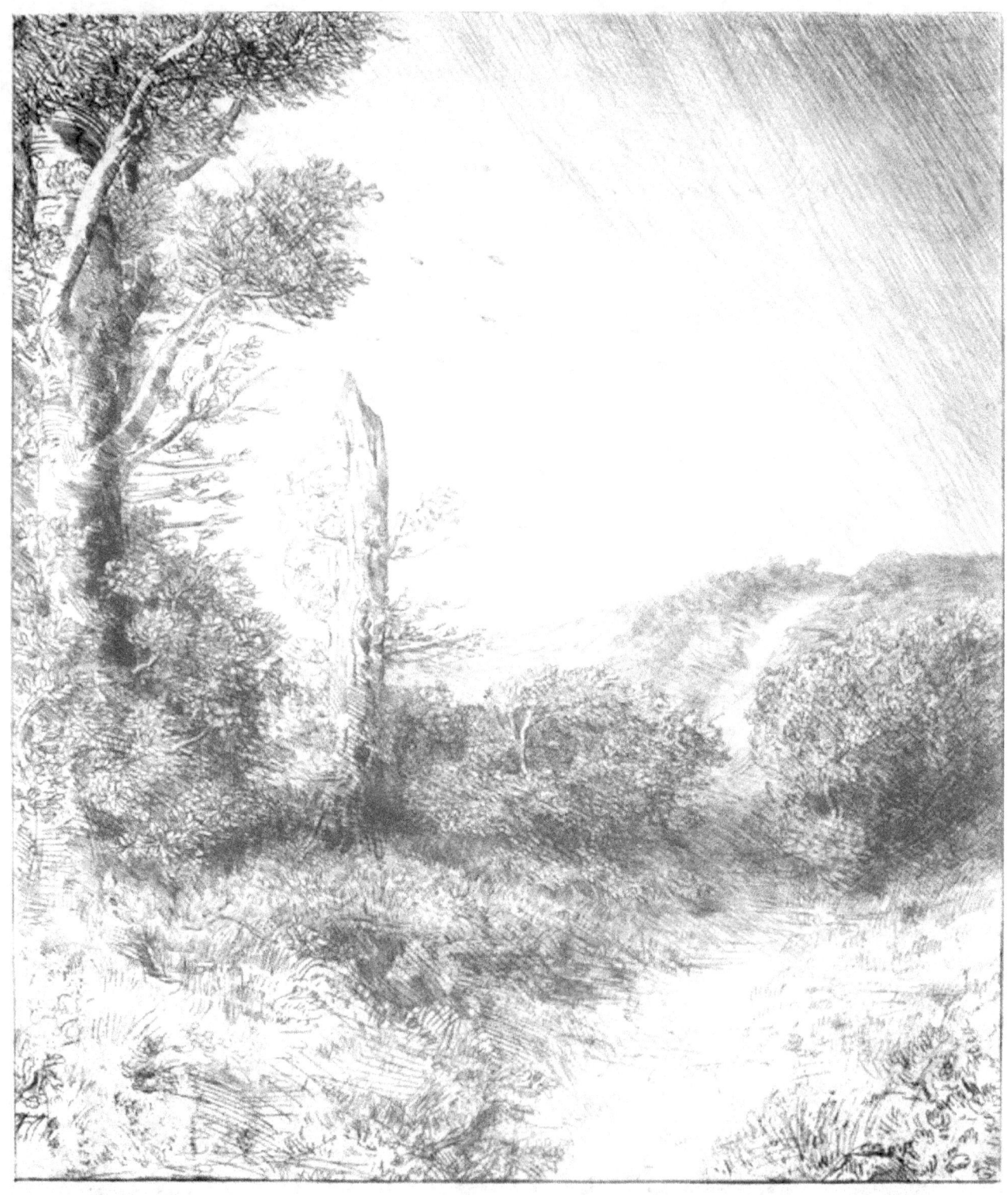

I can achieve

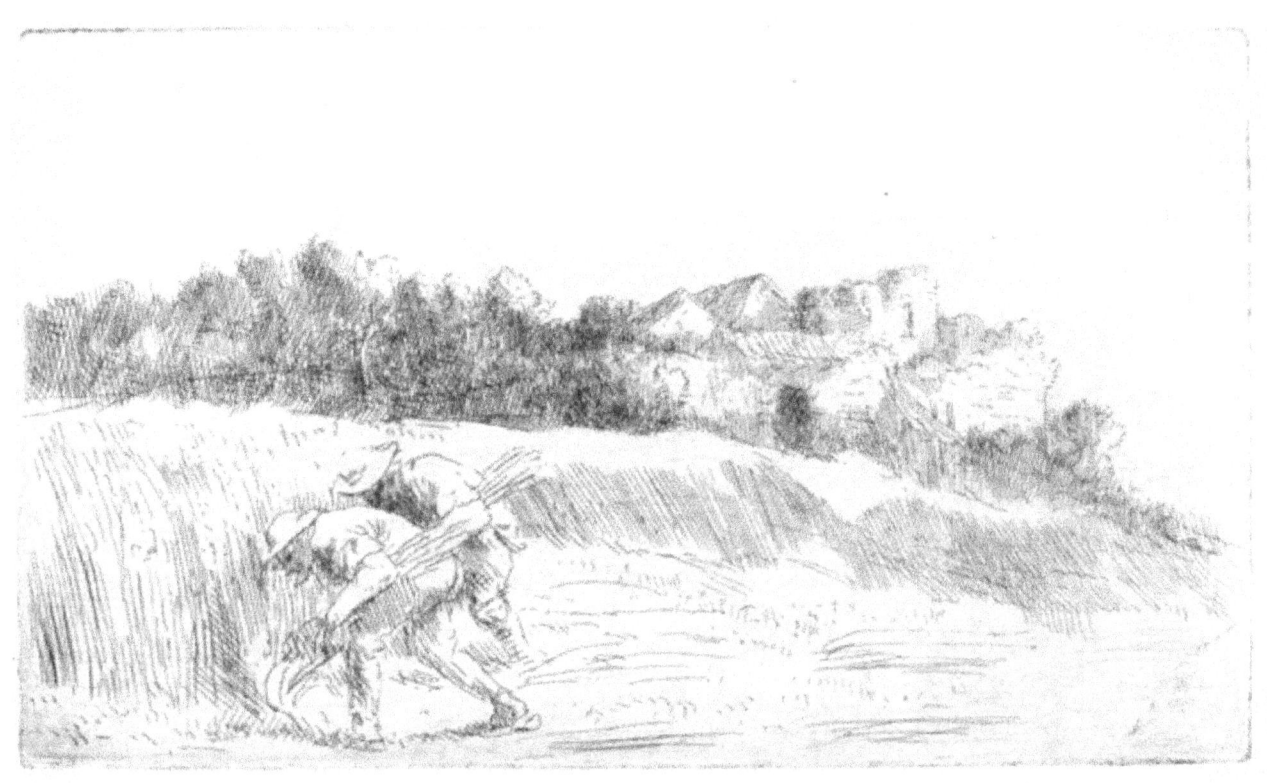

I am worthy of respect

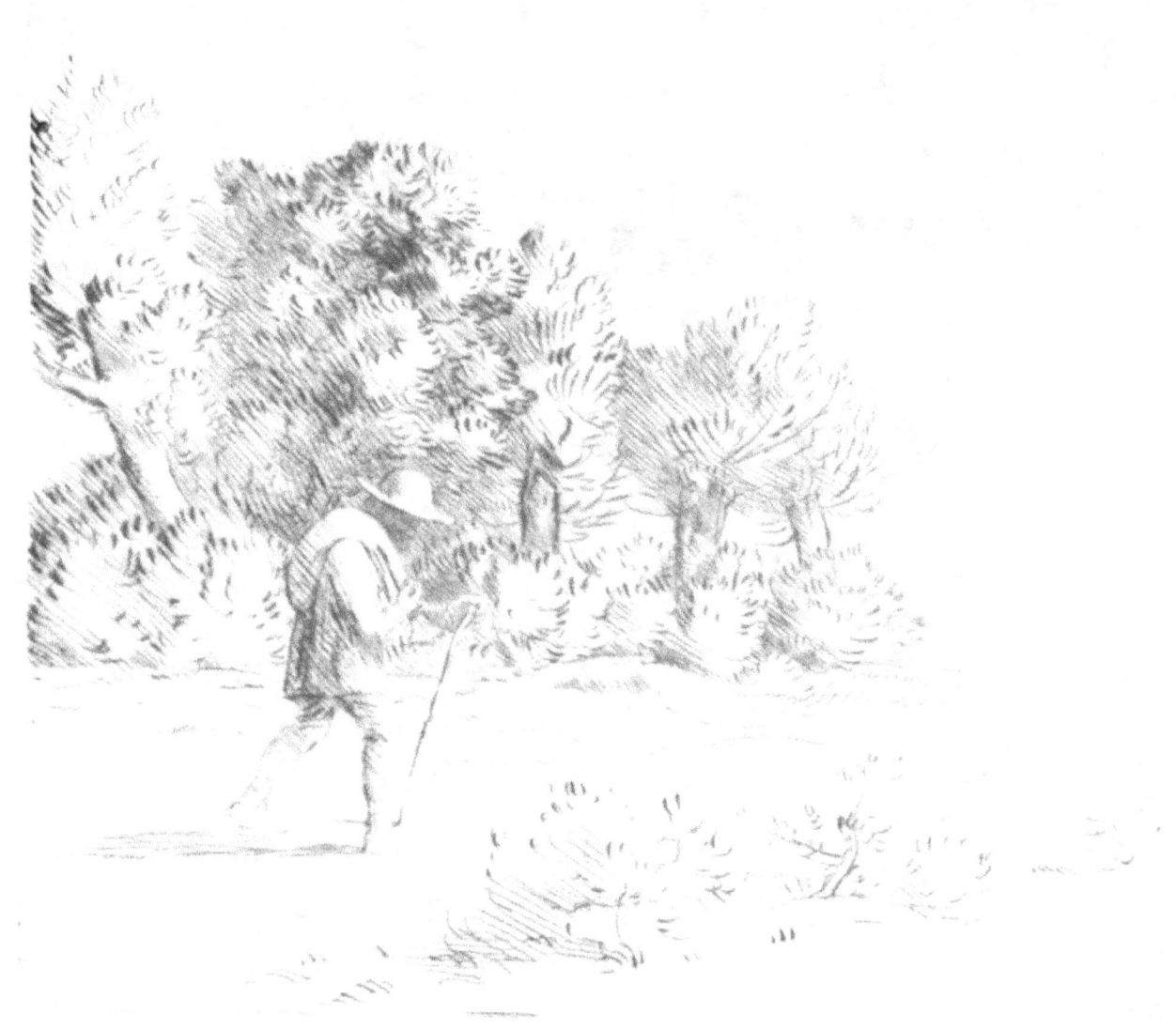

I can let go

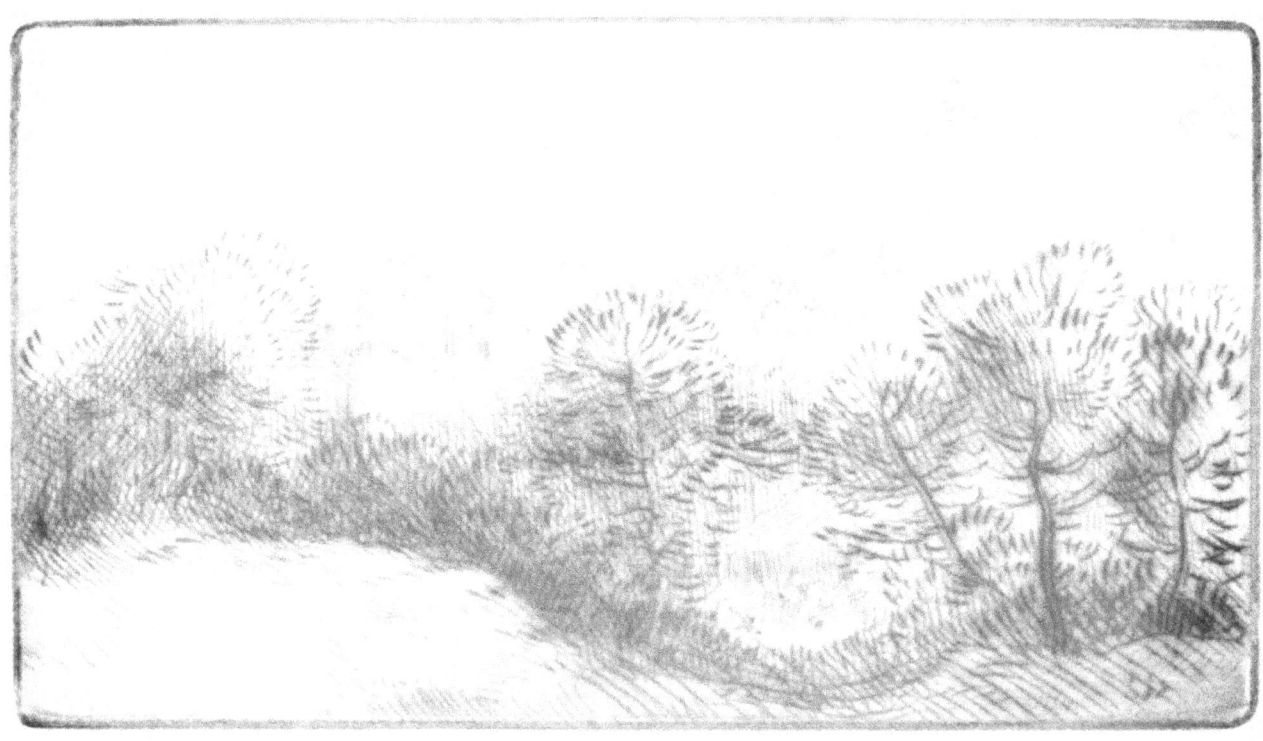

I lived

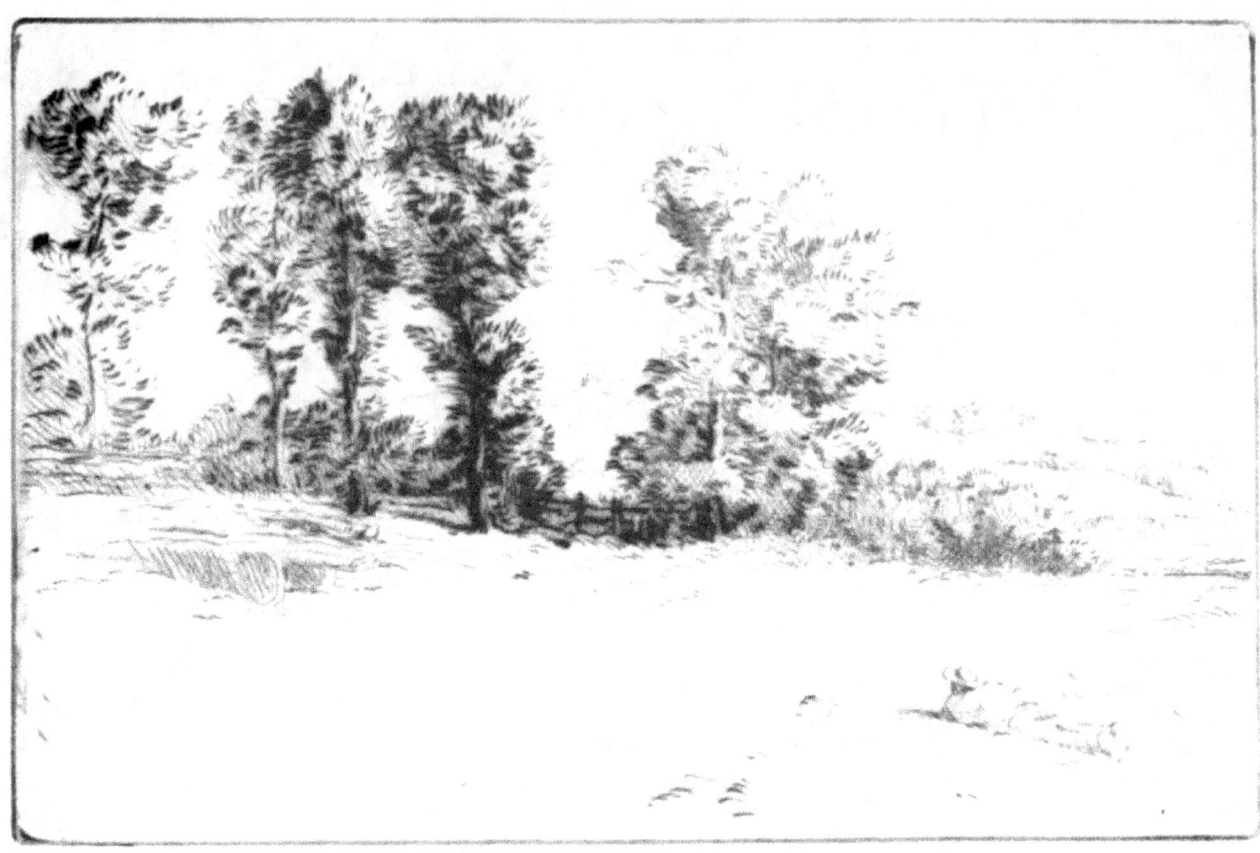

I am unique

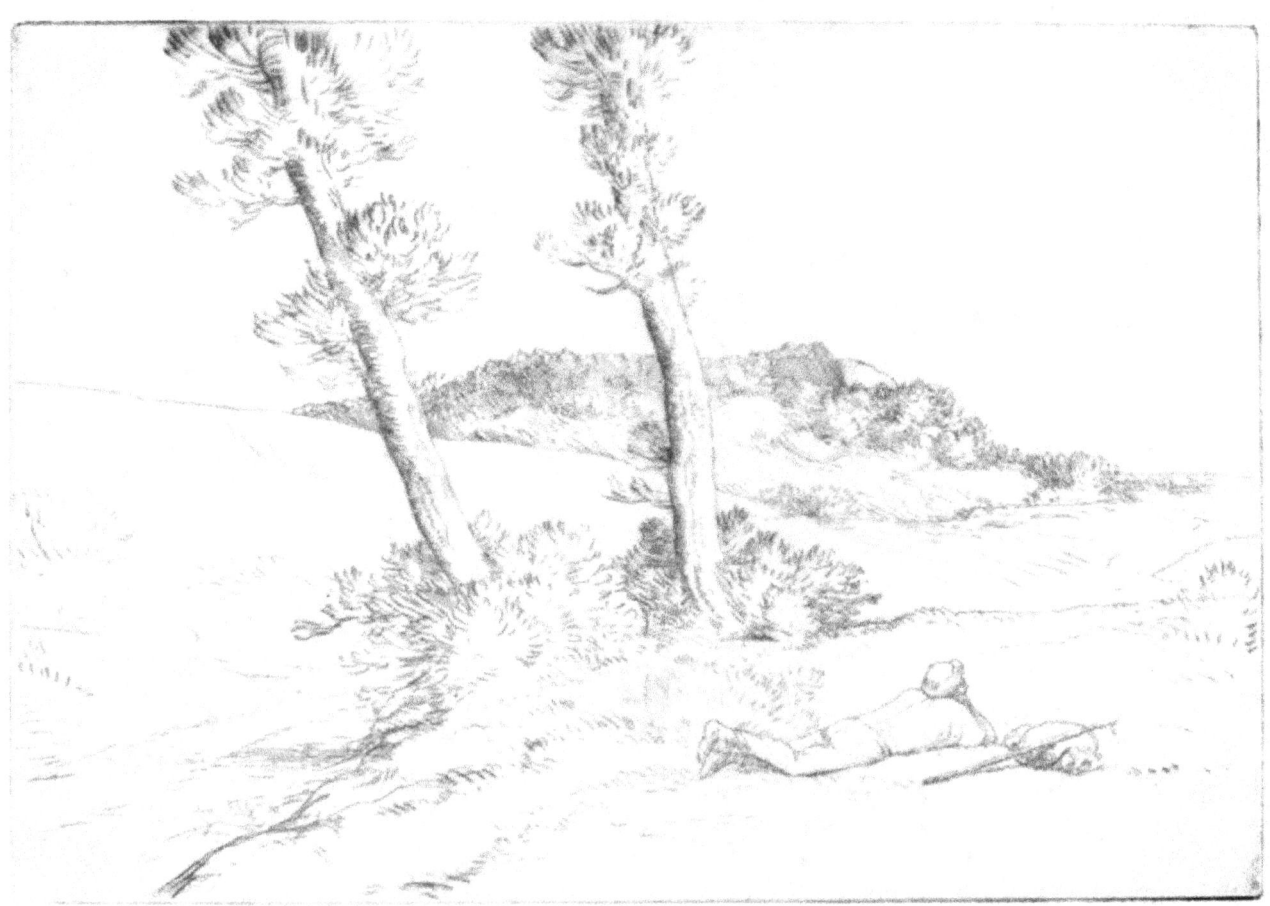

I can hold it together

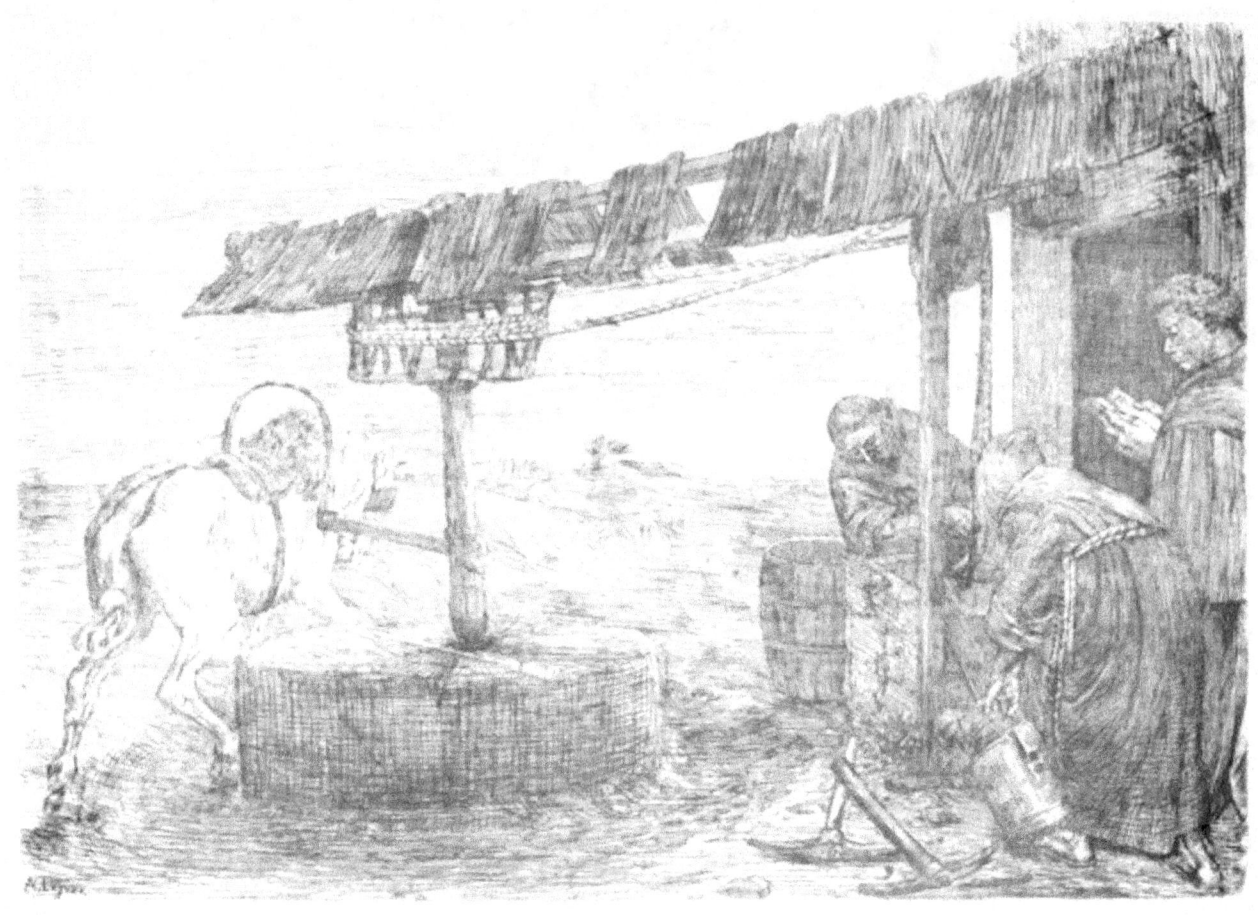

I can go with the flow

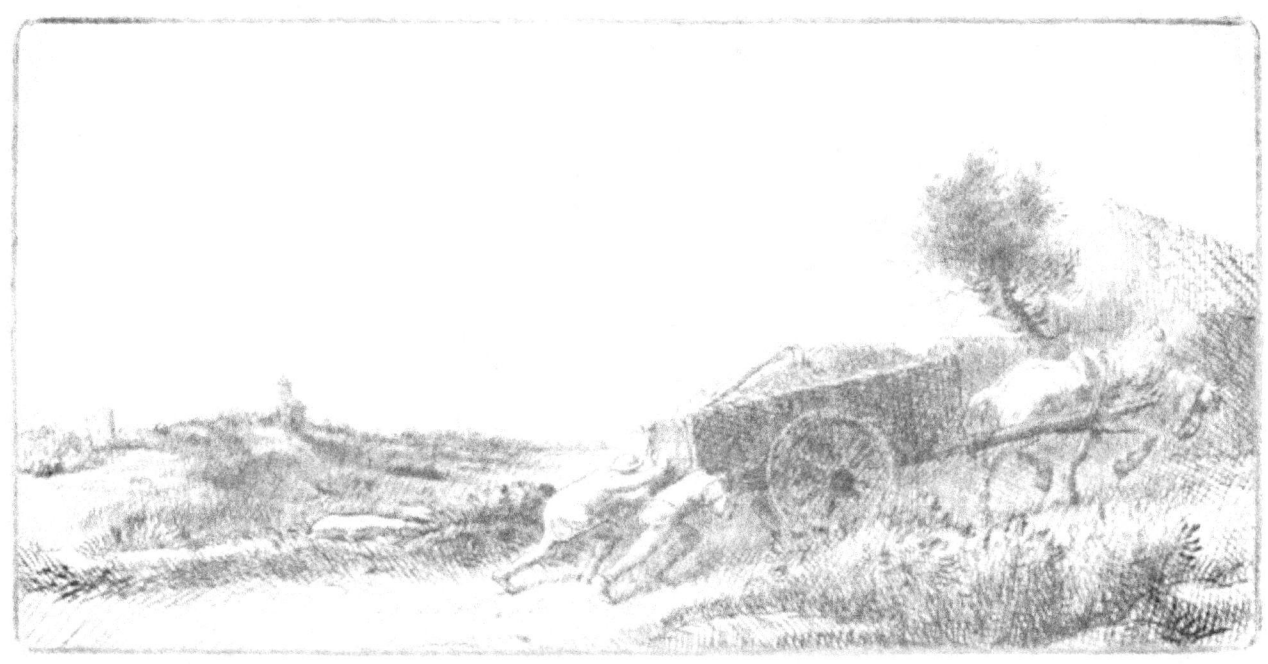

I deserve to be treated well

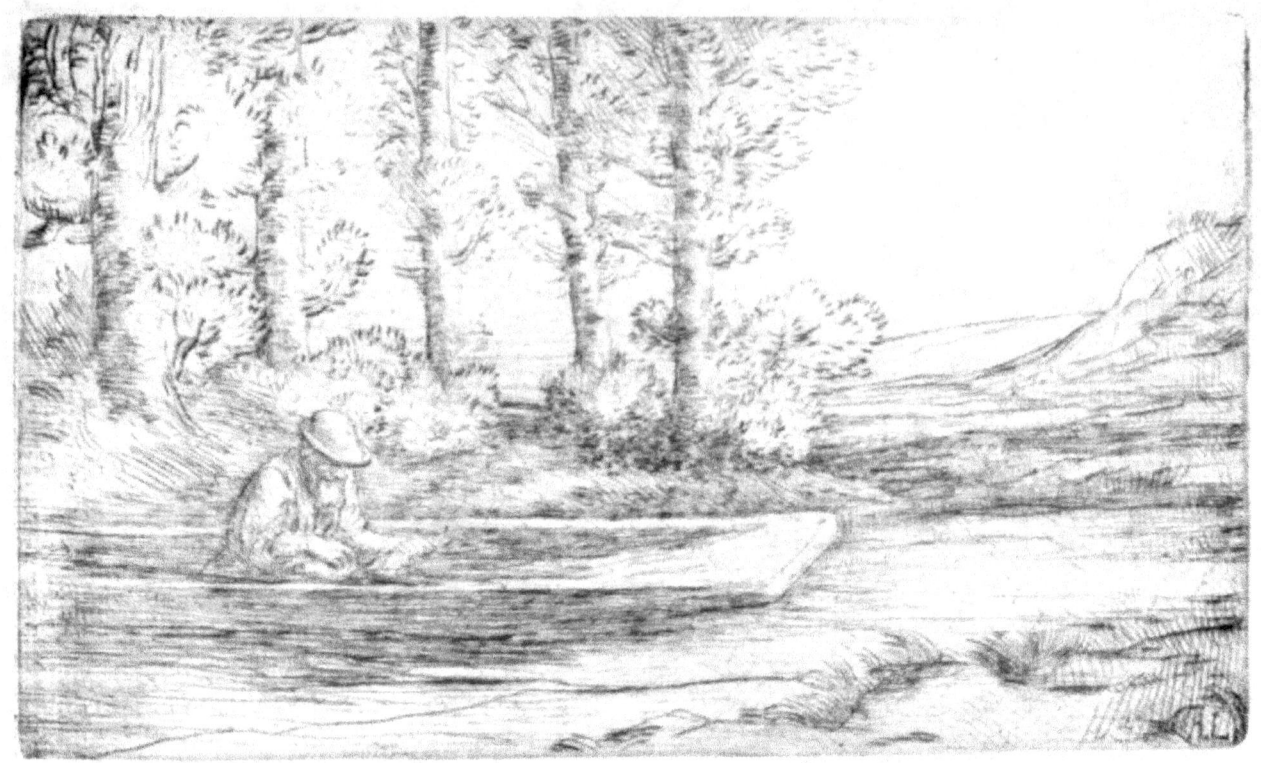

I am powerful

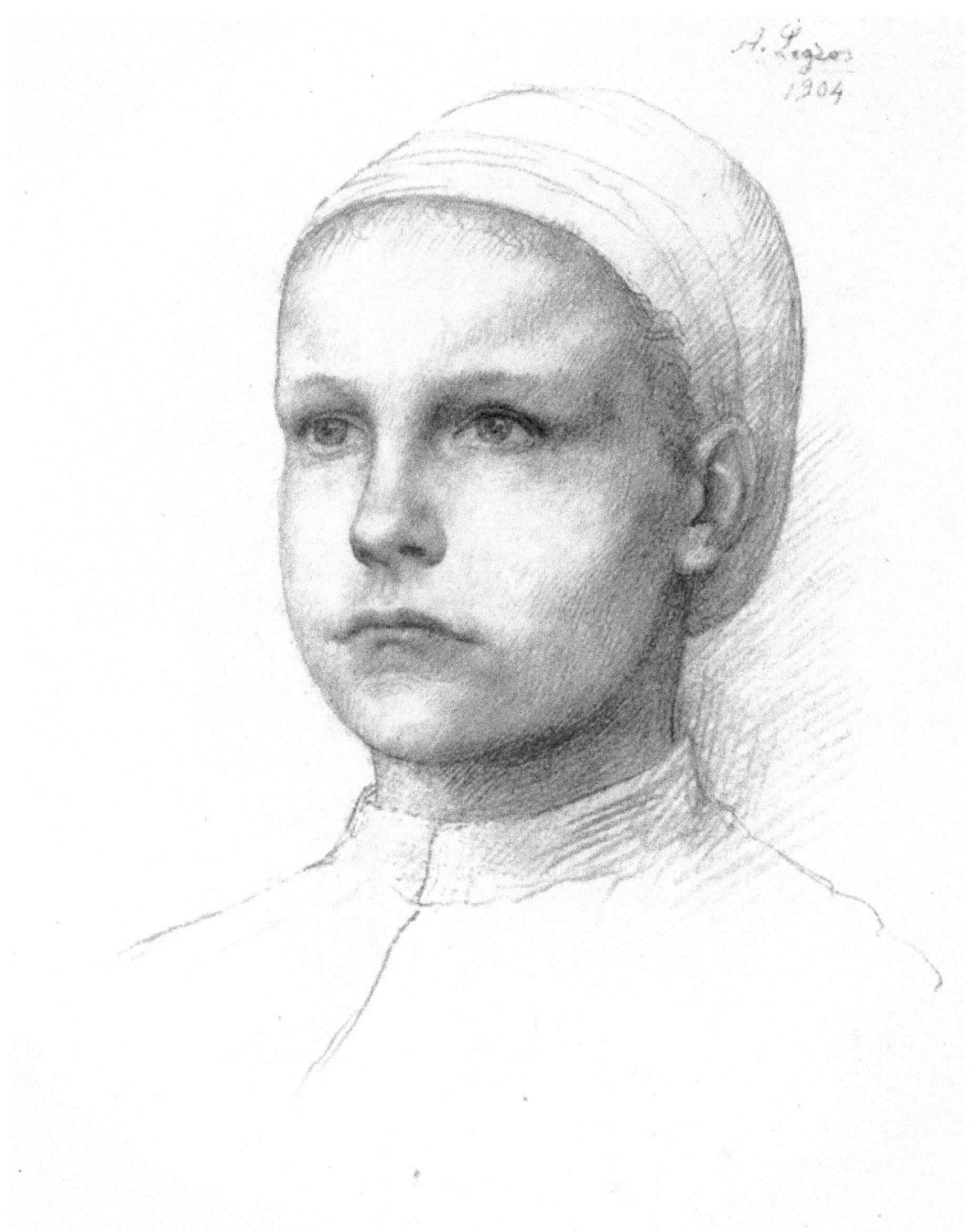

I can believe in myself

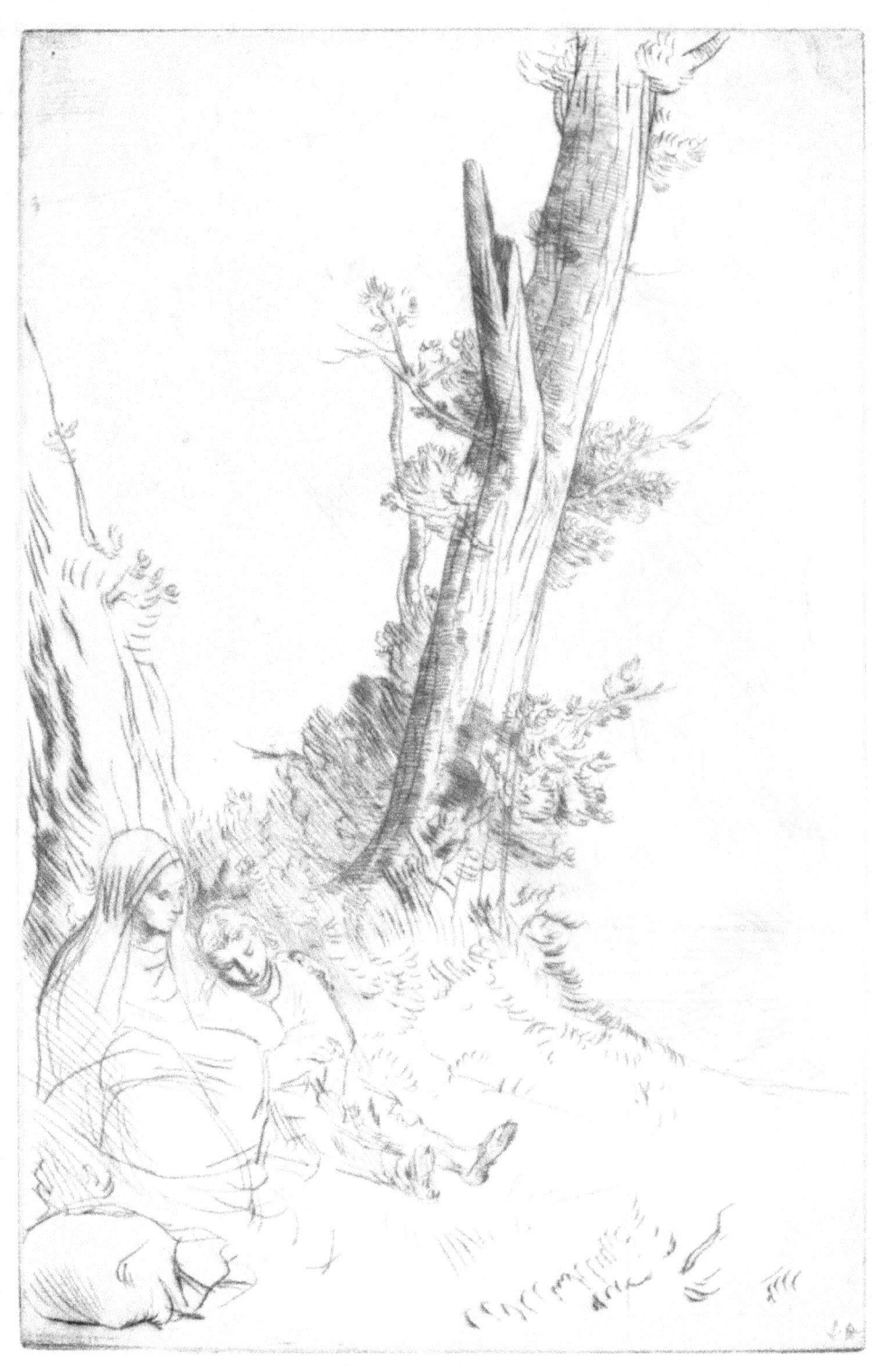

I am worthy of love

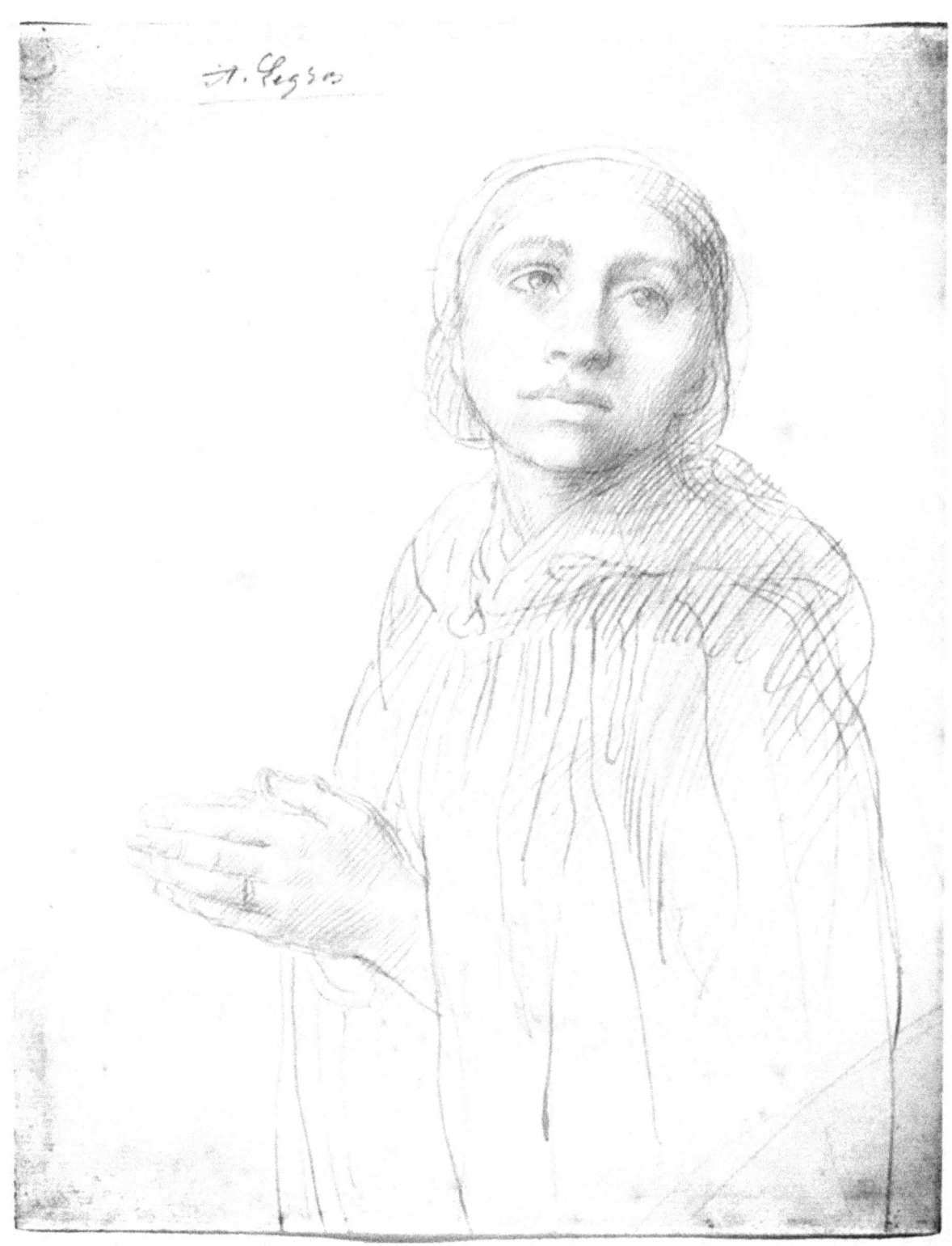

I am precious

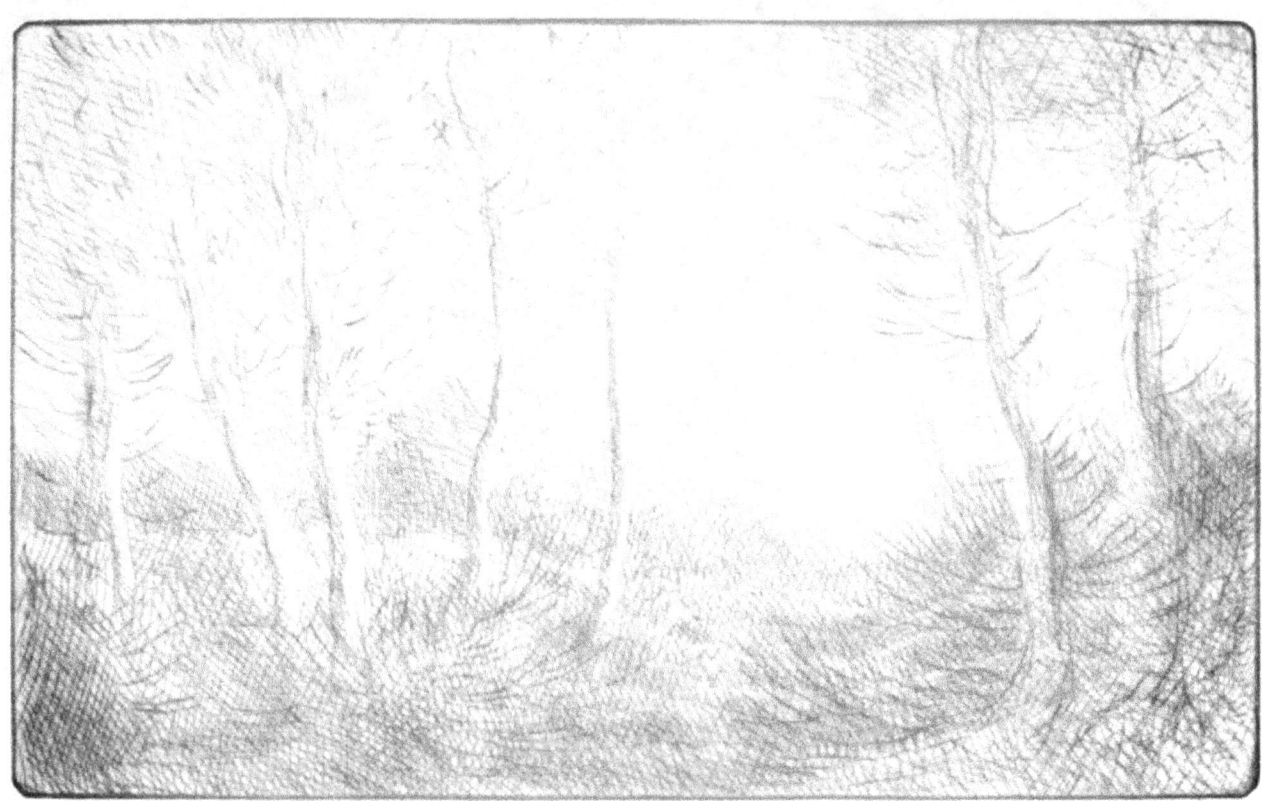

I am admirable

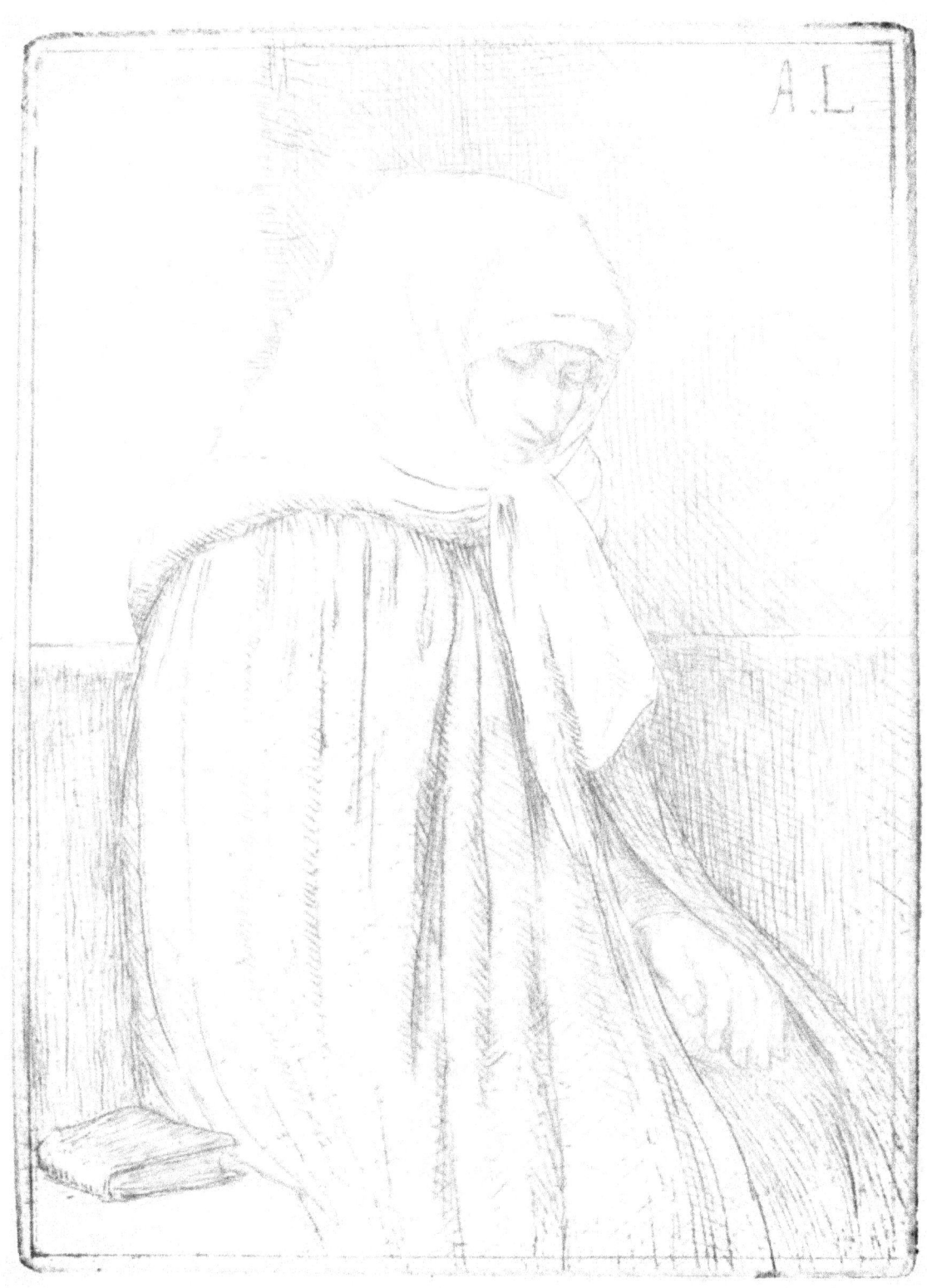

I am well

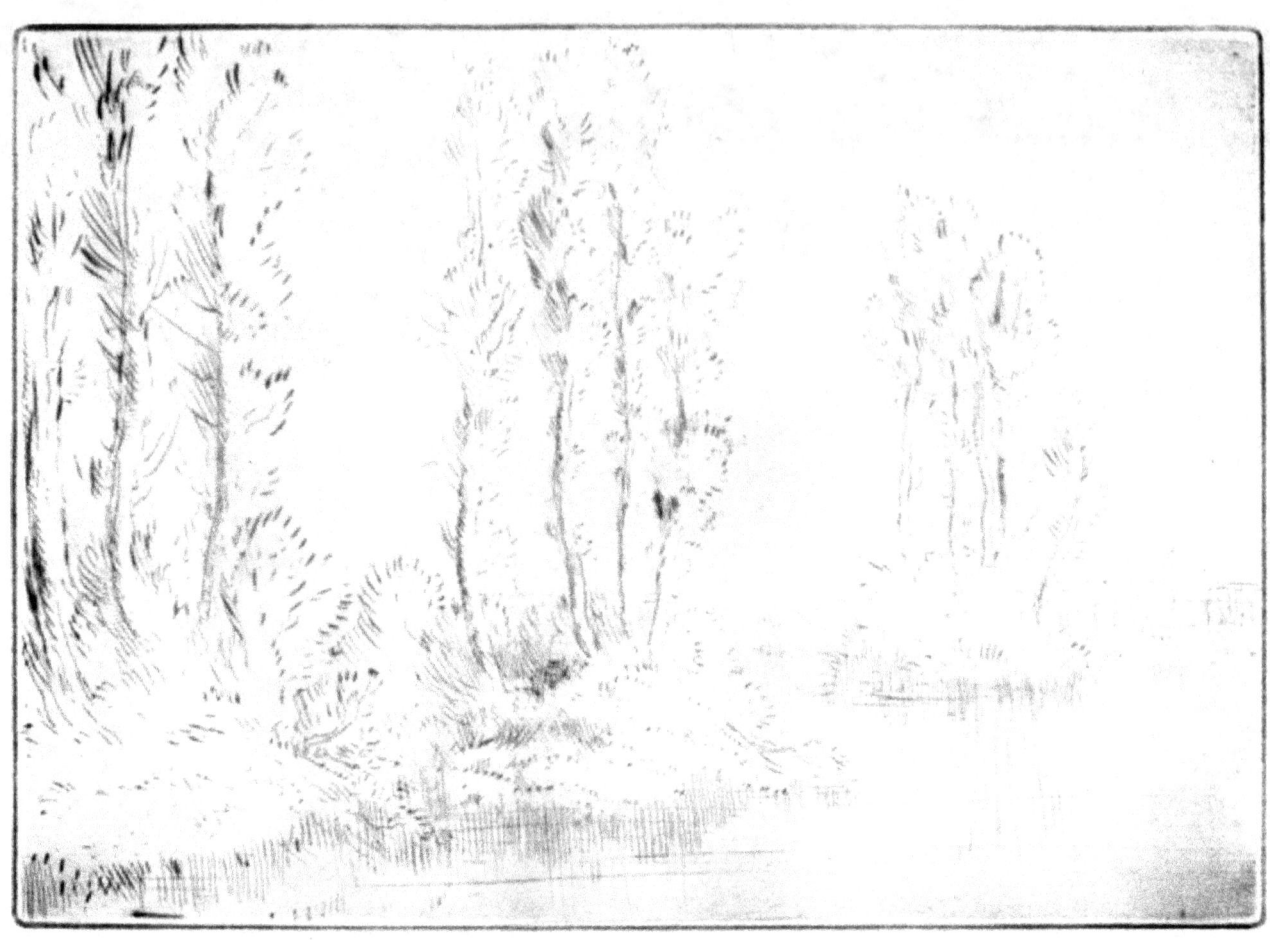

I can fulfill my purpose

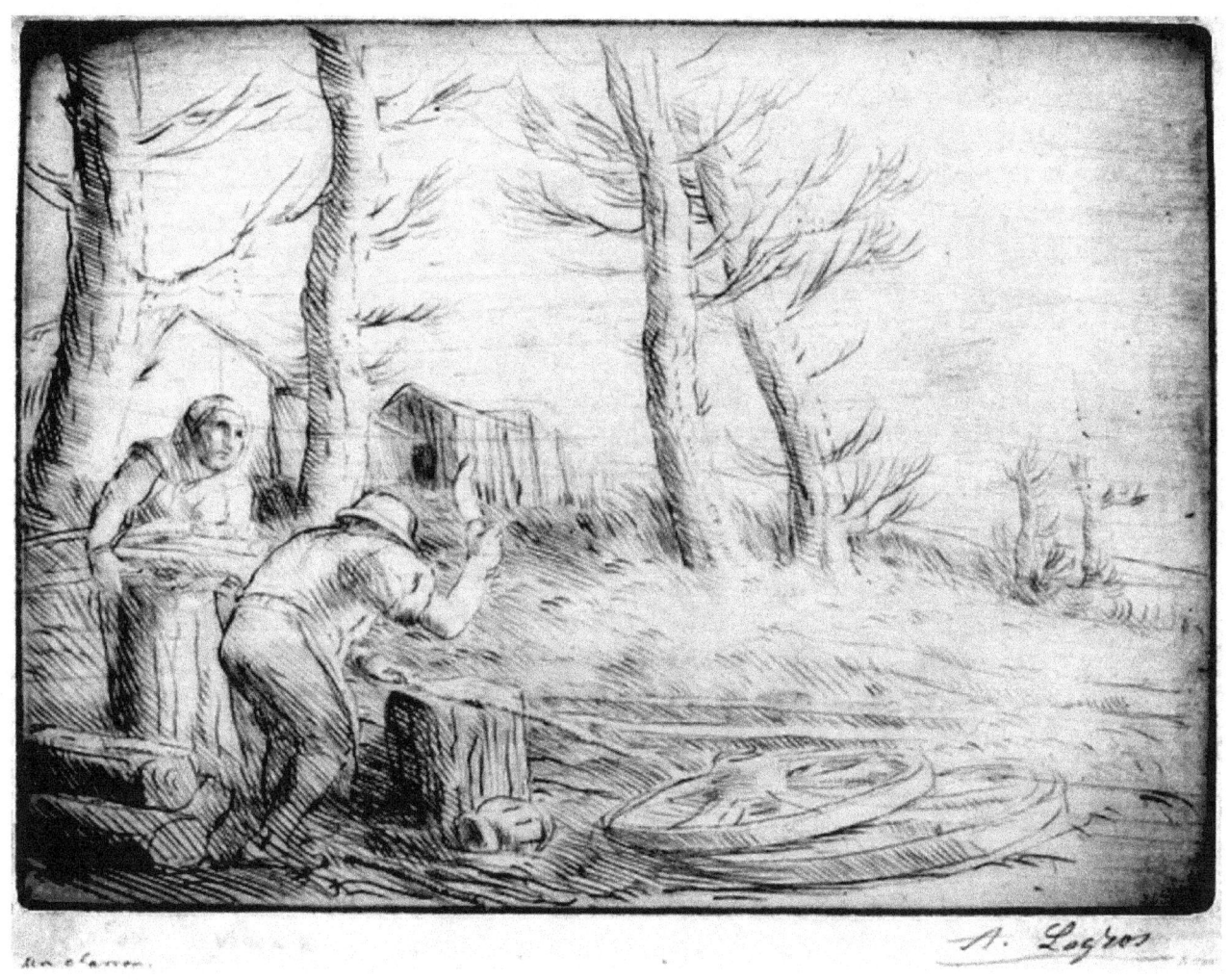

I am worthy of peace

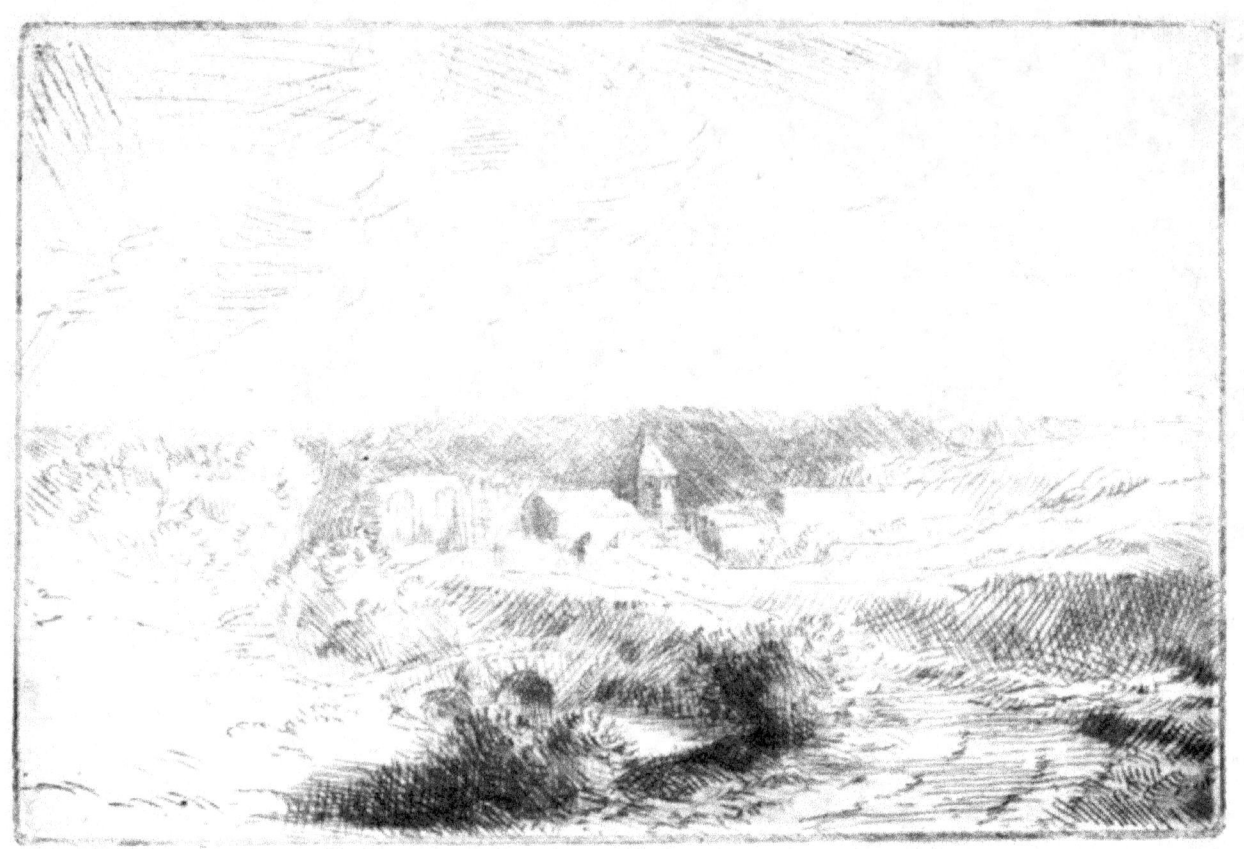

I am competent

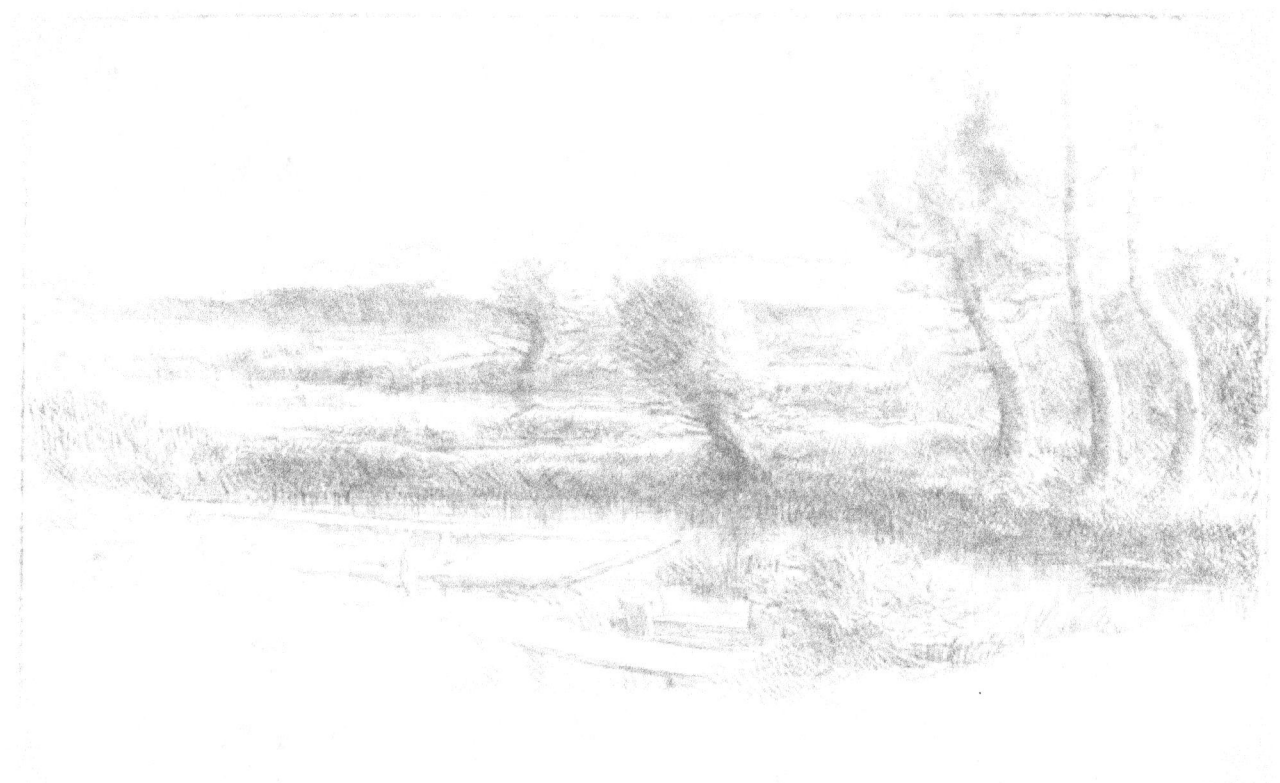

I can discover my purpose

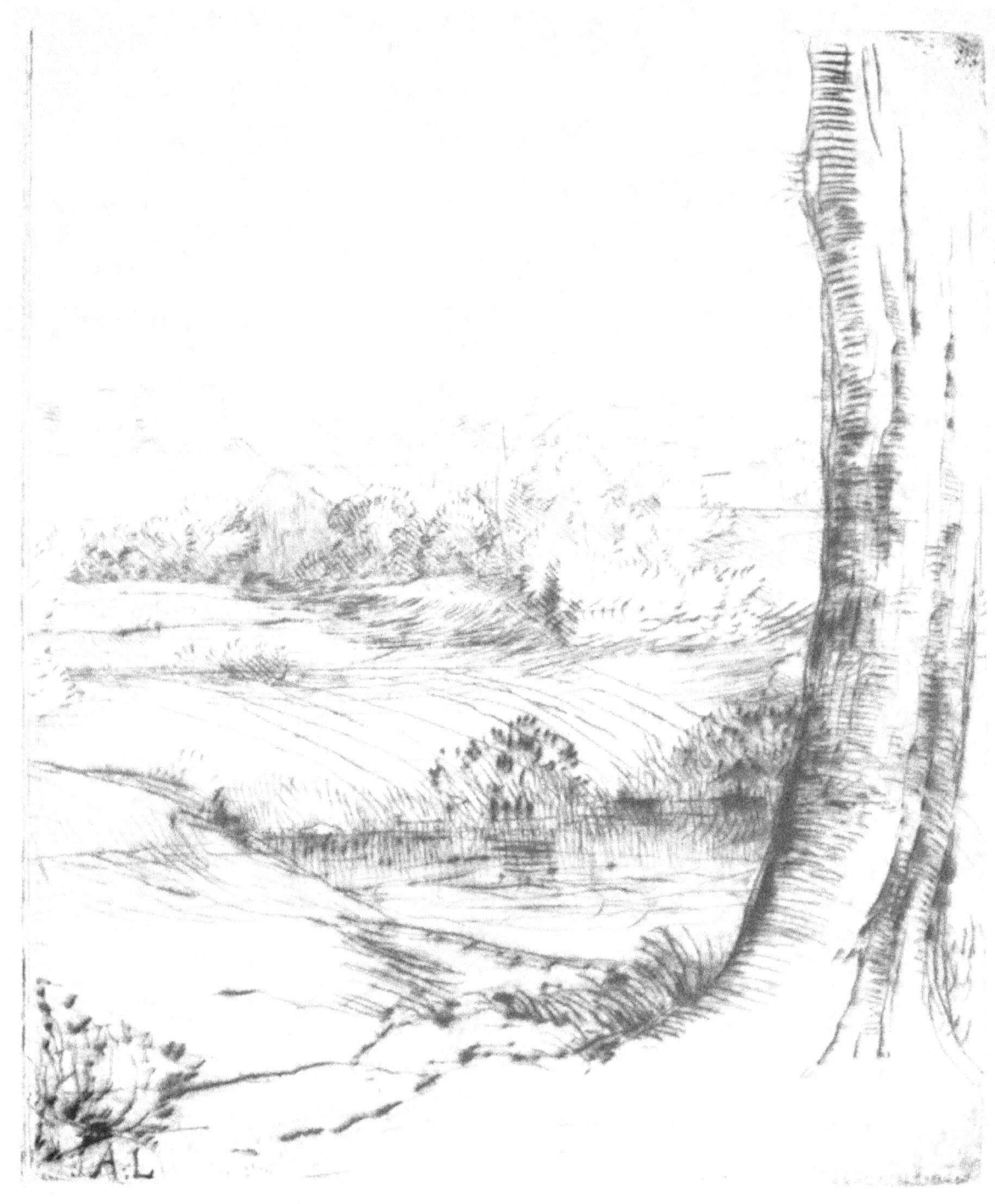

I can live with uncertainty

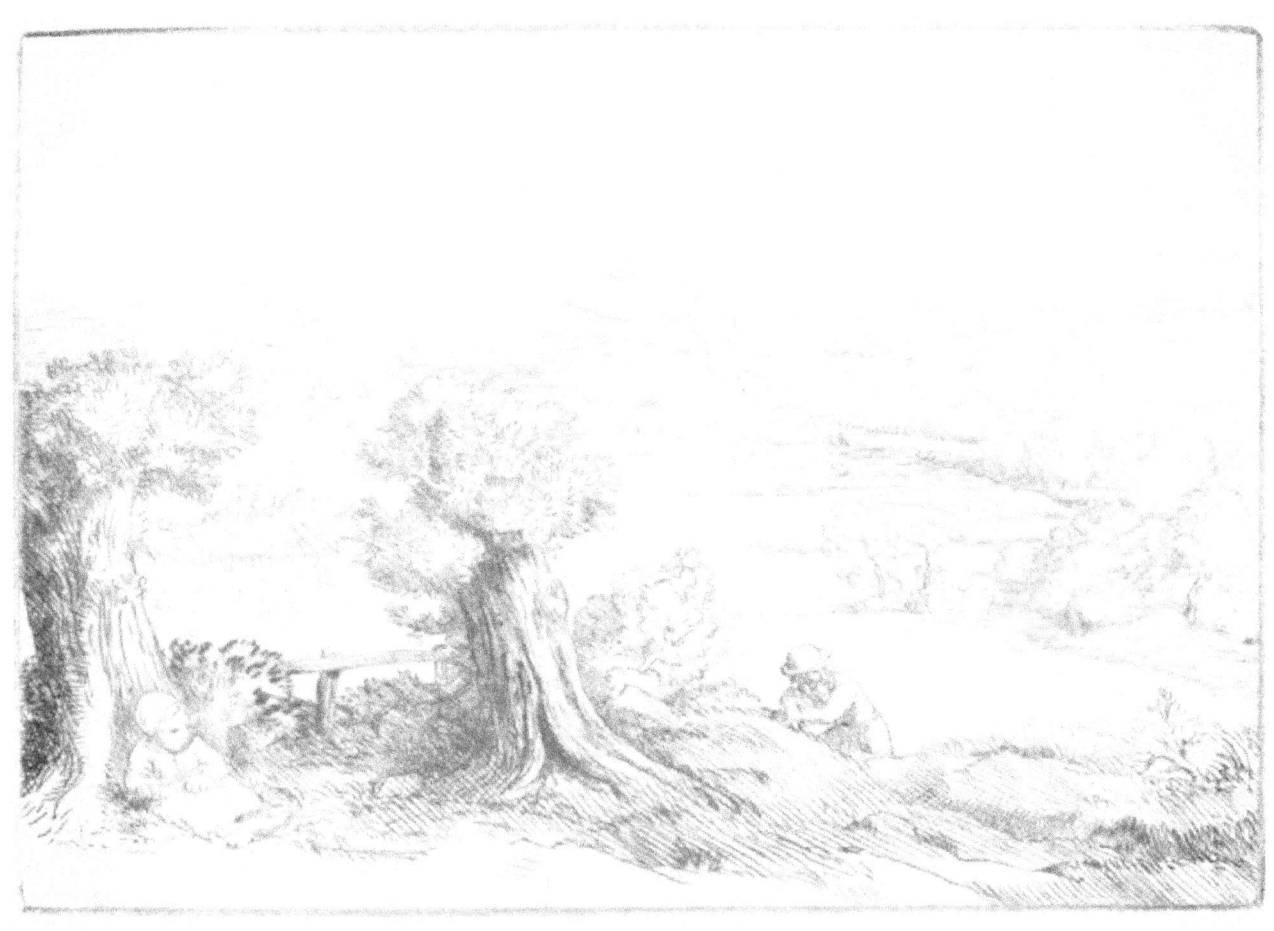

I can be flexible

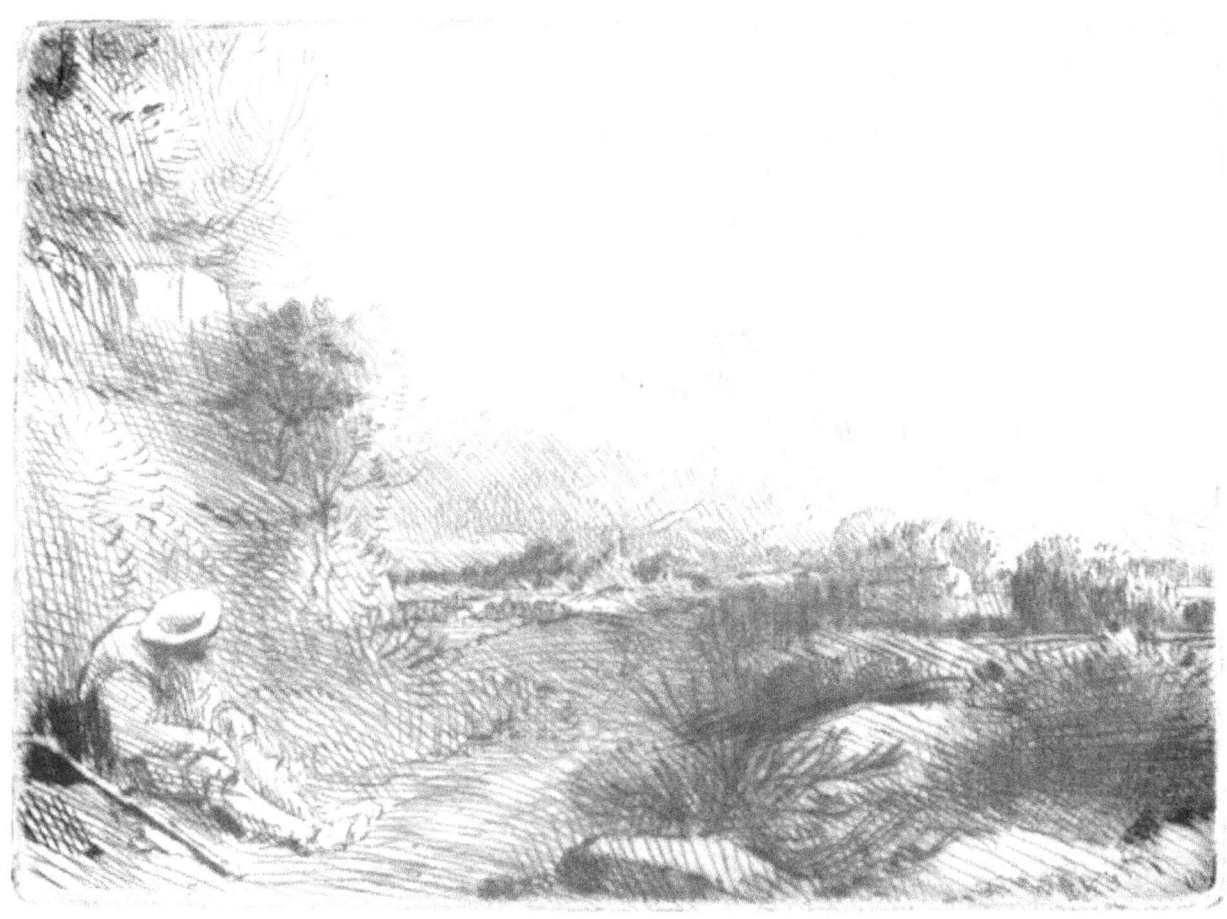

I am free

I can hold on

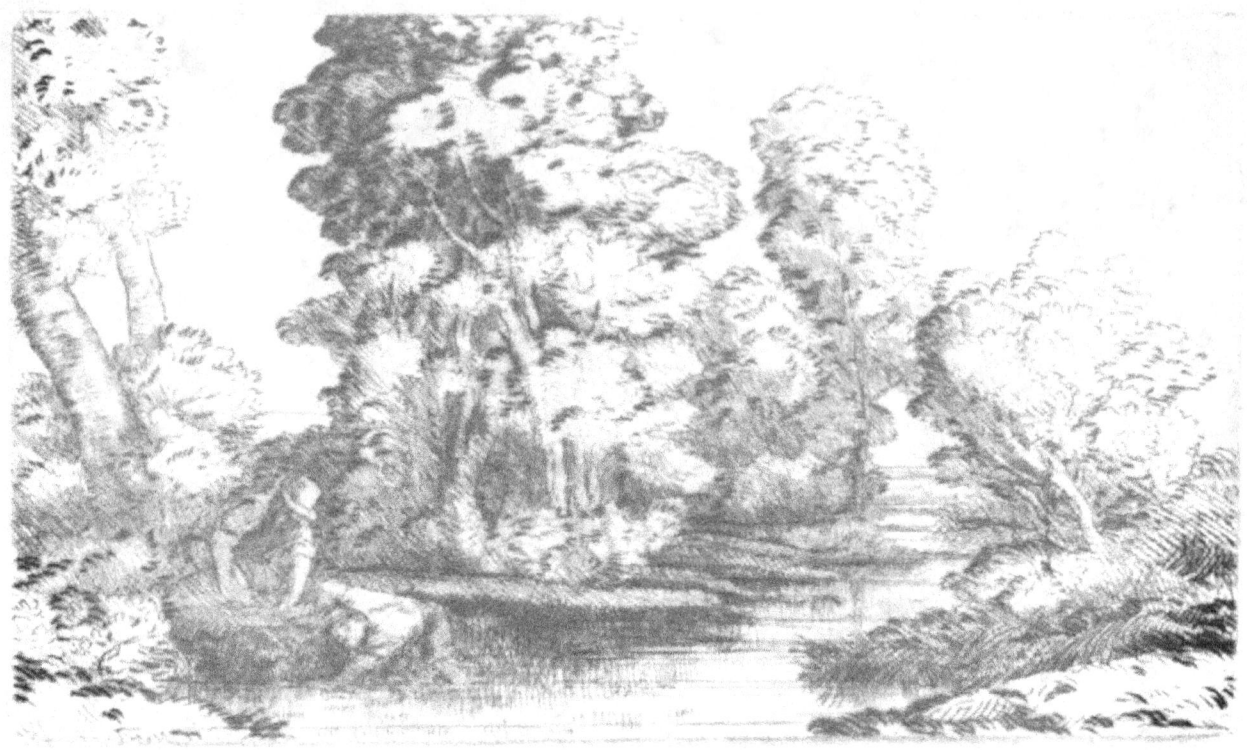

I deserve to exist

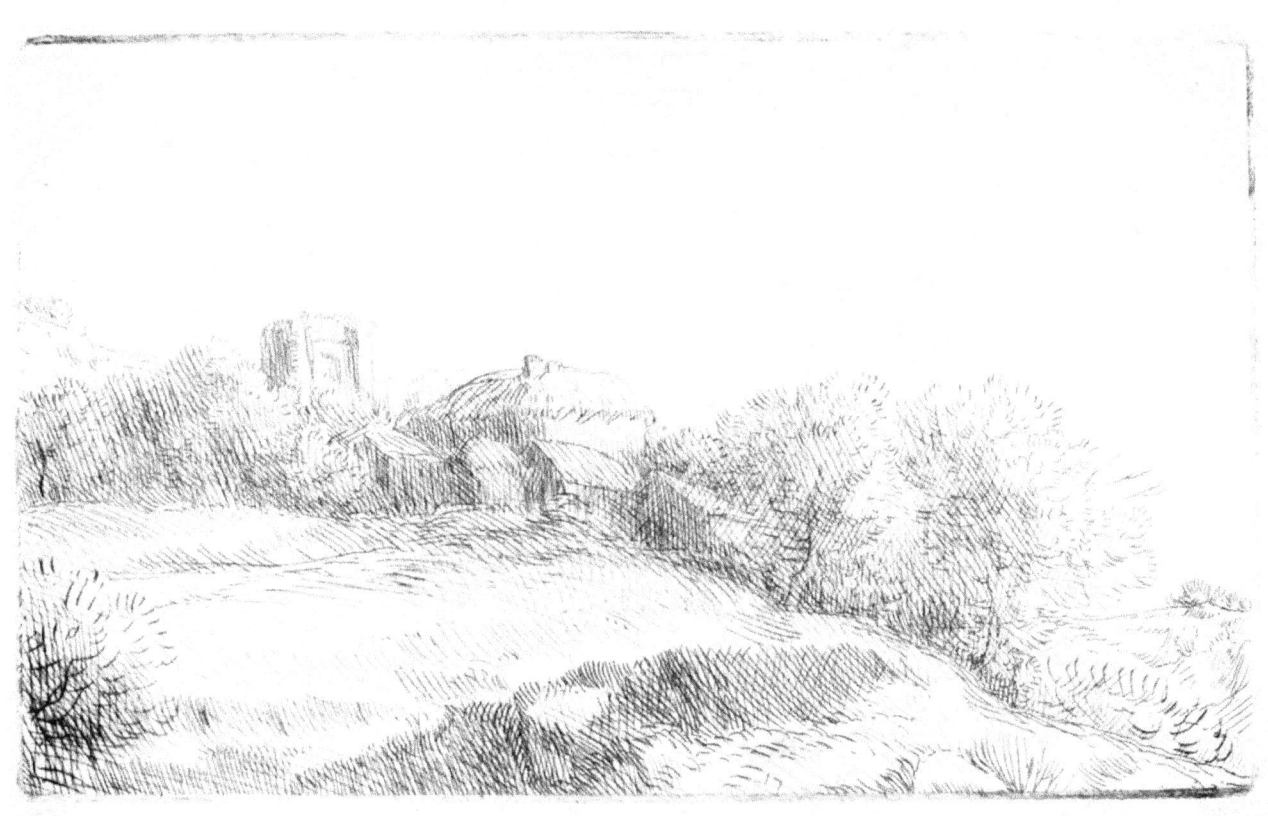

I am acceptable

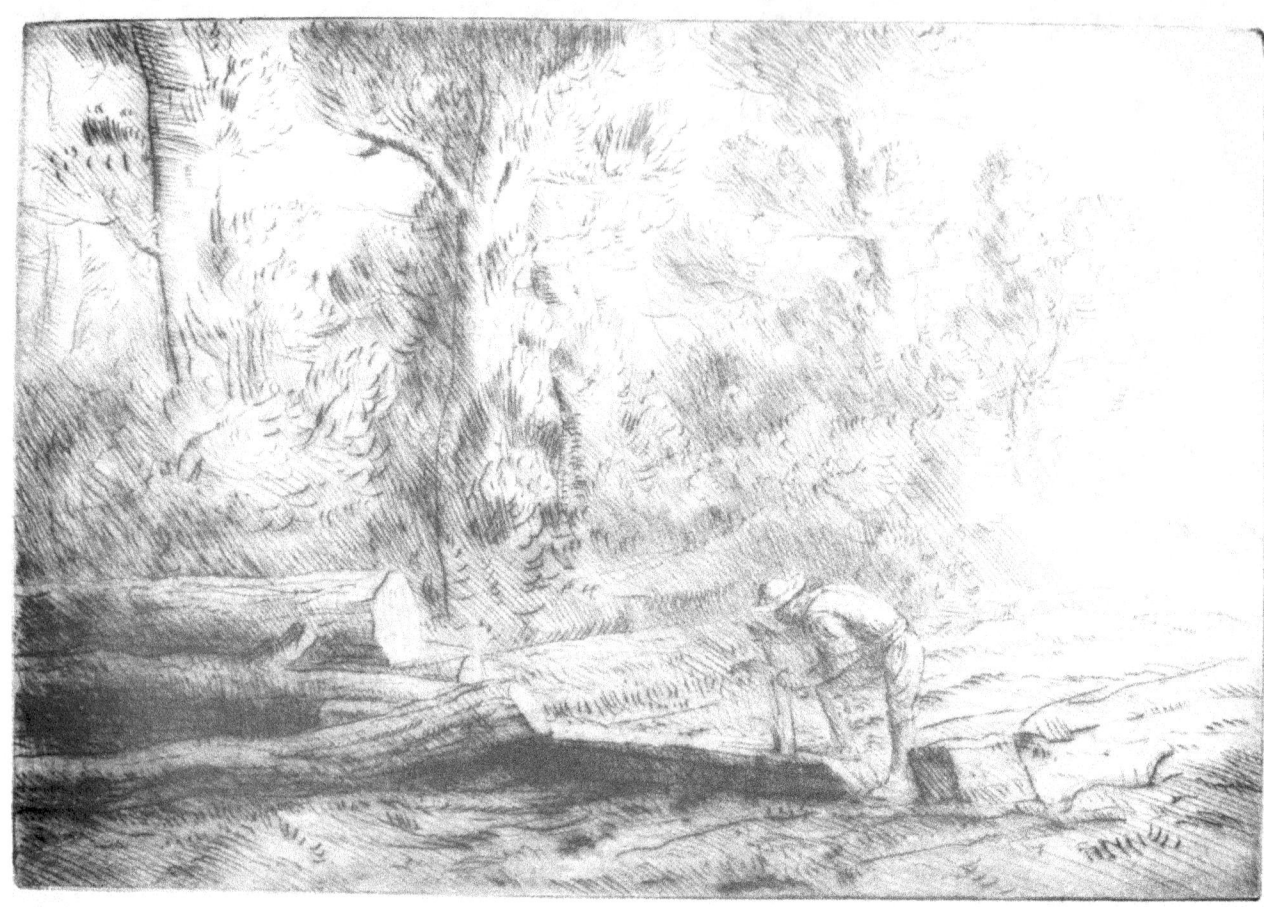

I am a person of character

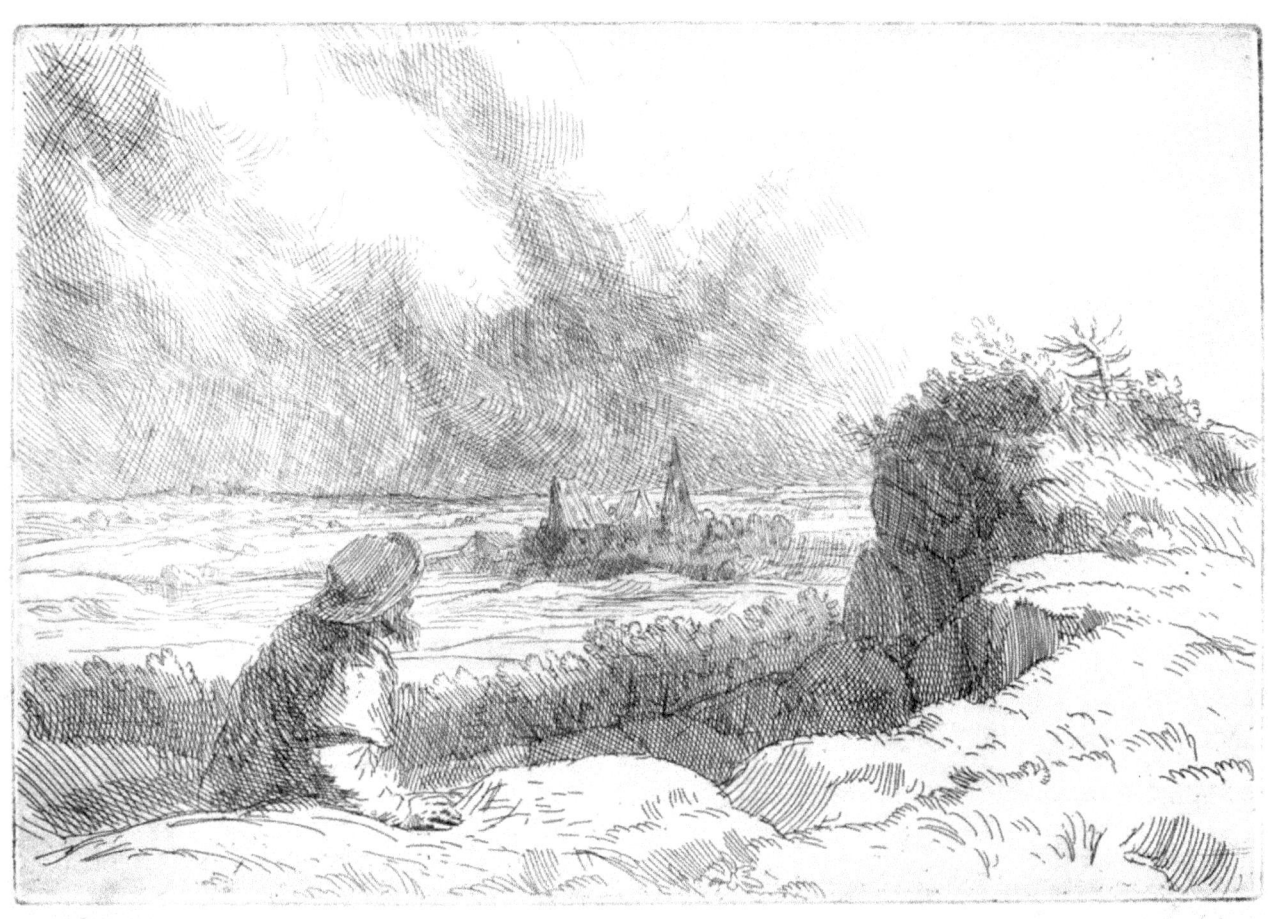

I can change

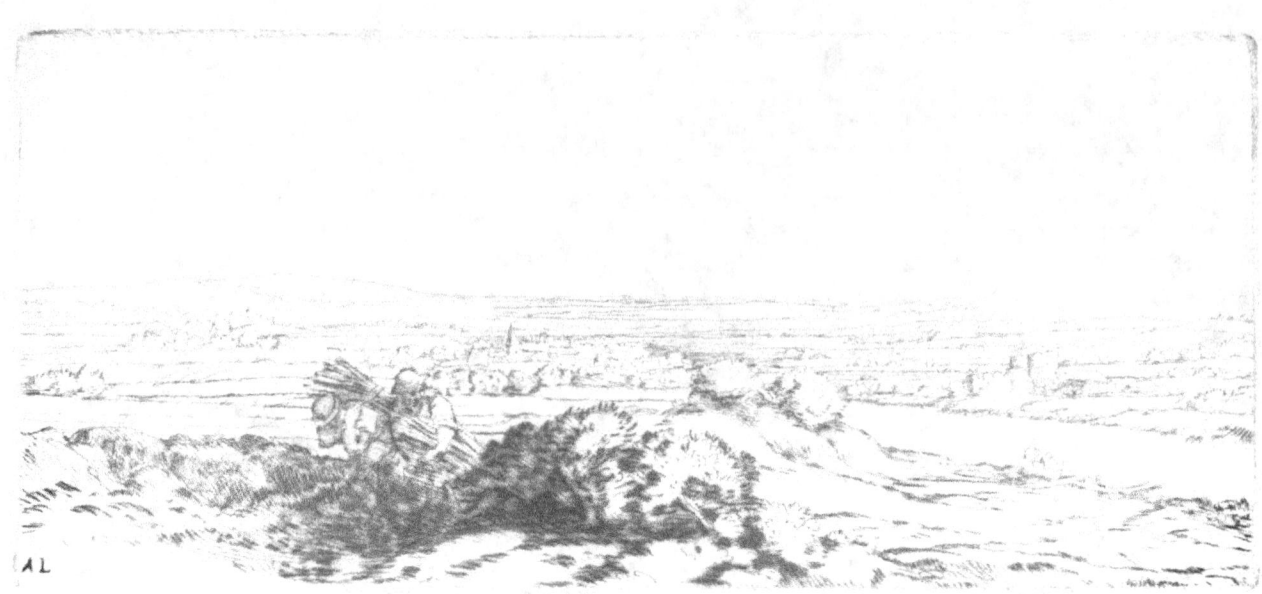

I am complete

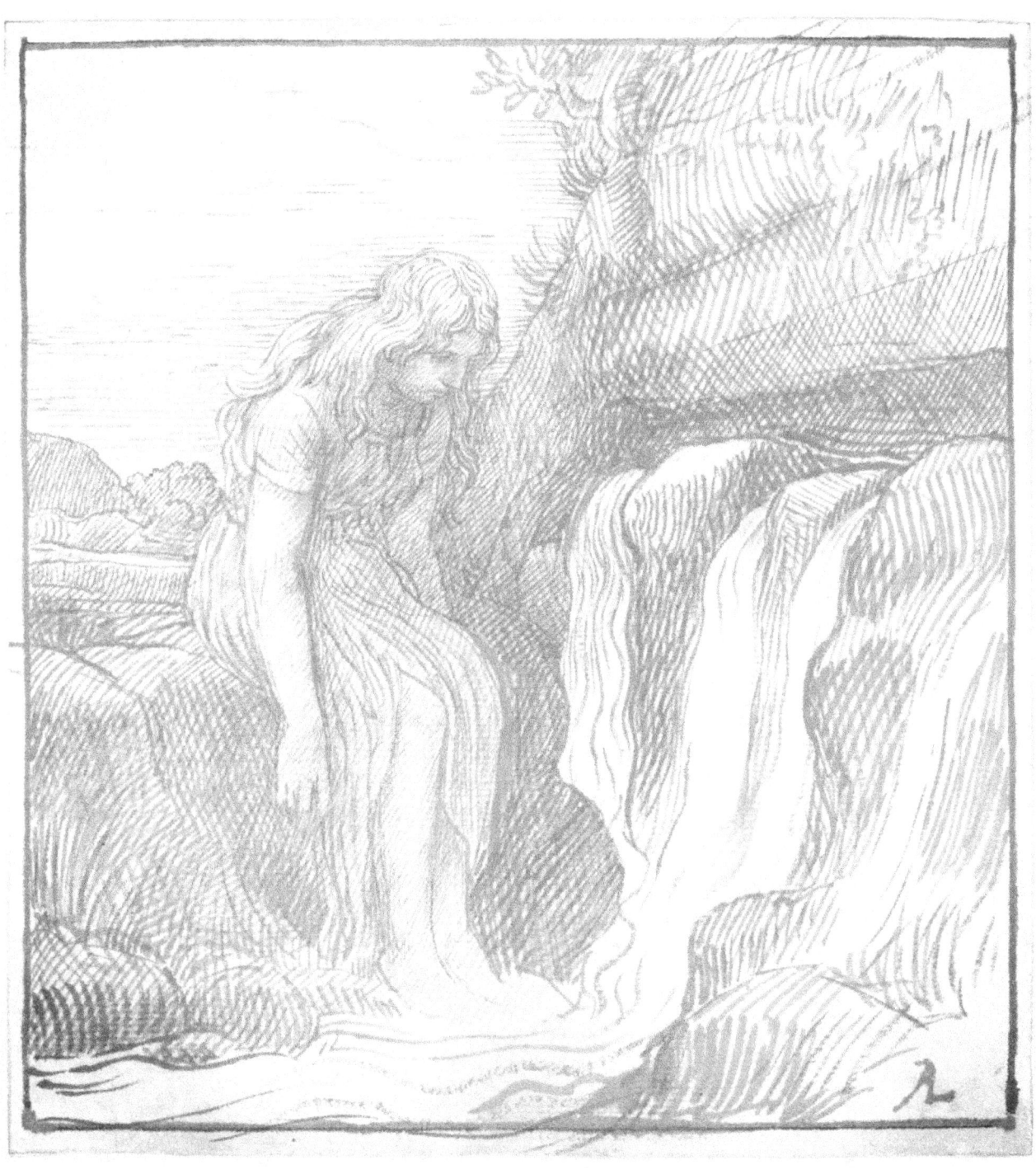

I am worthy of good relationships

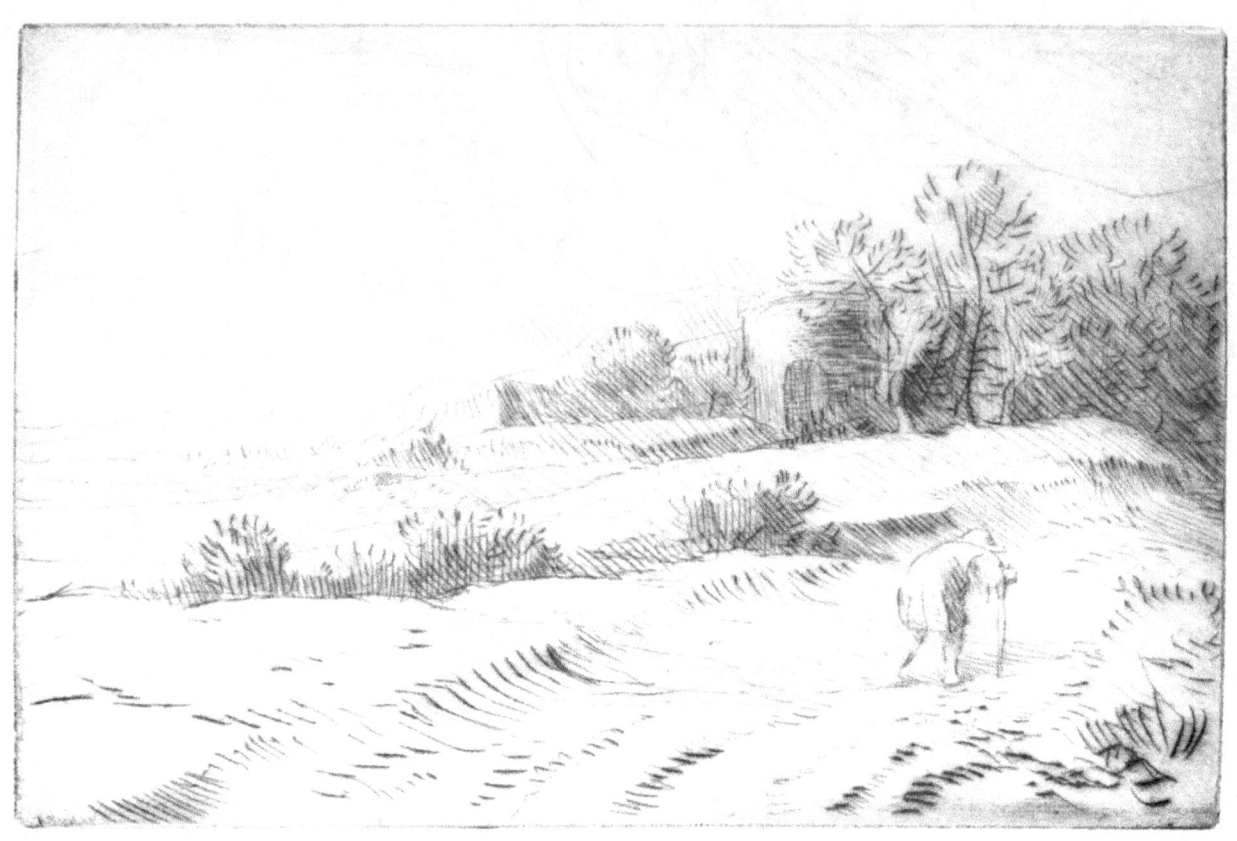

I am wise

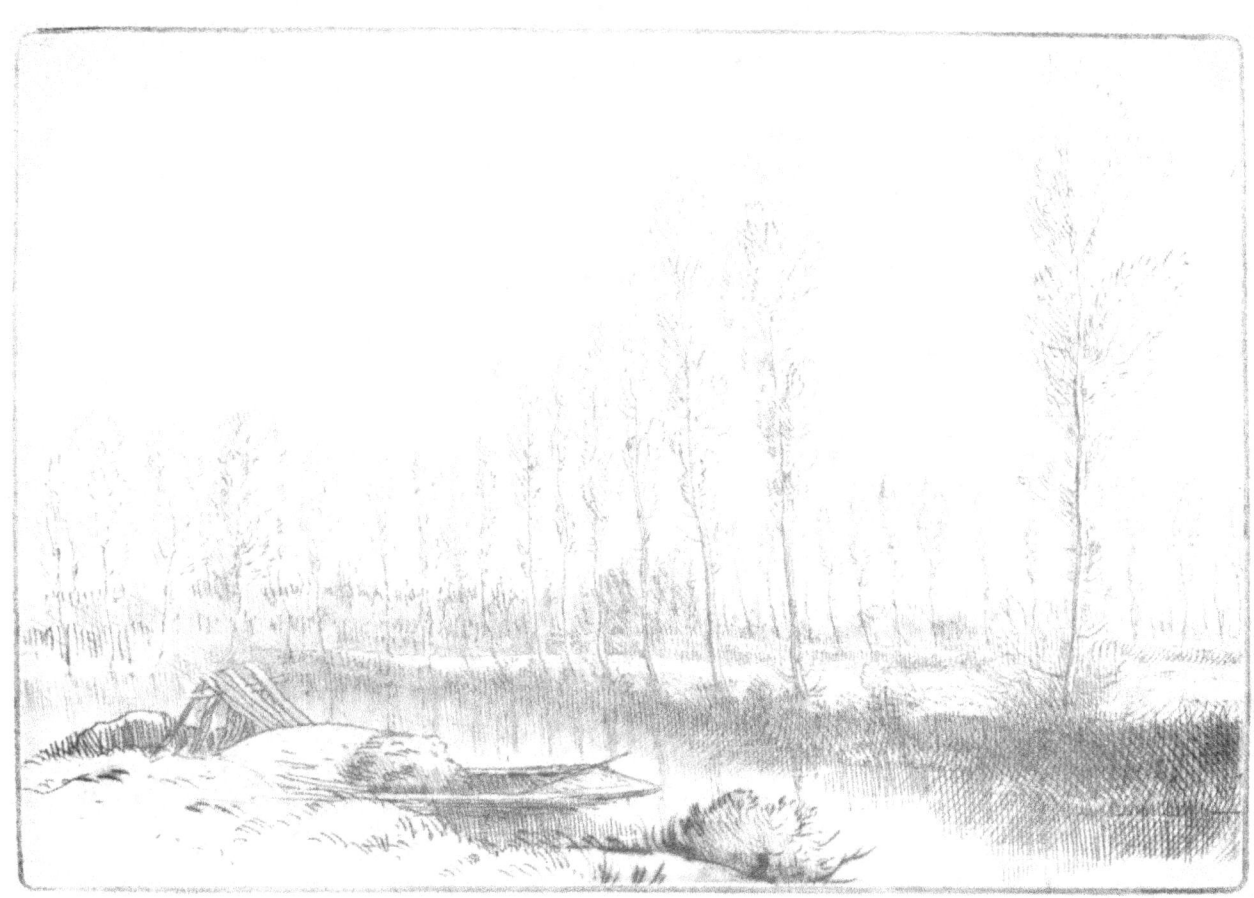

I am meaningful

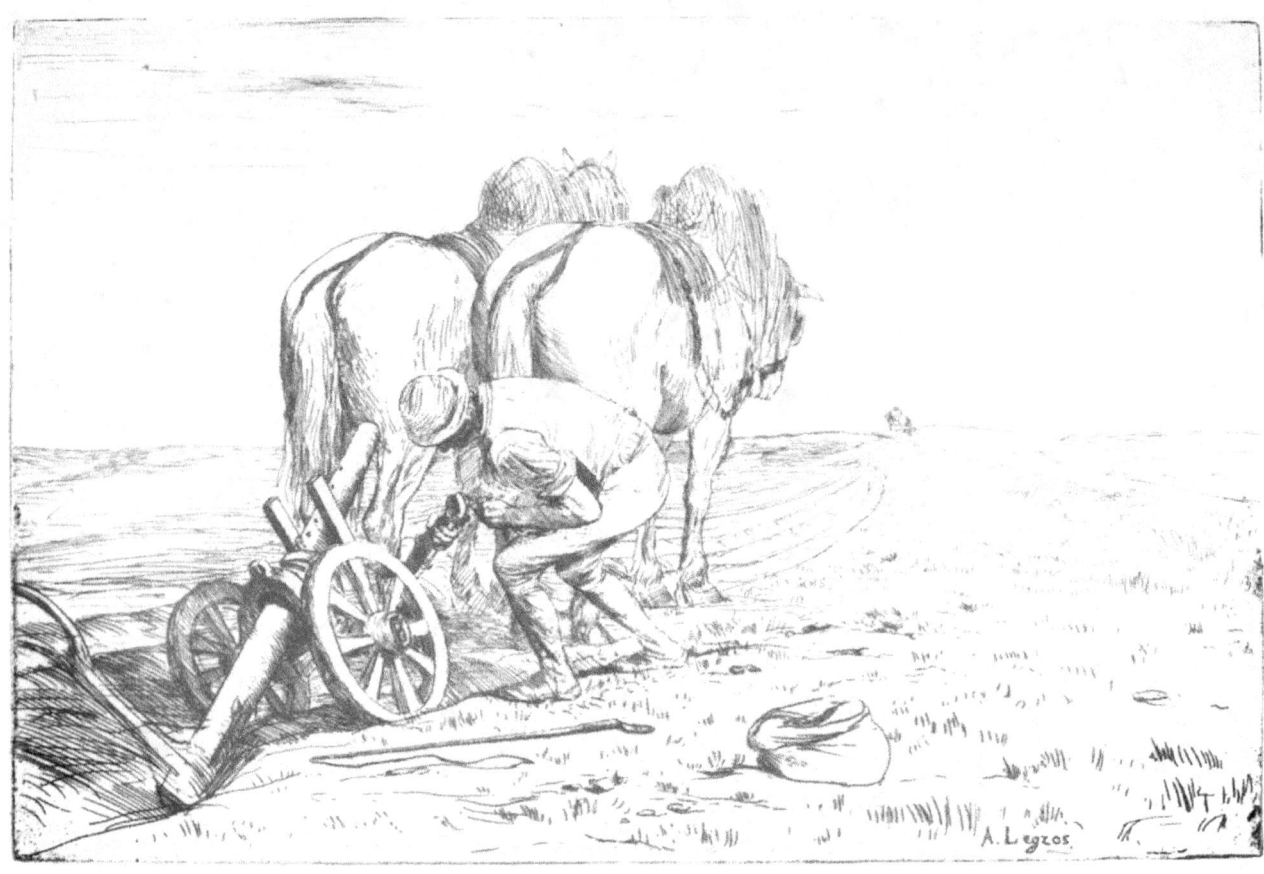

I am secure now

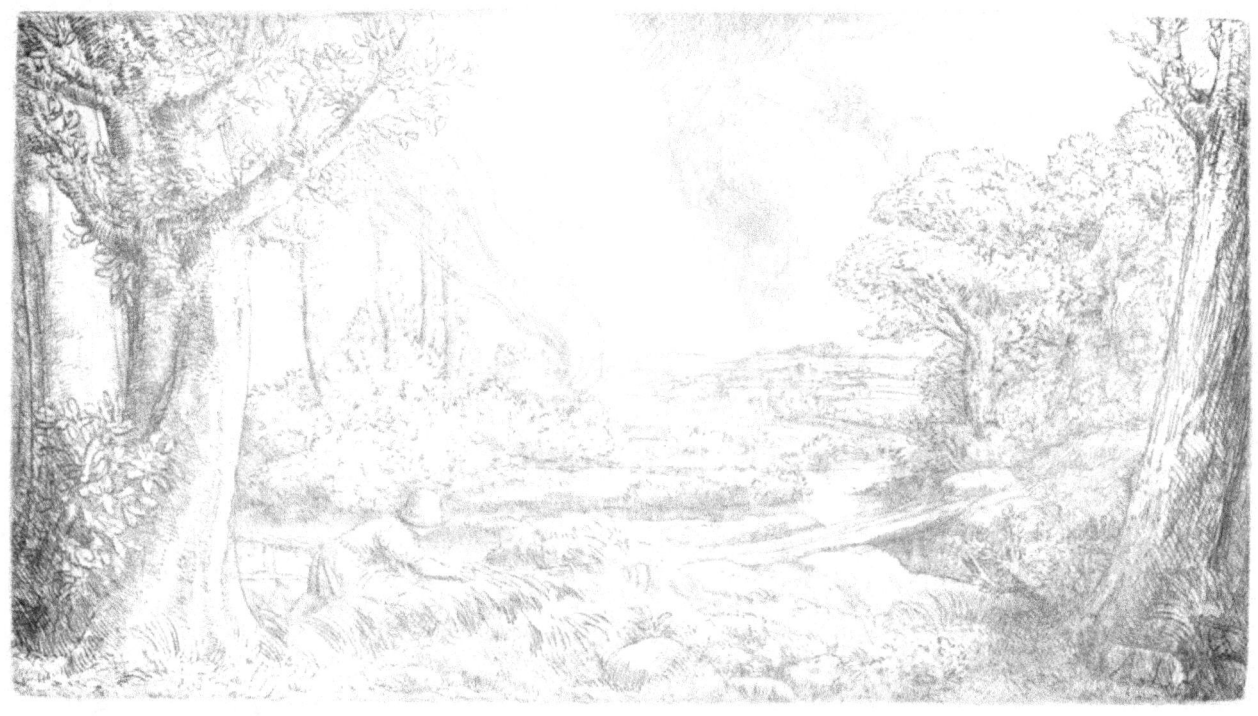

I can be authentic

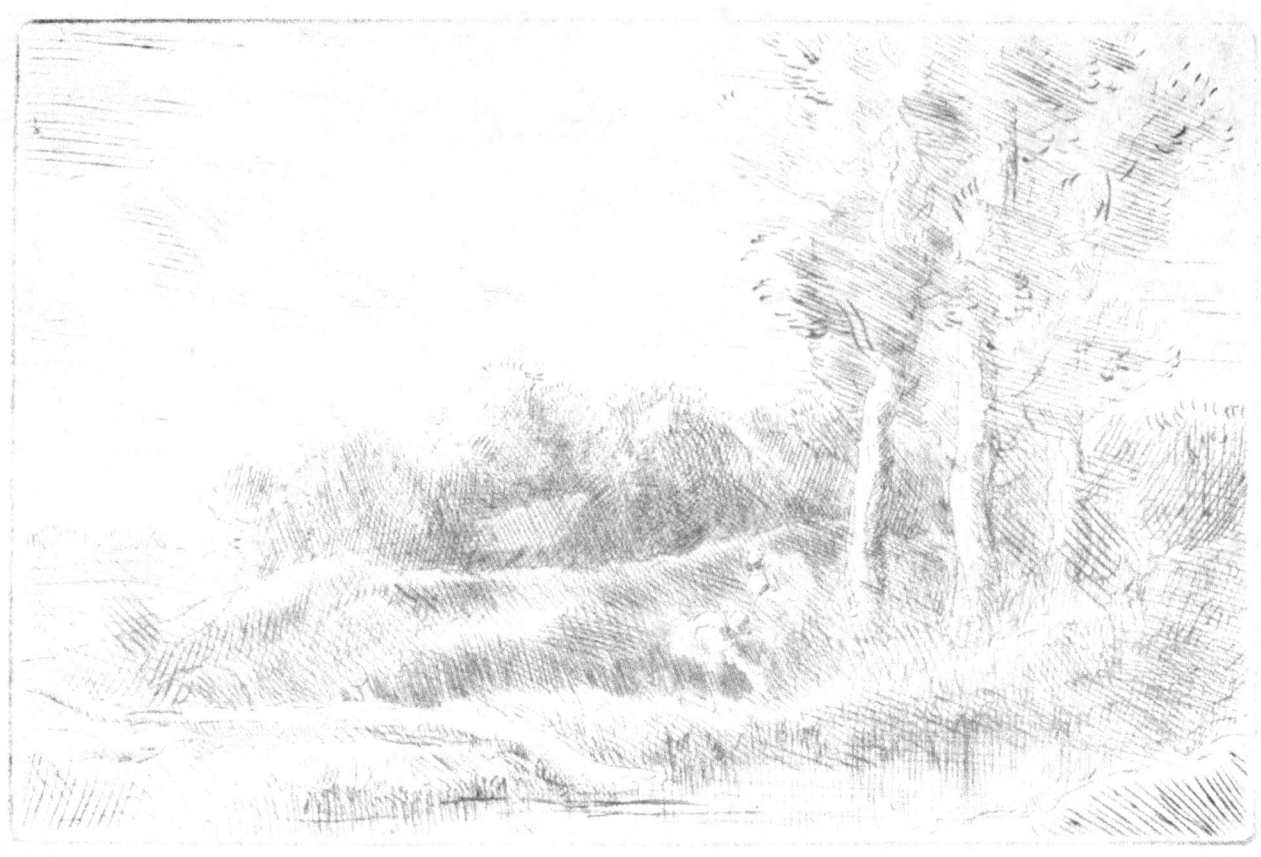

It is finished

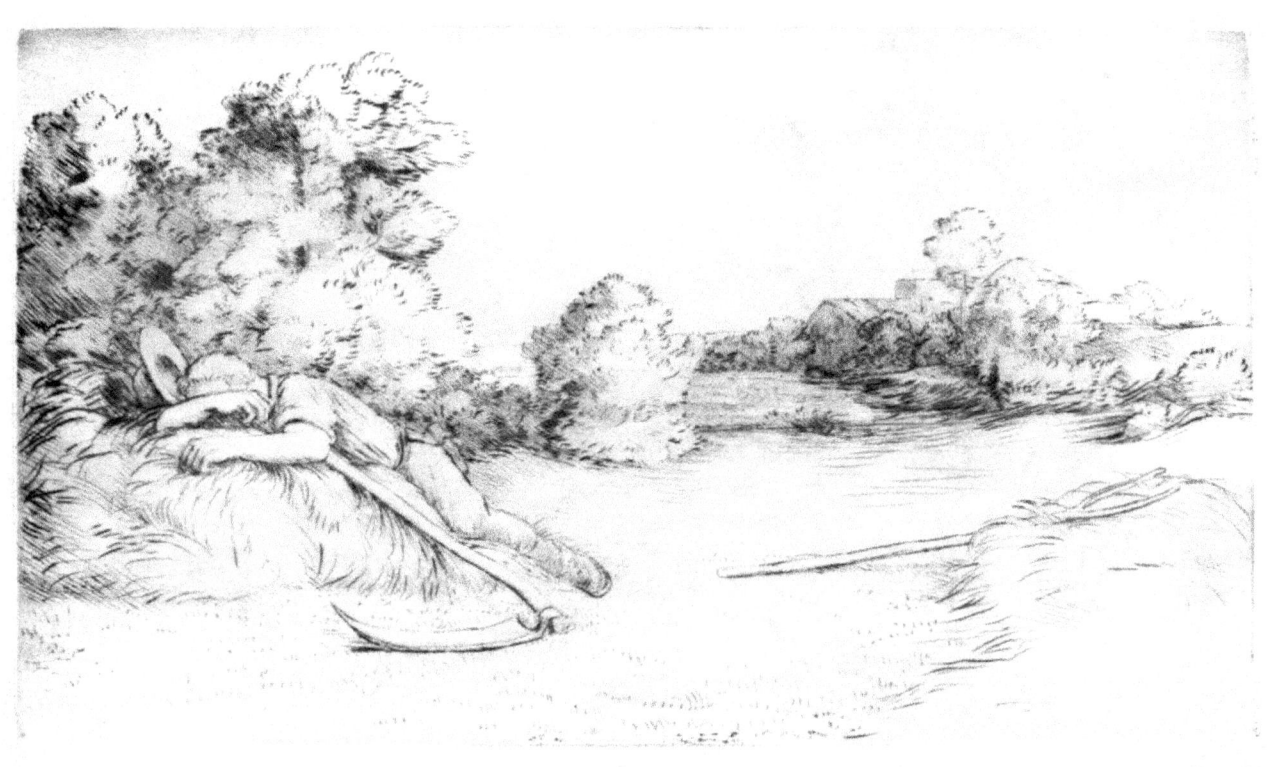

I can just notice

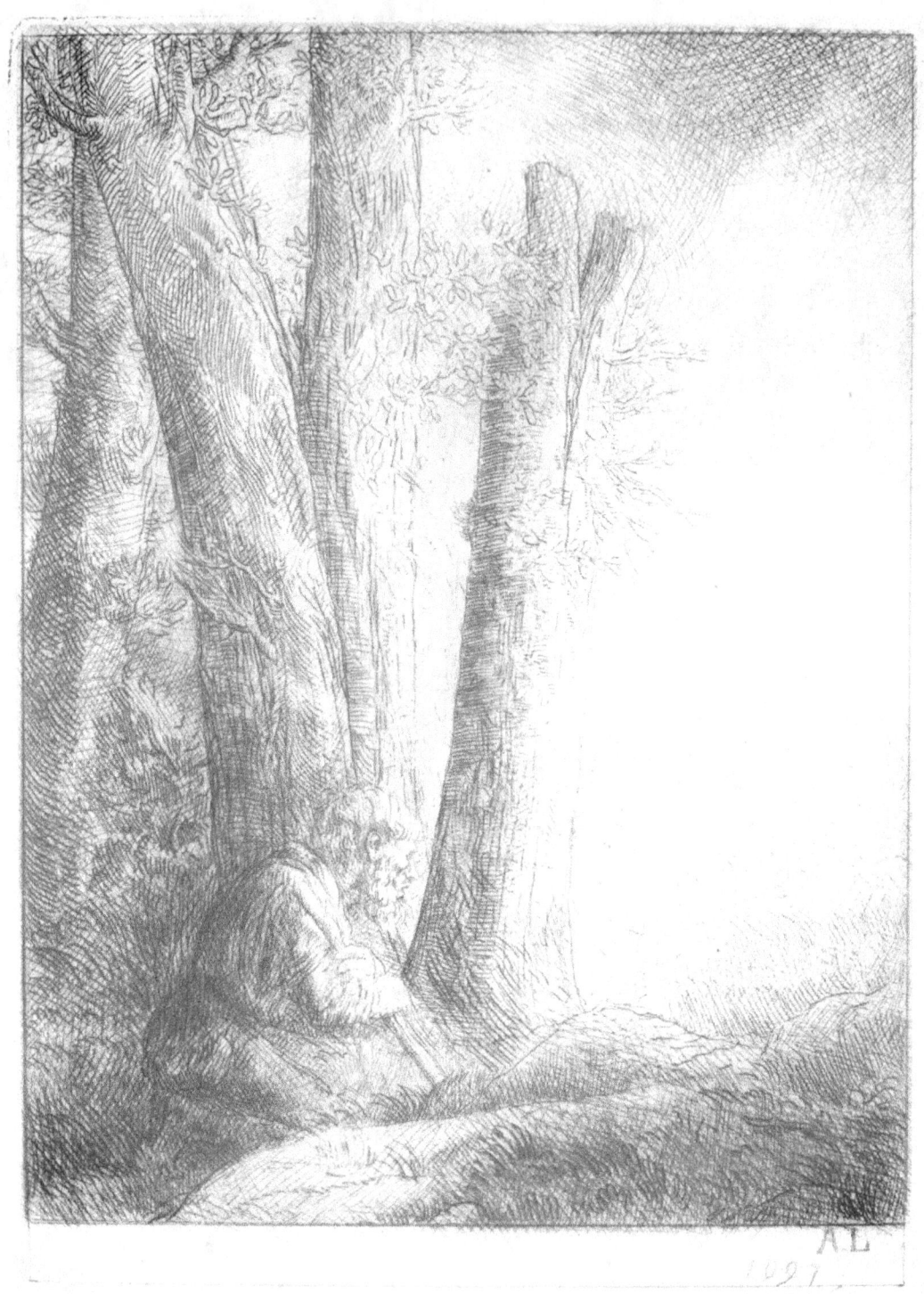

I am wholesome

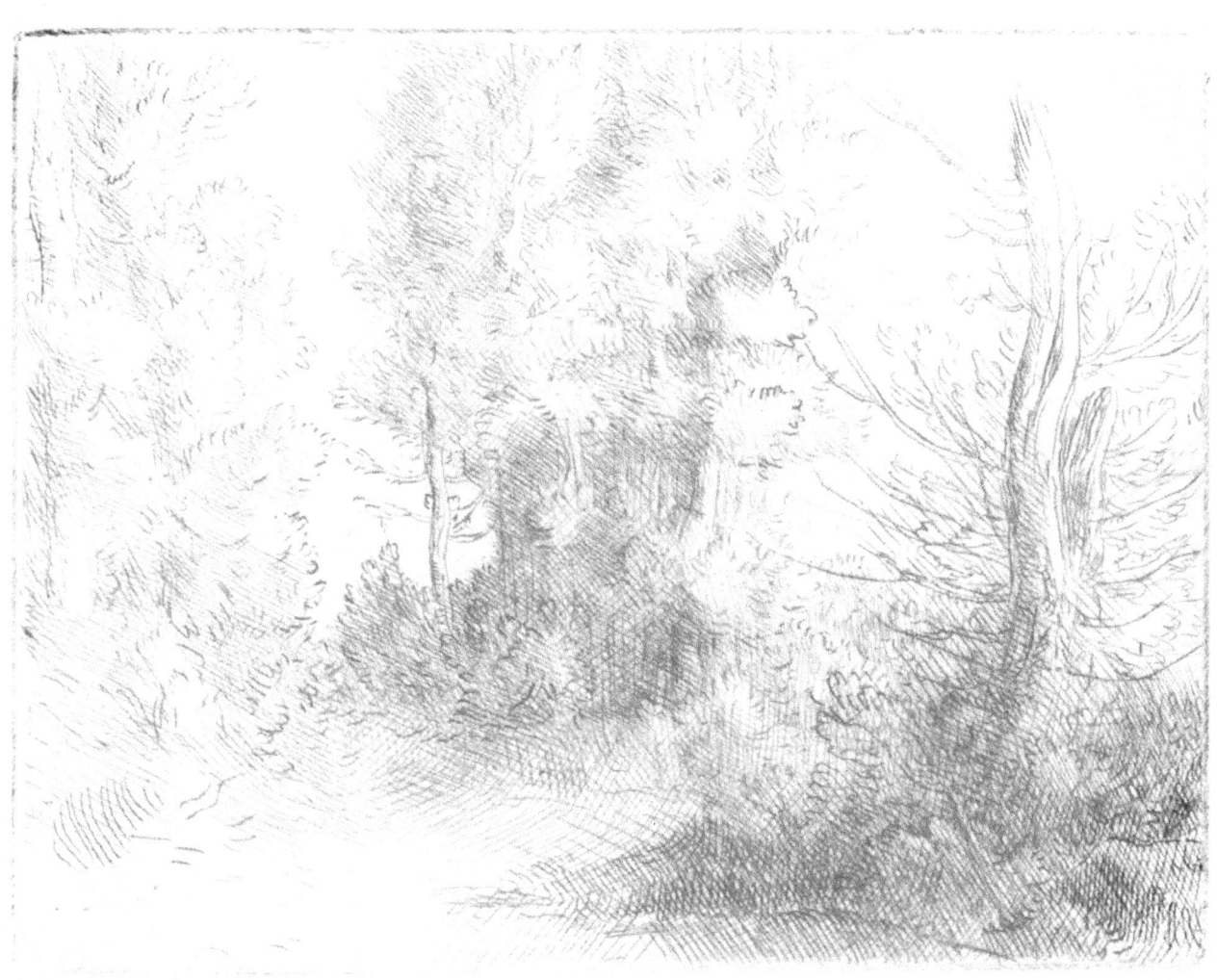

I can be imperfect

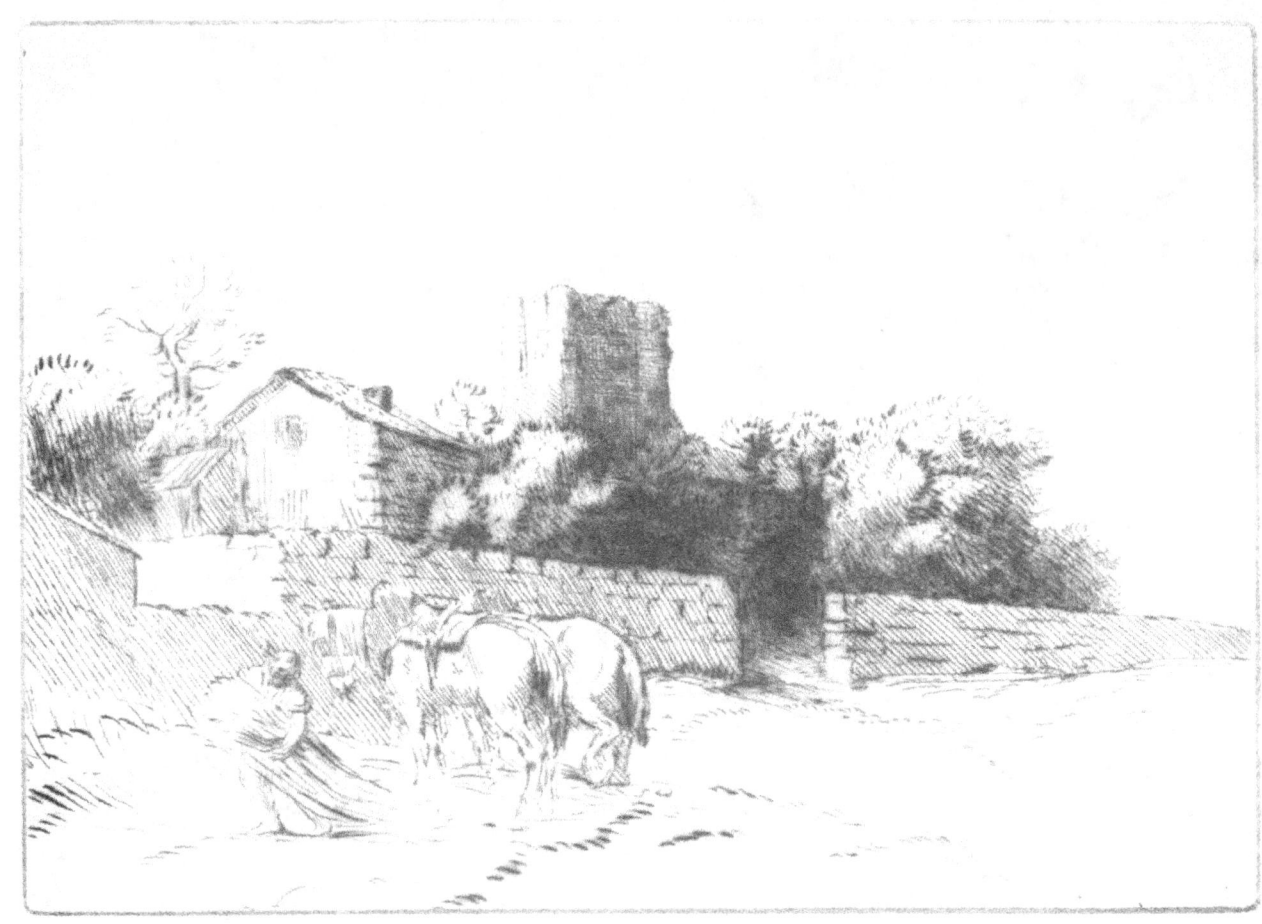

I can be present

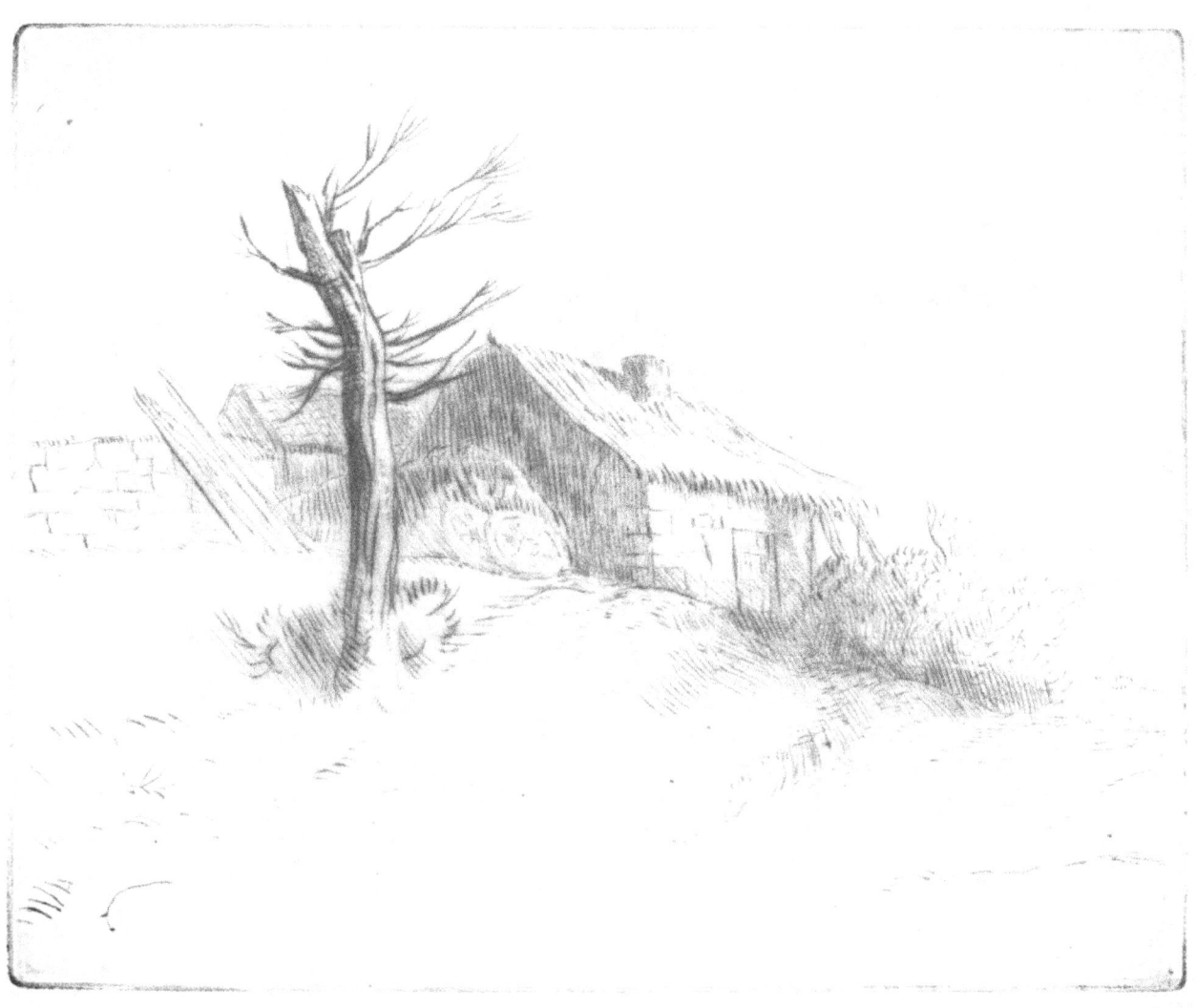

I am stronger than I used to be

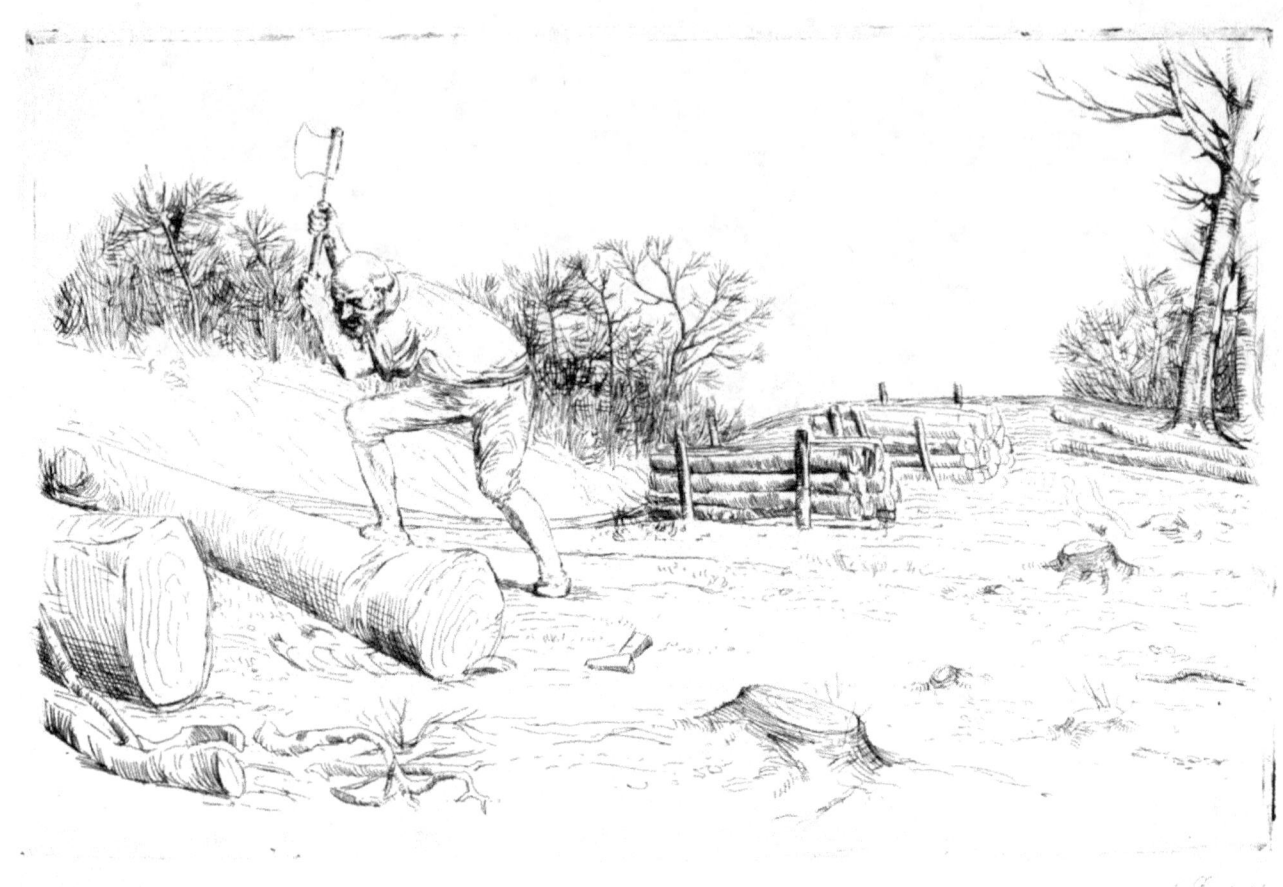

I can find meaning

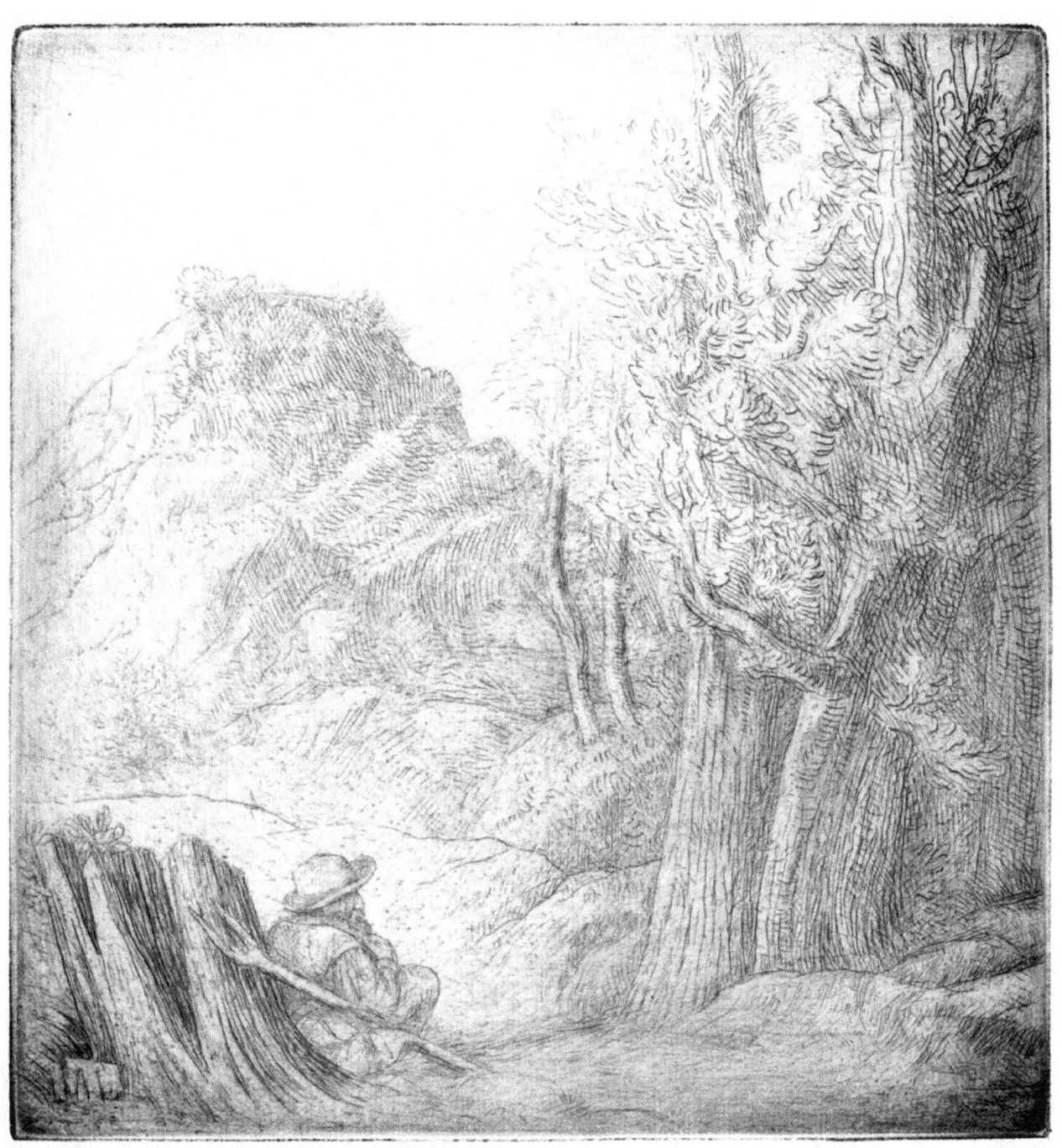

My situation is different now

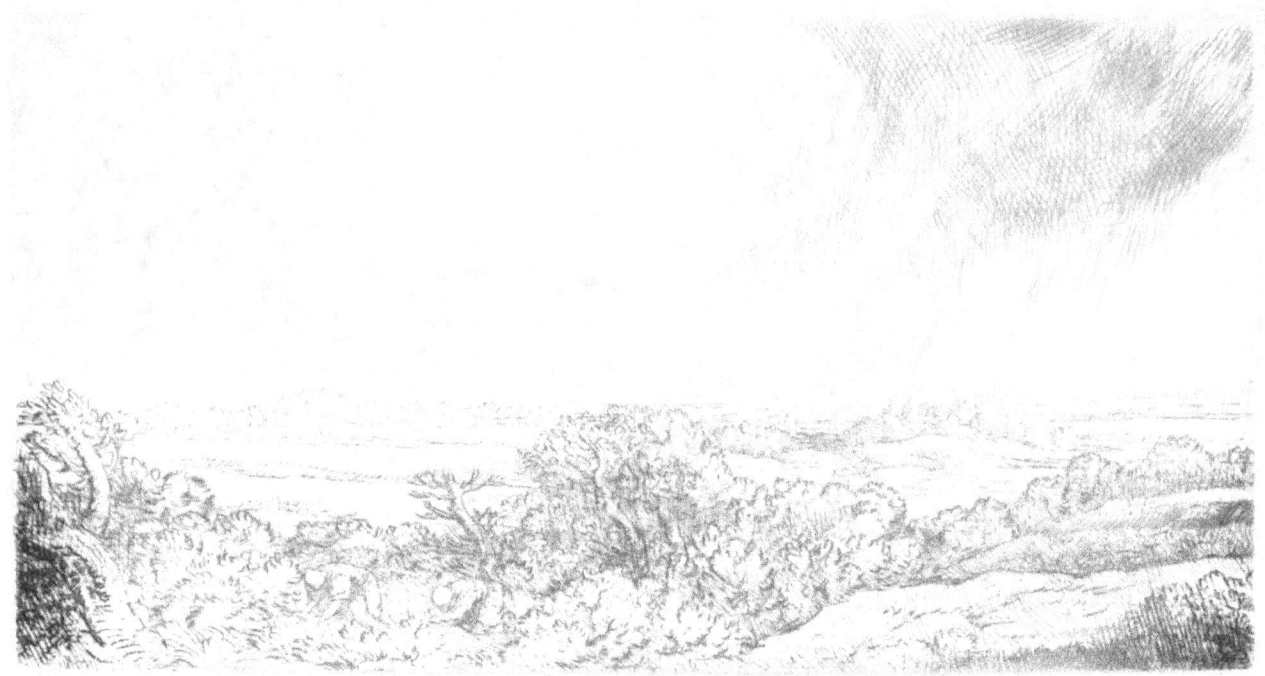

I do not need to have all the answers

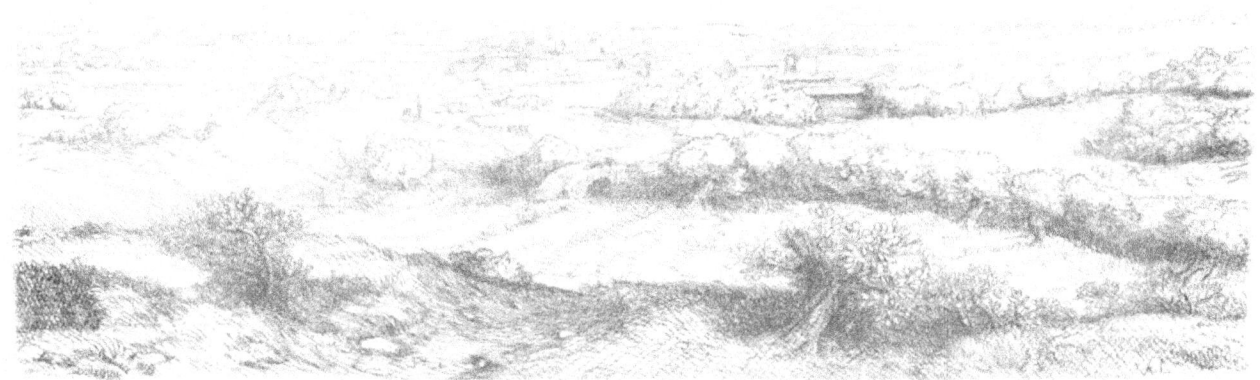

I can be transformed

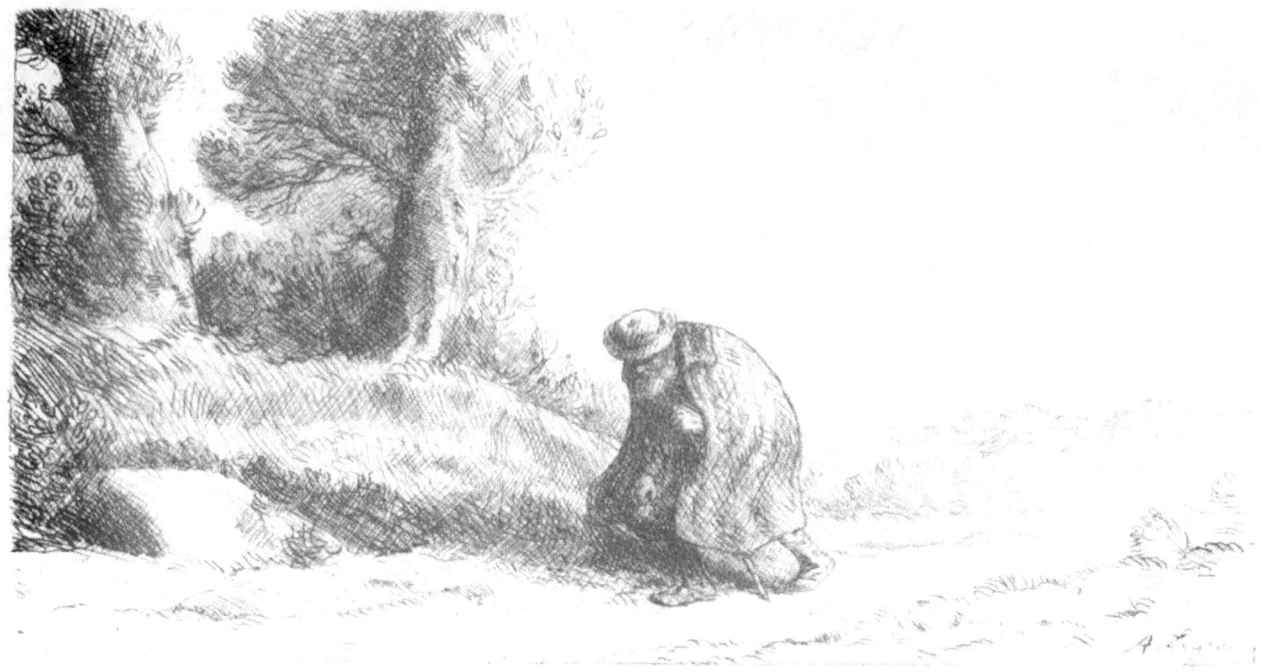

I did what I could

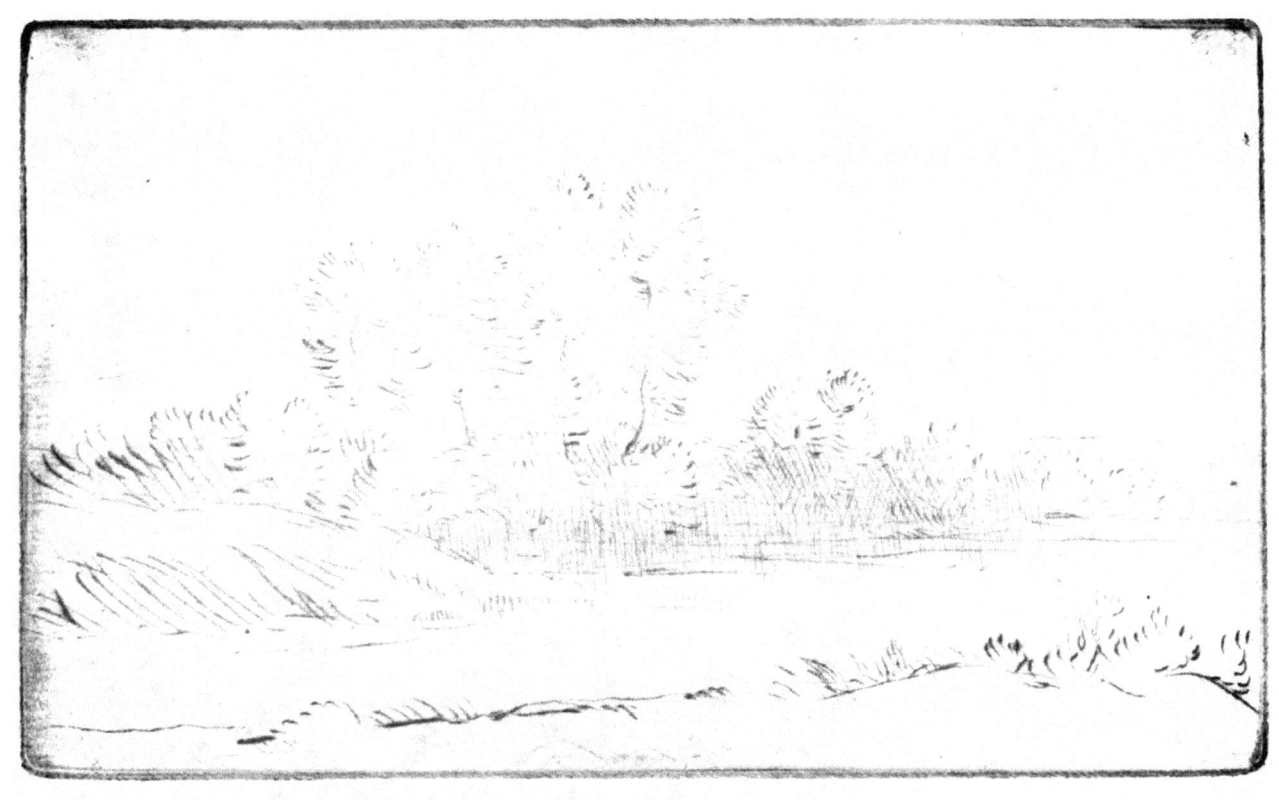

What happened does not define me

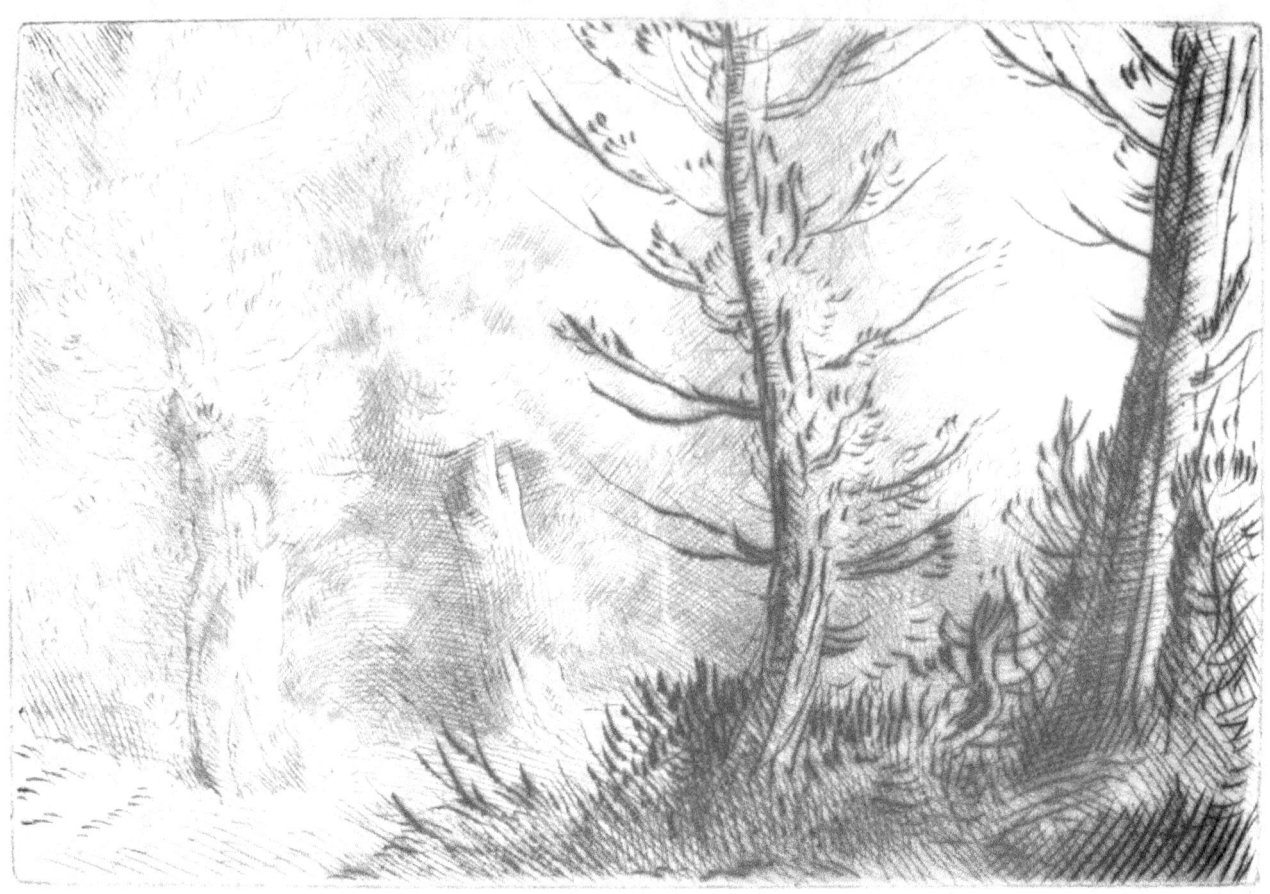

I can learn to make my needs known

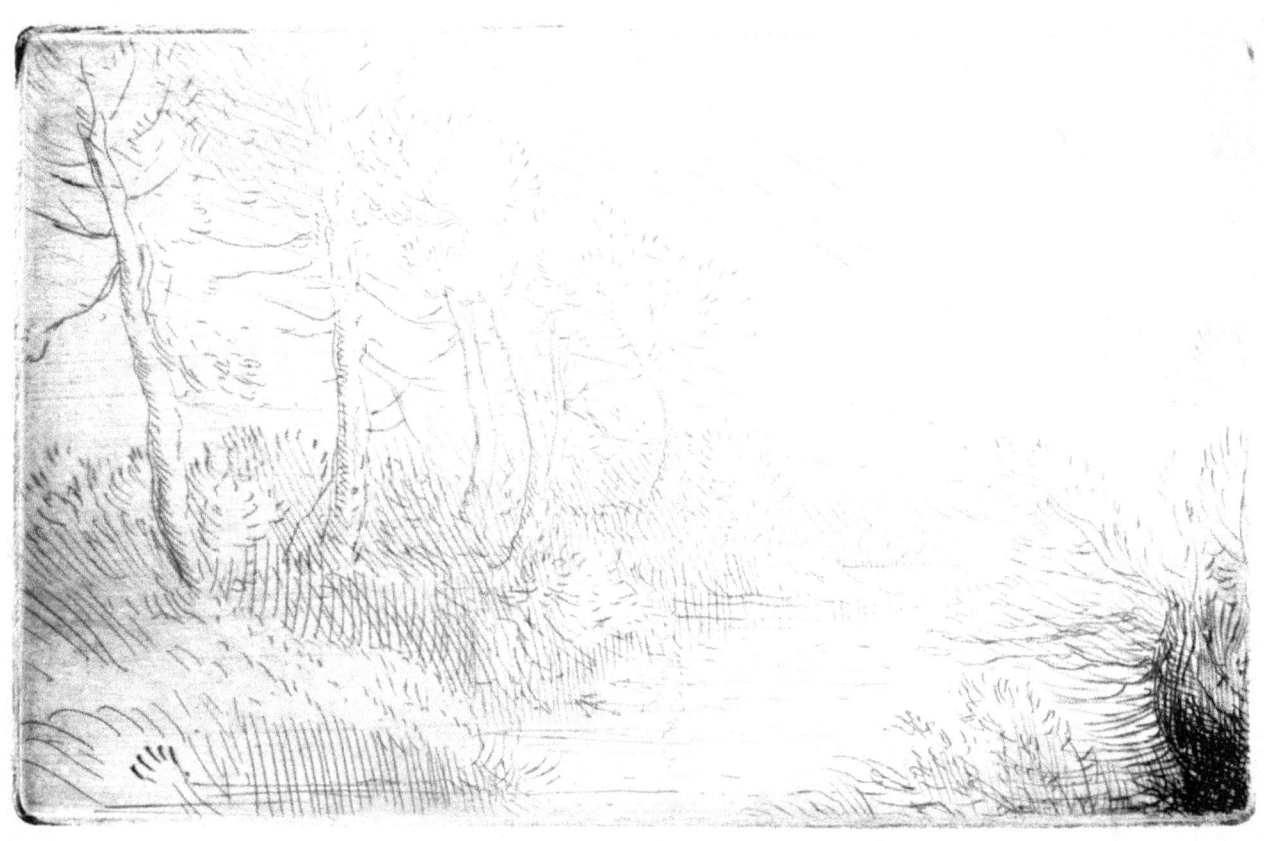

I can live with paradox

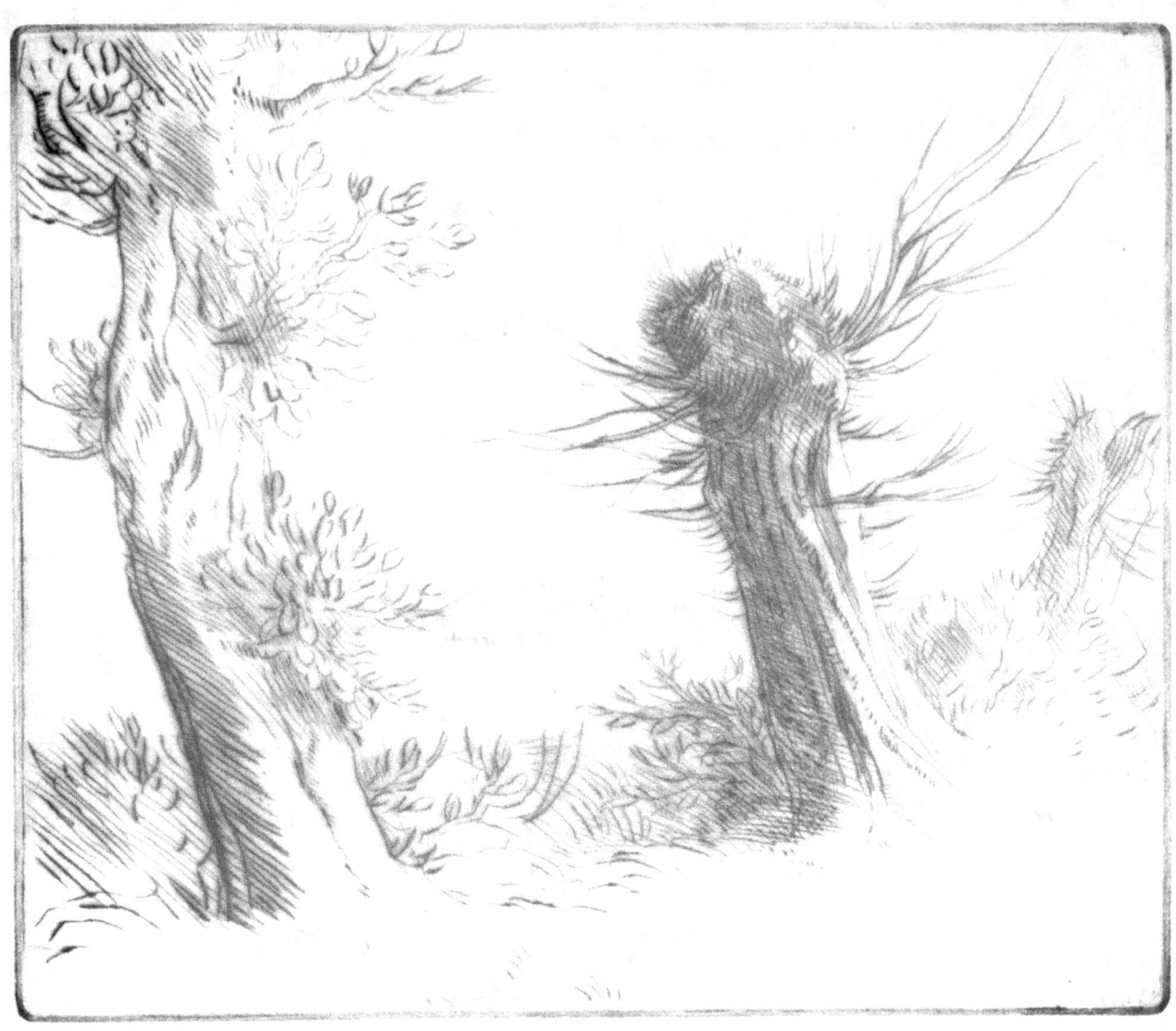

I now have better judgment

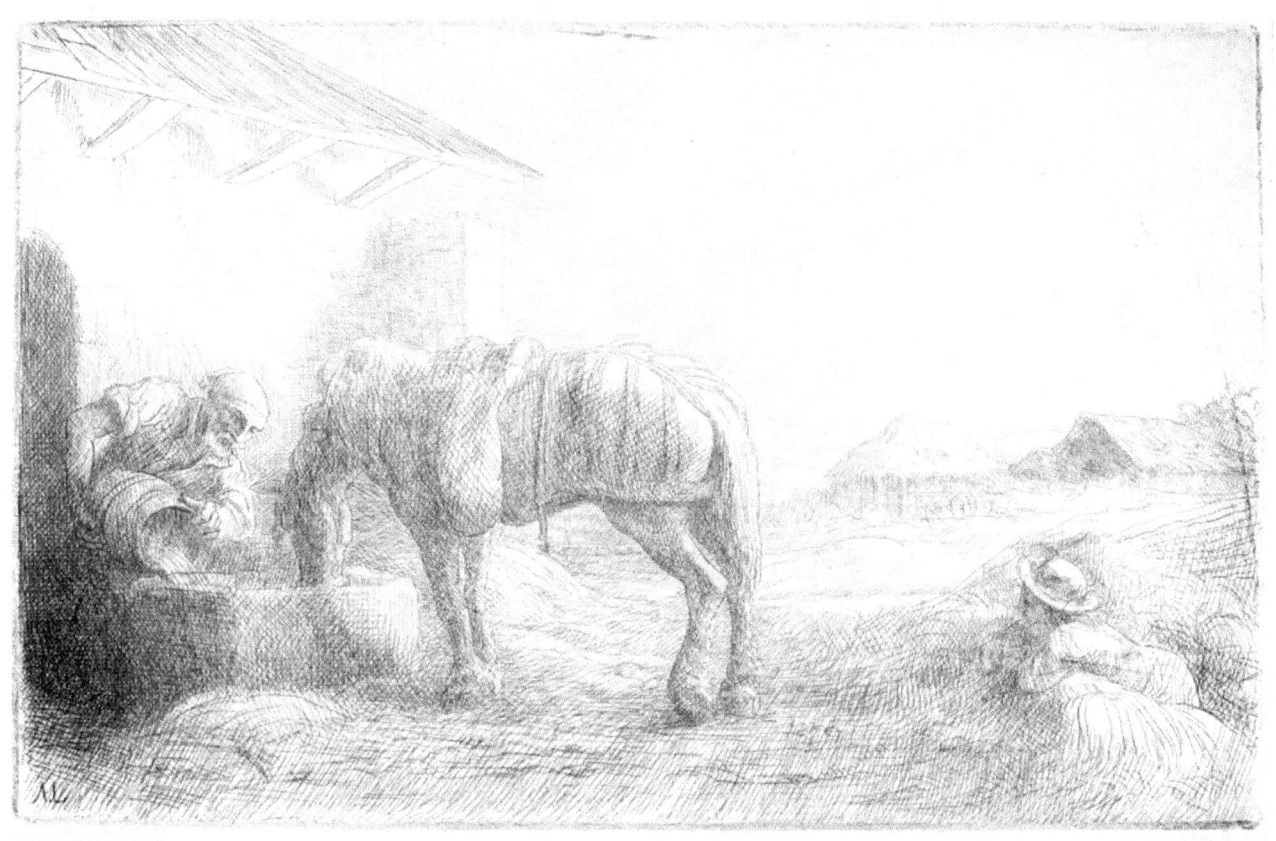

I can learn to be honest

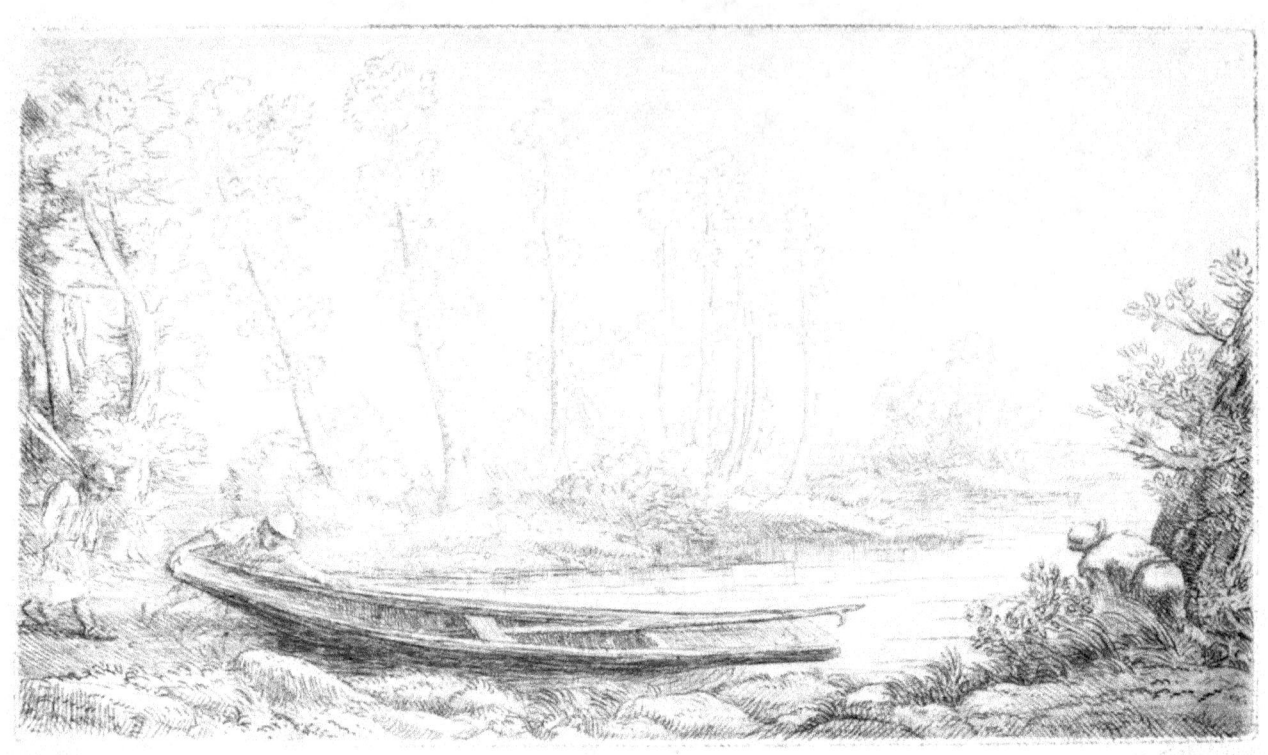

I know enough

I am worth it

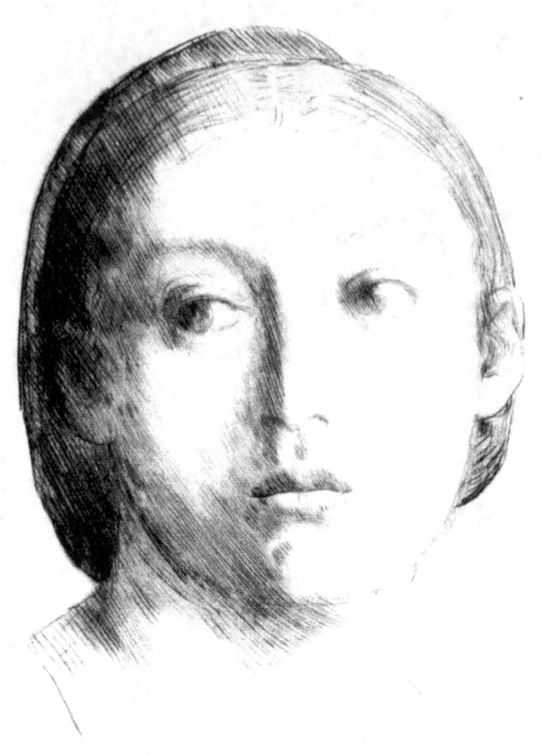

My heart was in the right place

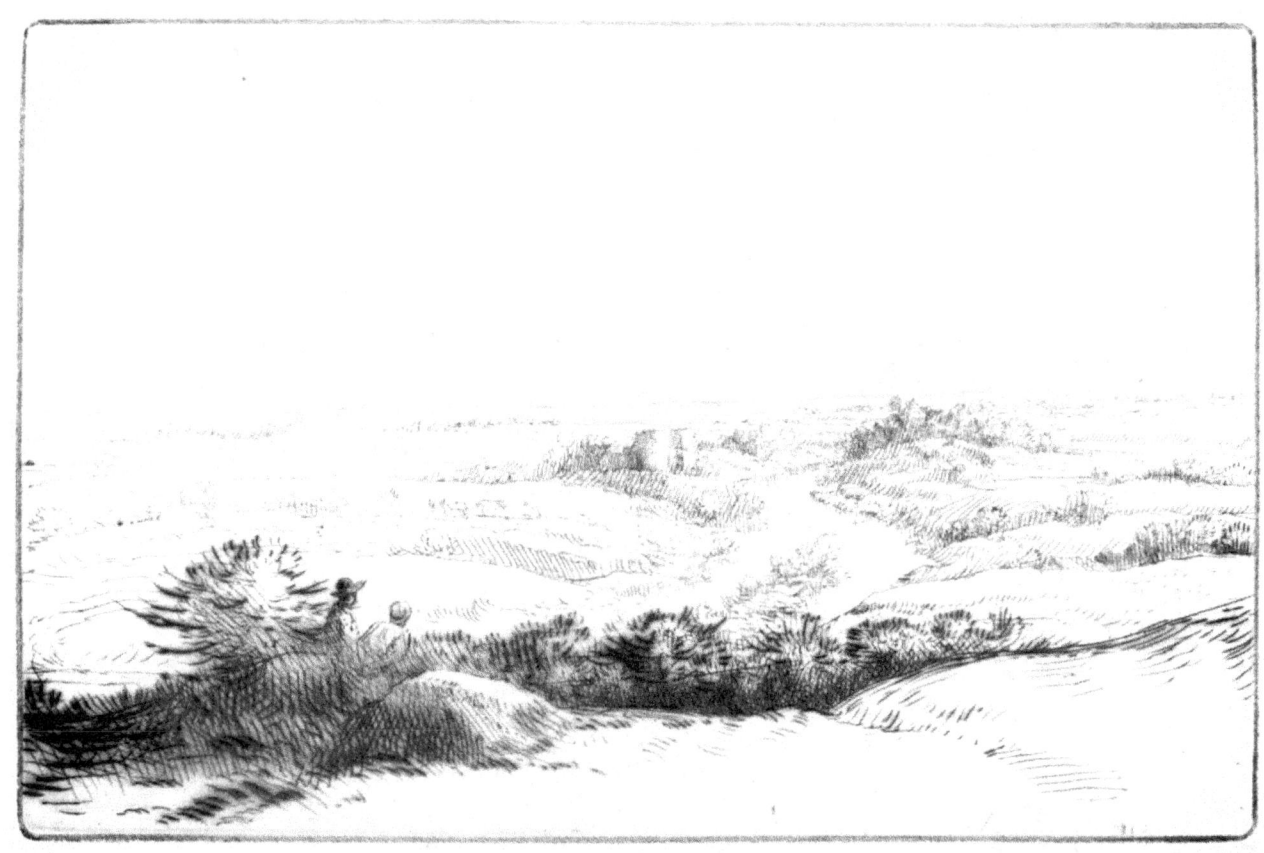

I can be transformed

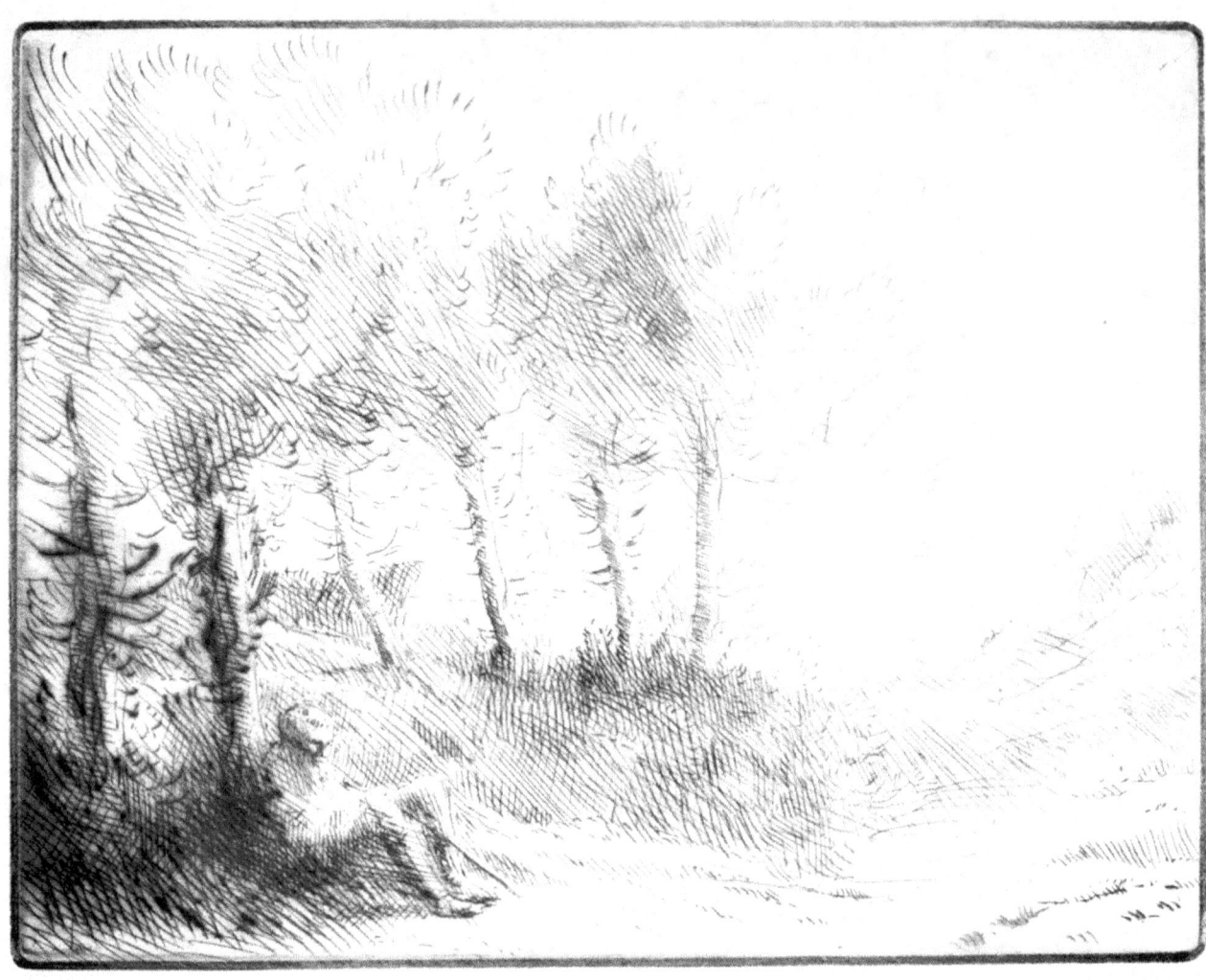

I am one of a kind

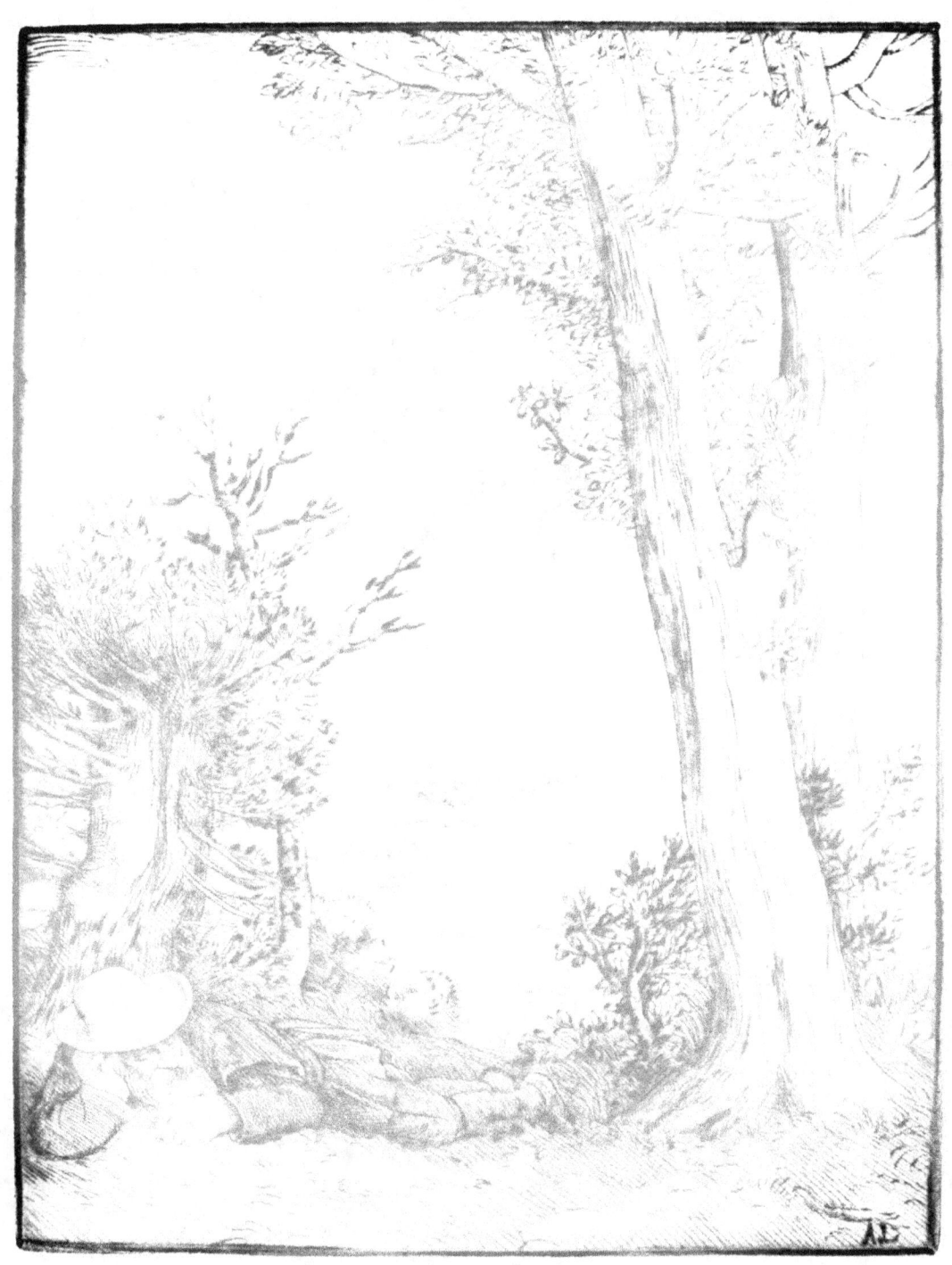

I can do what I need to do

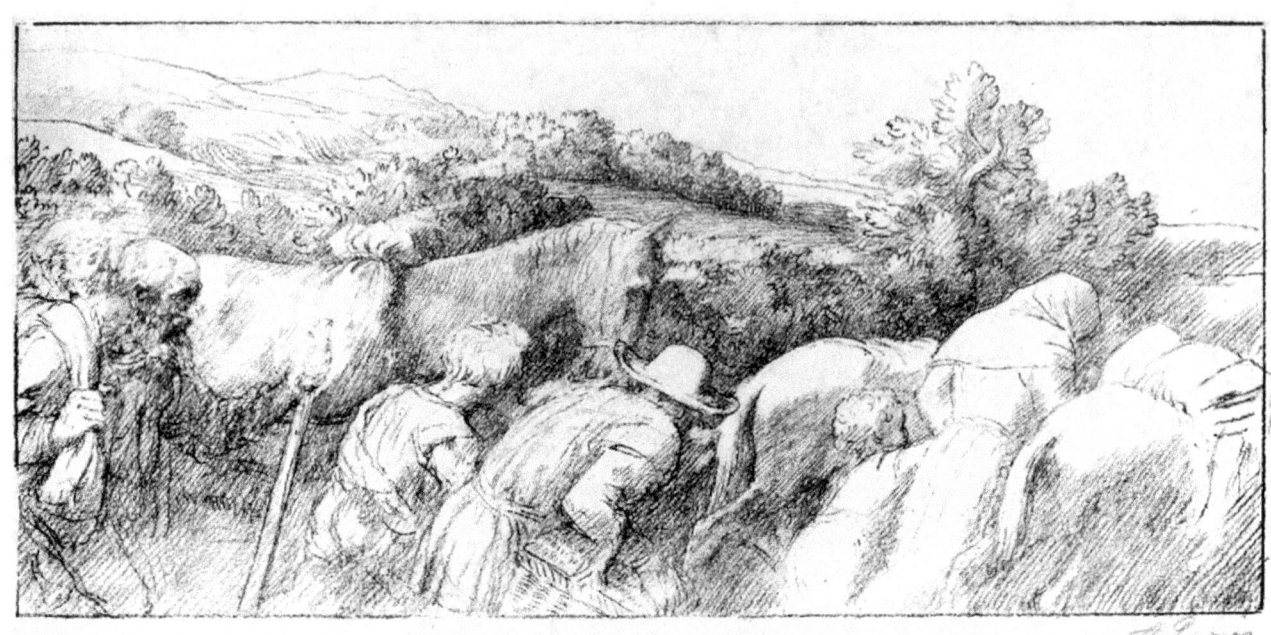

I can be honest

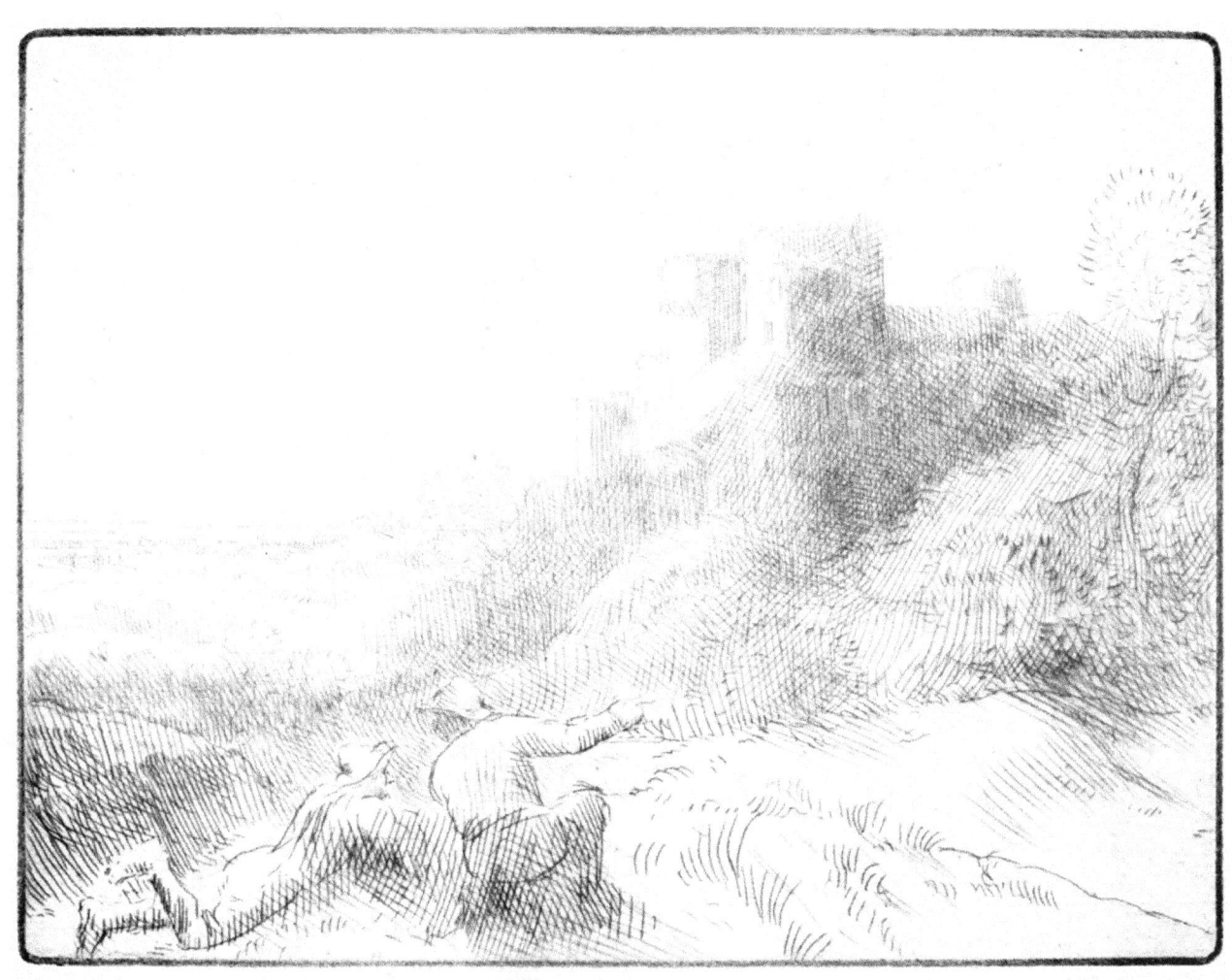

I am just right

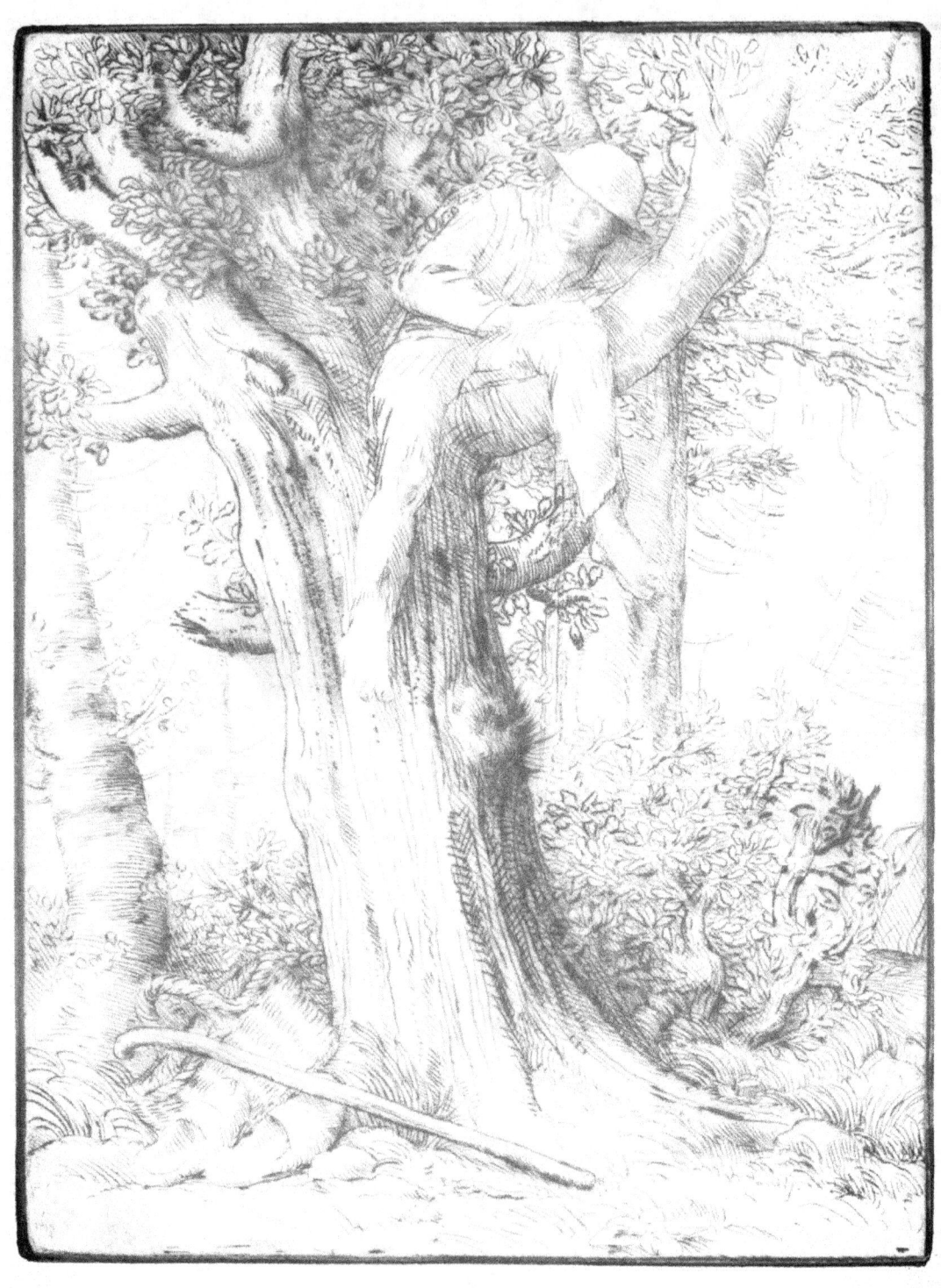

I can be healthier

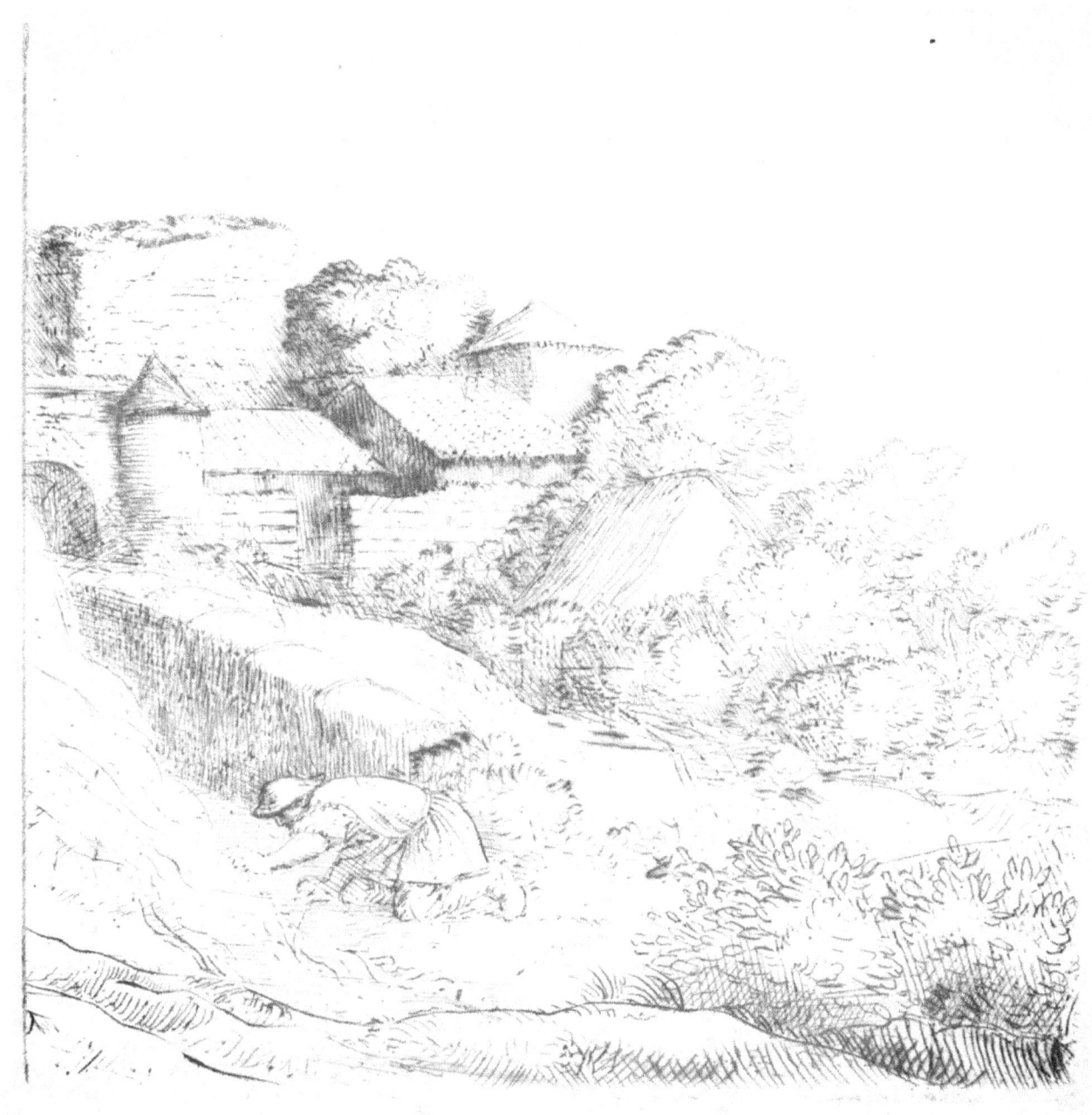

I am special

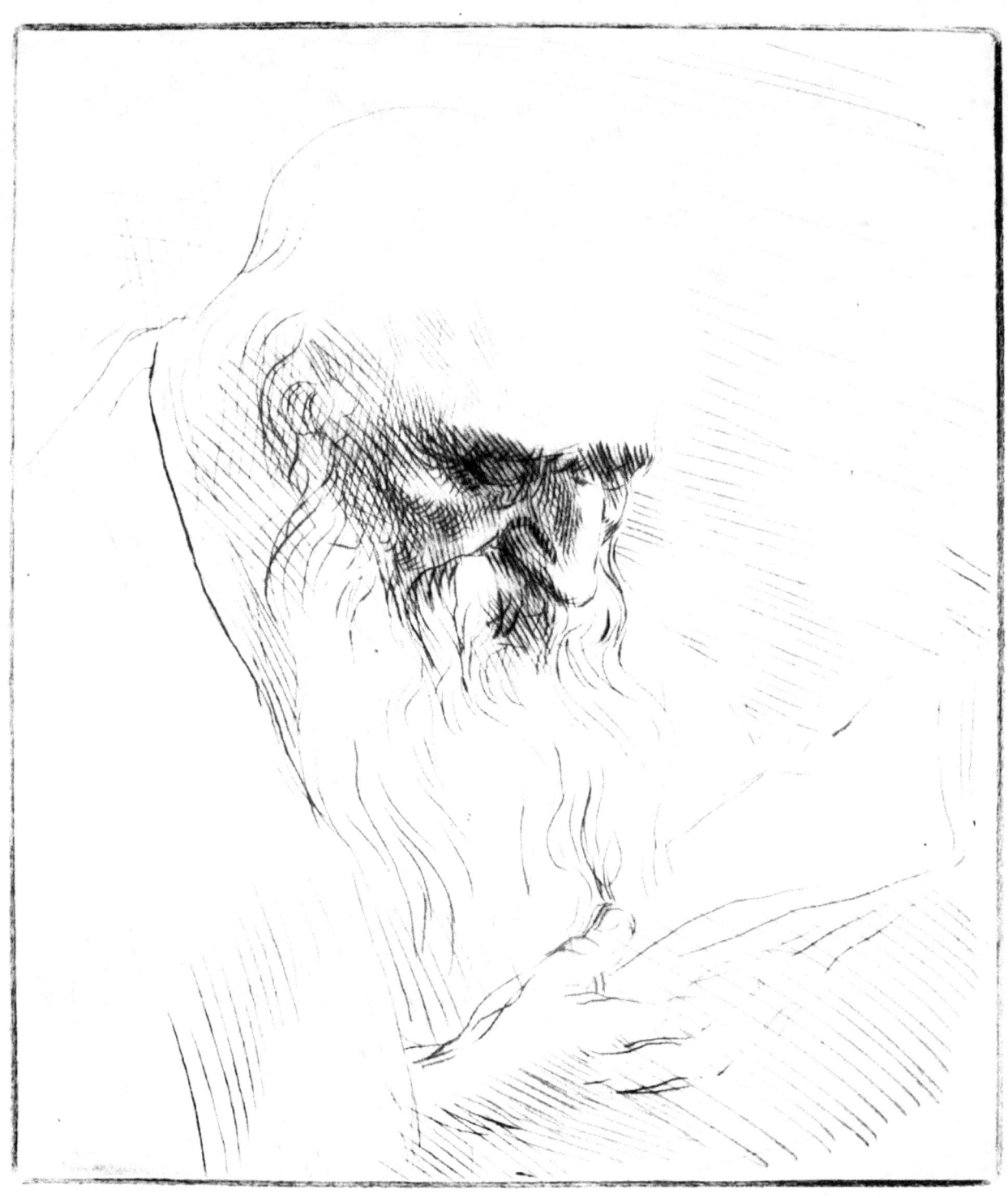

I now have more choices

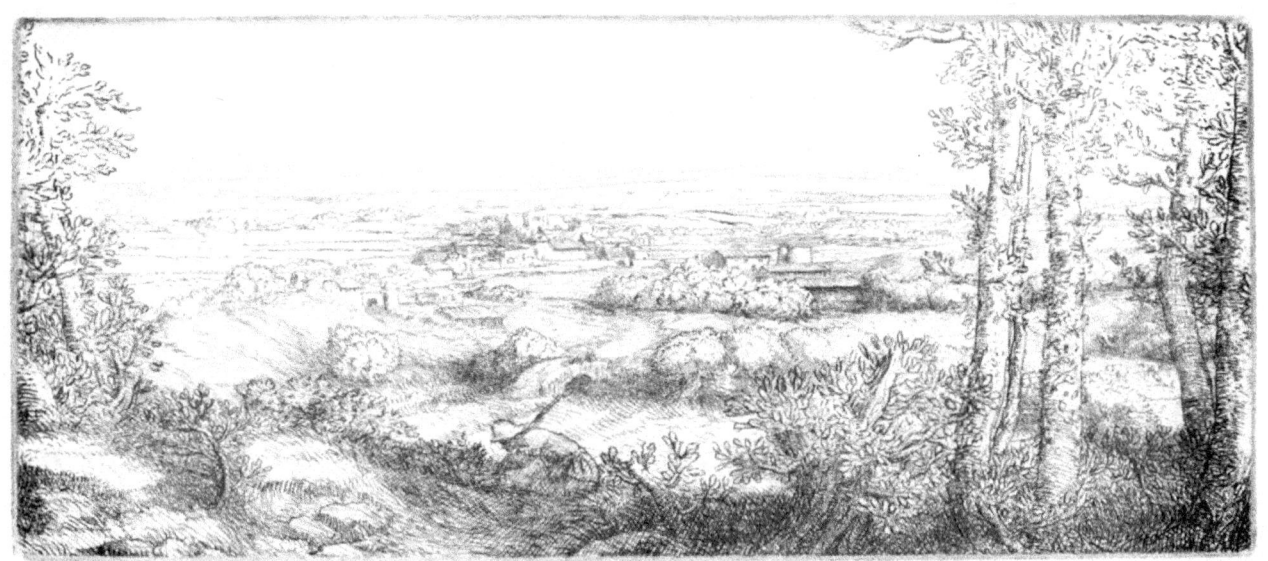

I am full of heart

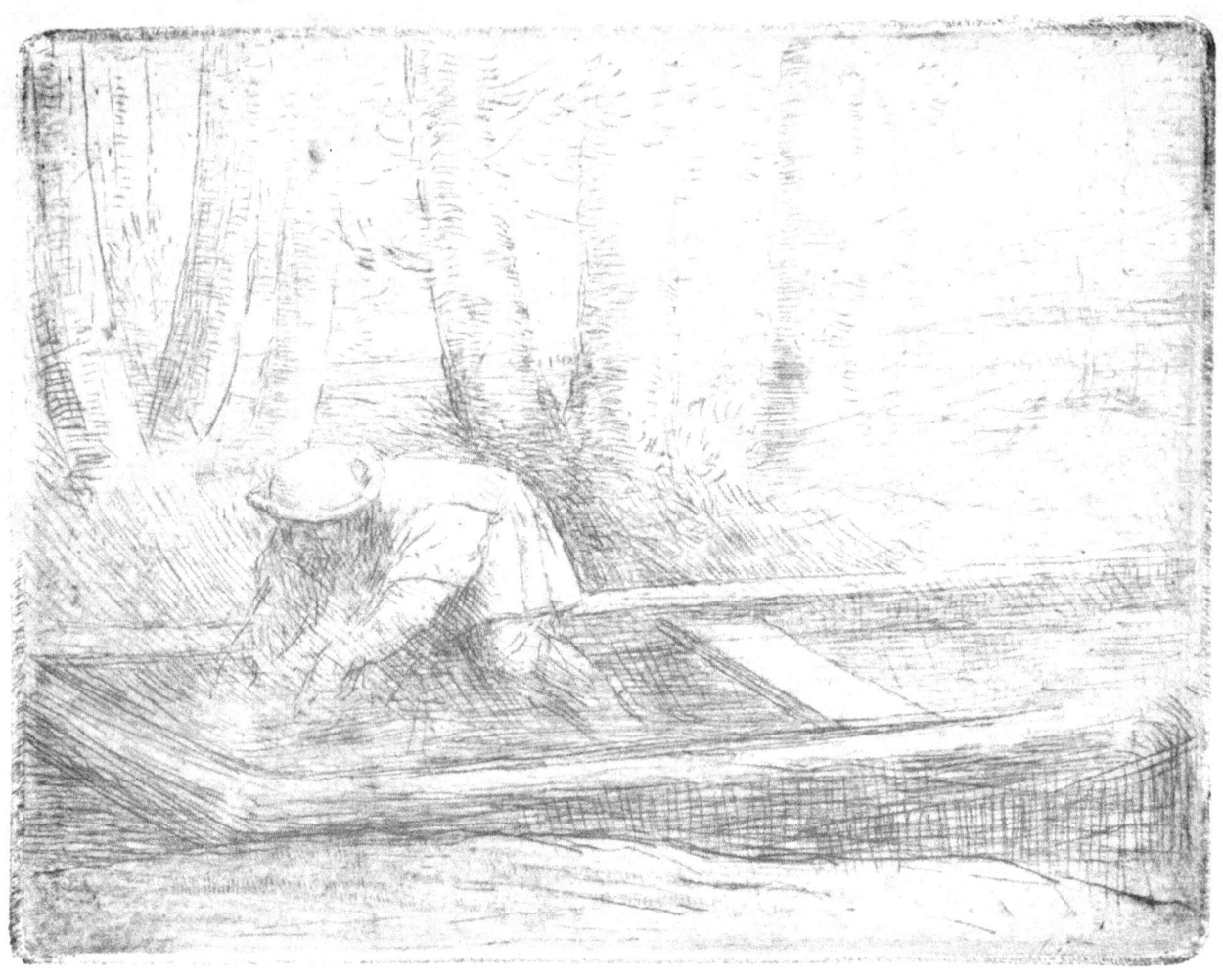

I can learn to be myself

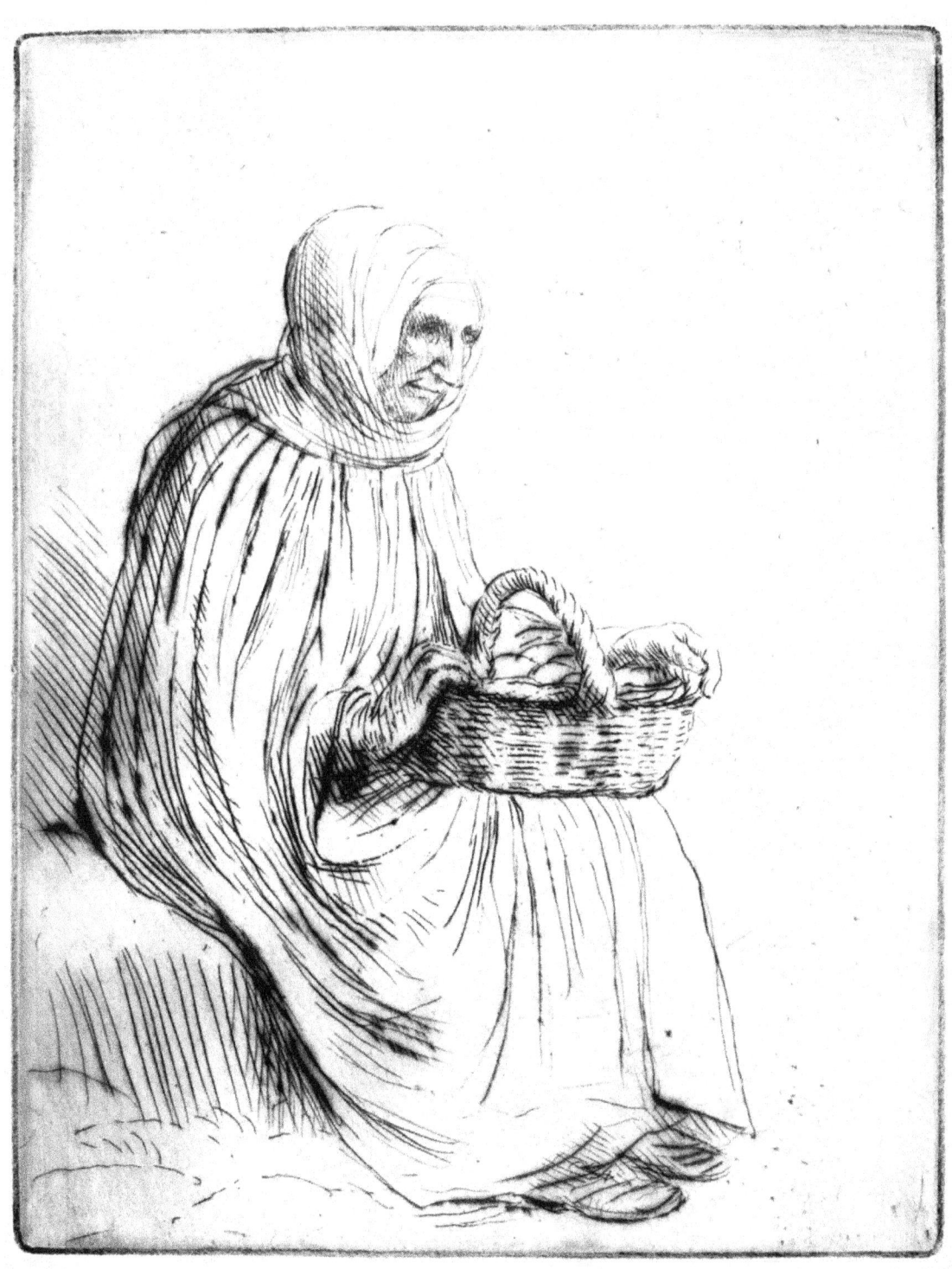

I have been made new

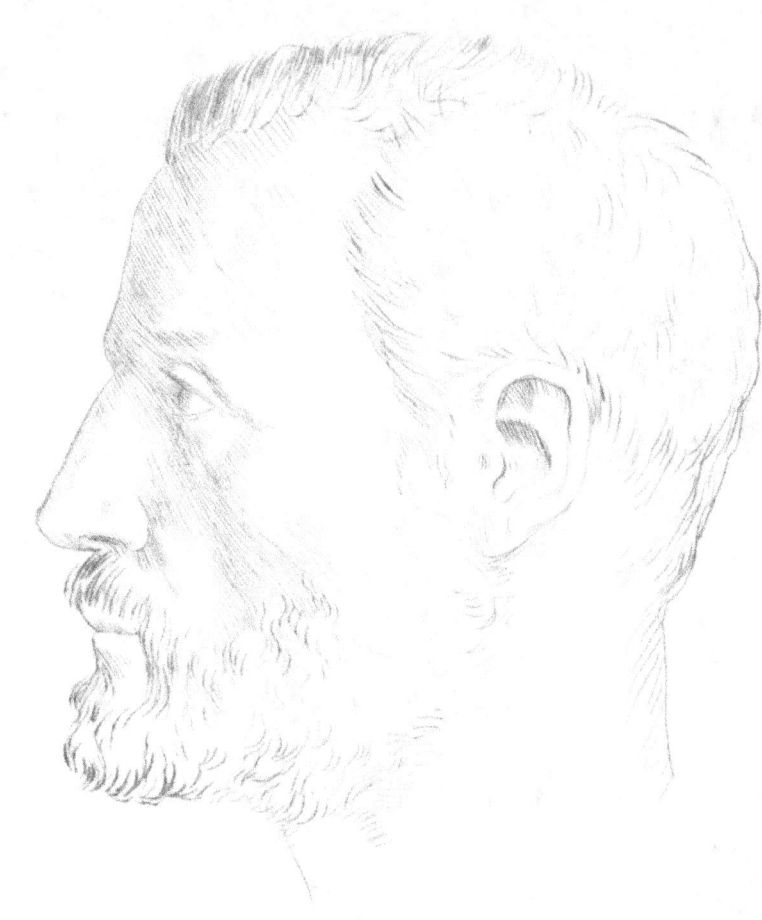

I can learn to succeed

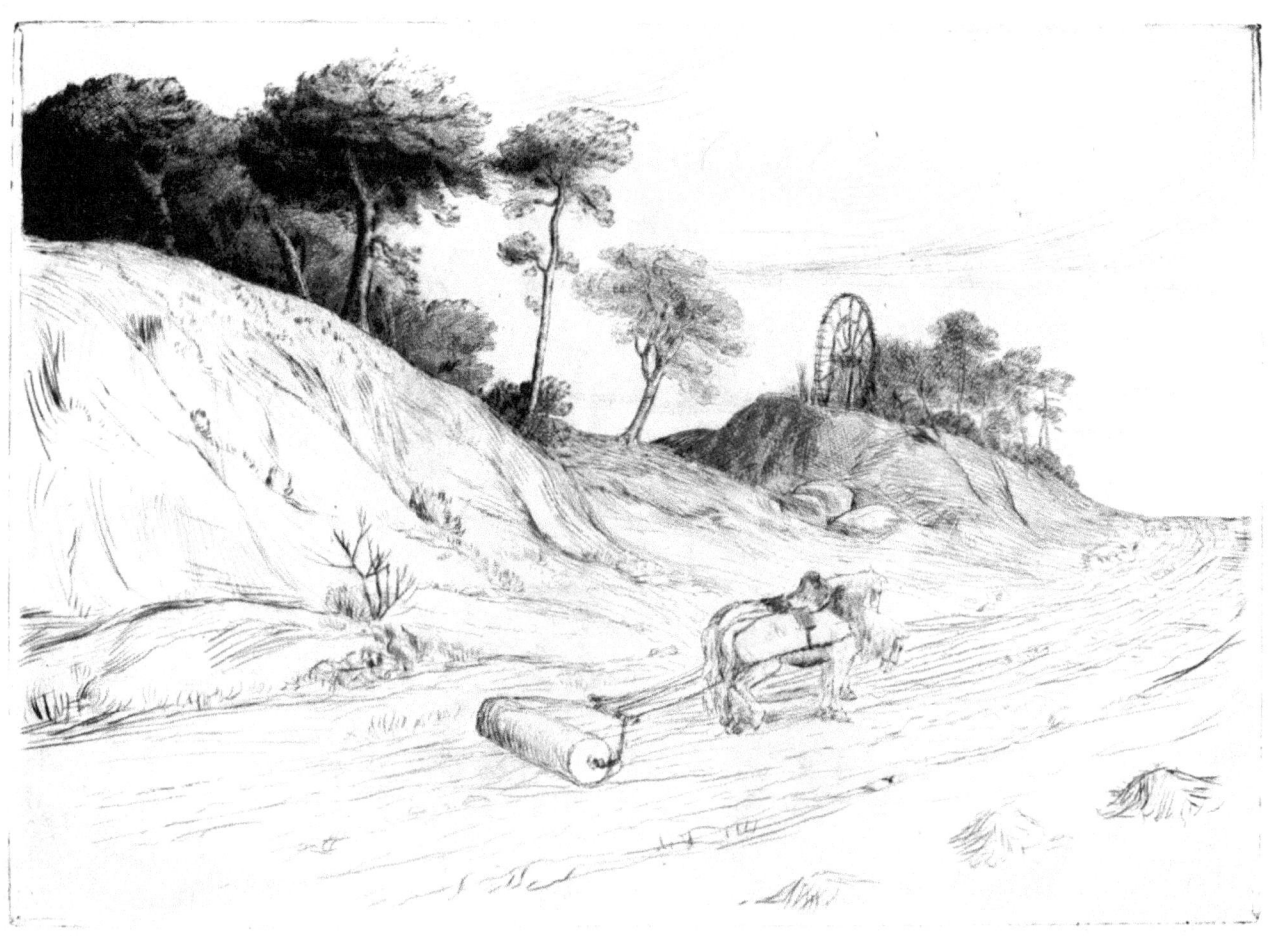

I am better now

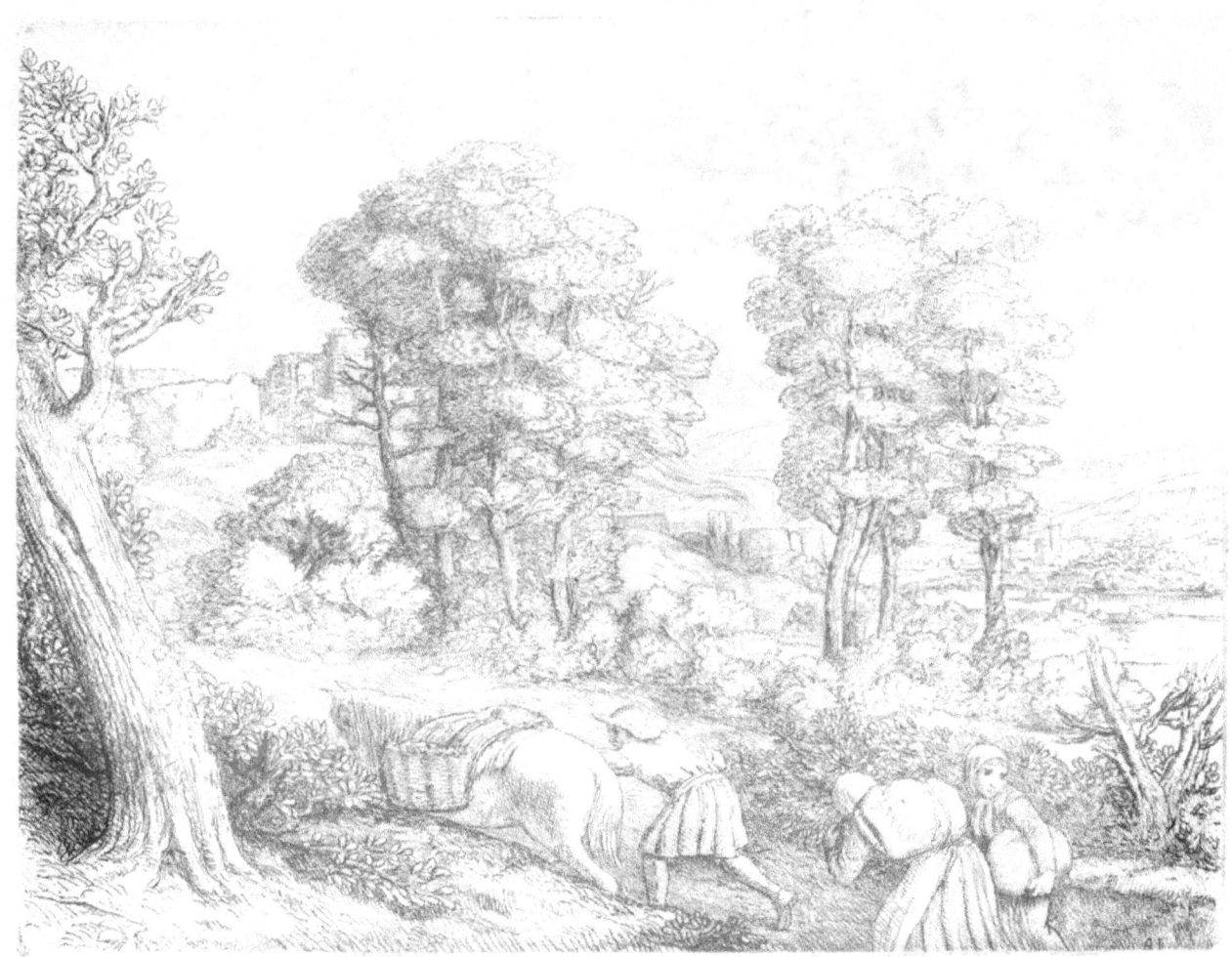

I am a person of principle

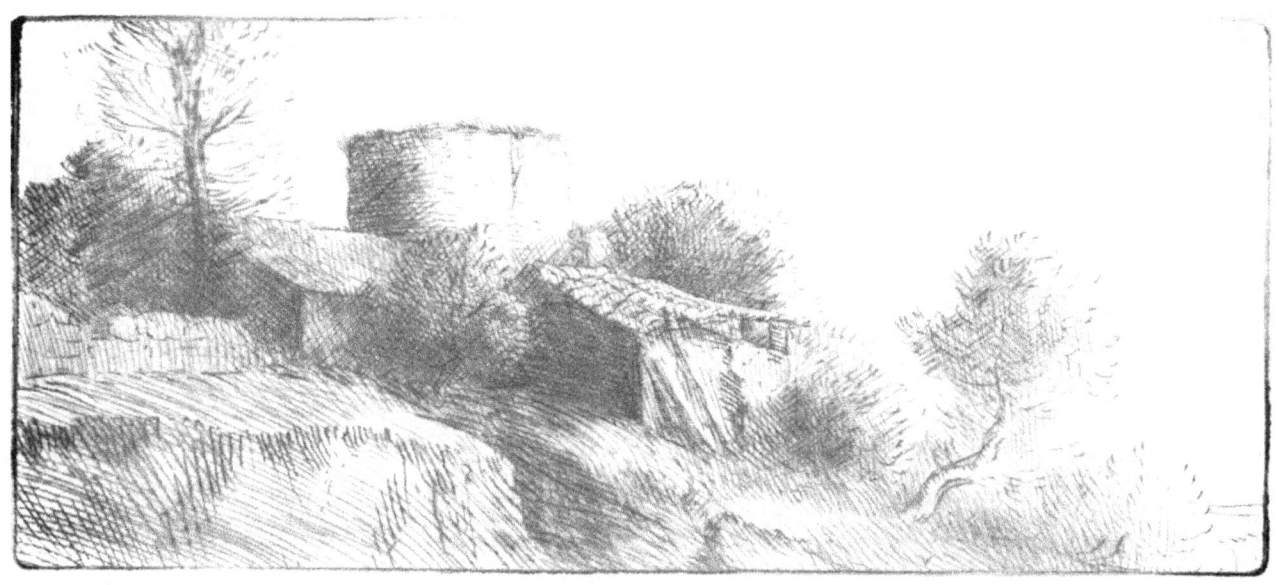

The worst is over

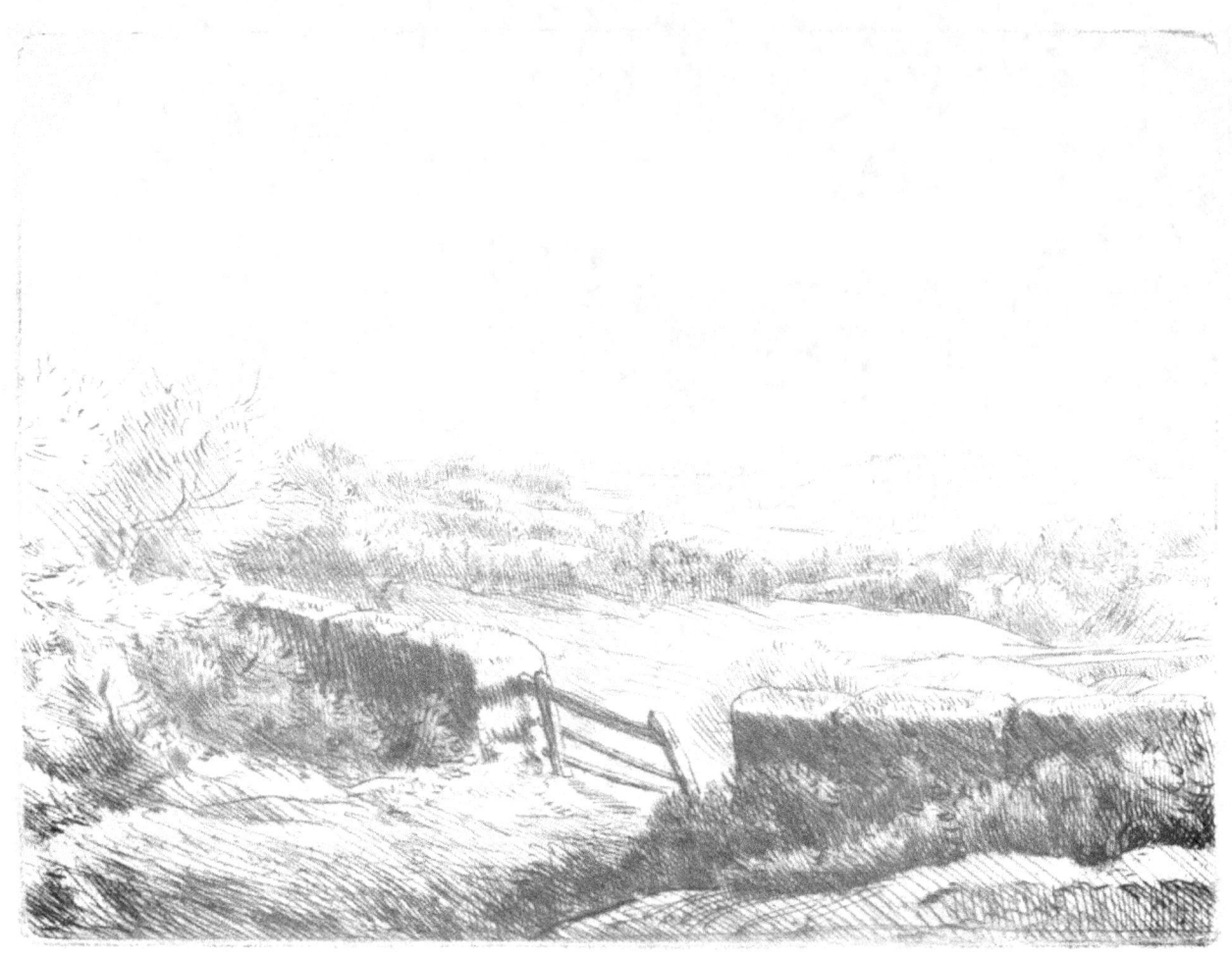

I am transformed

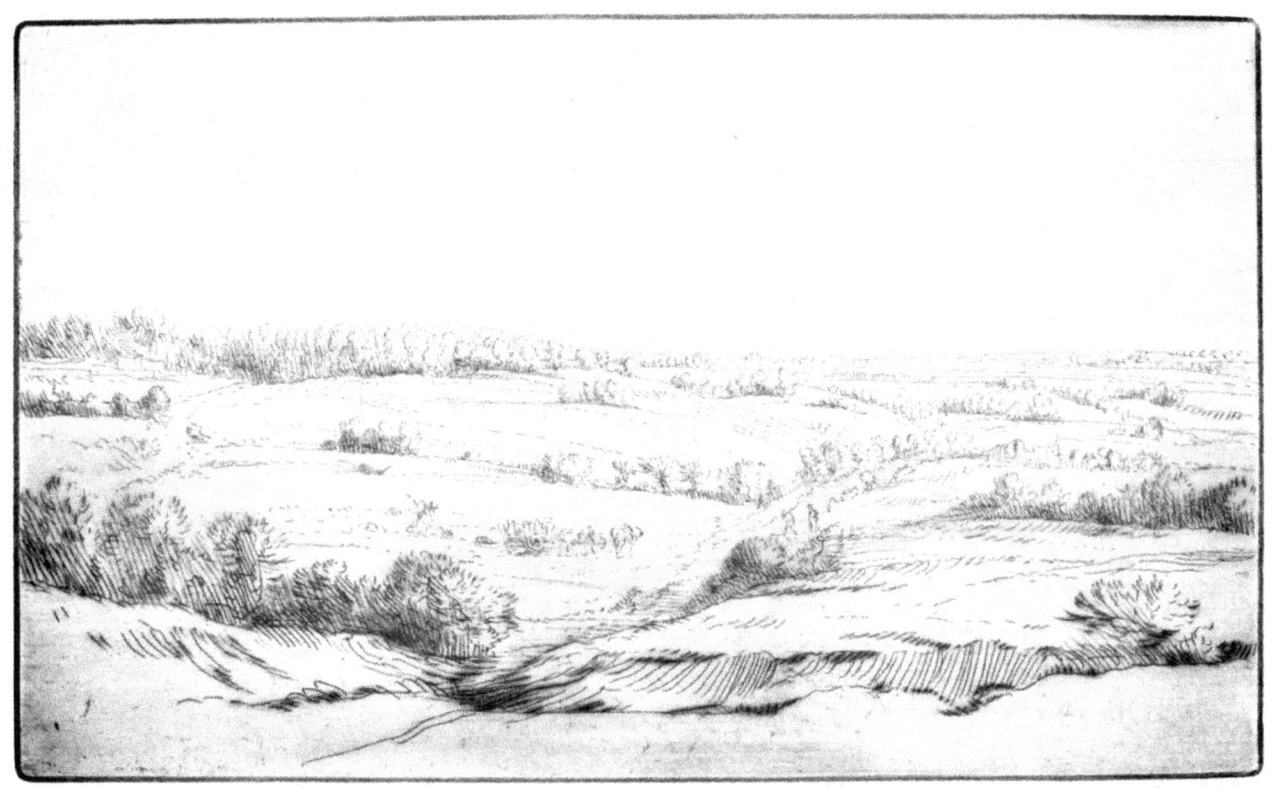

I now have more control

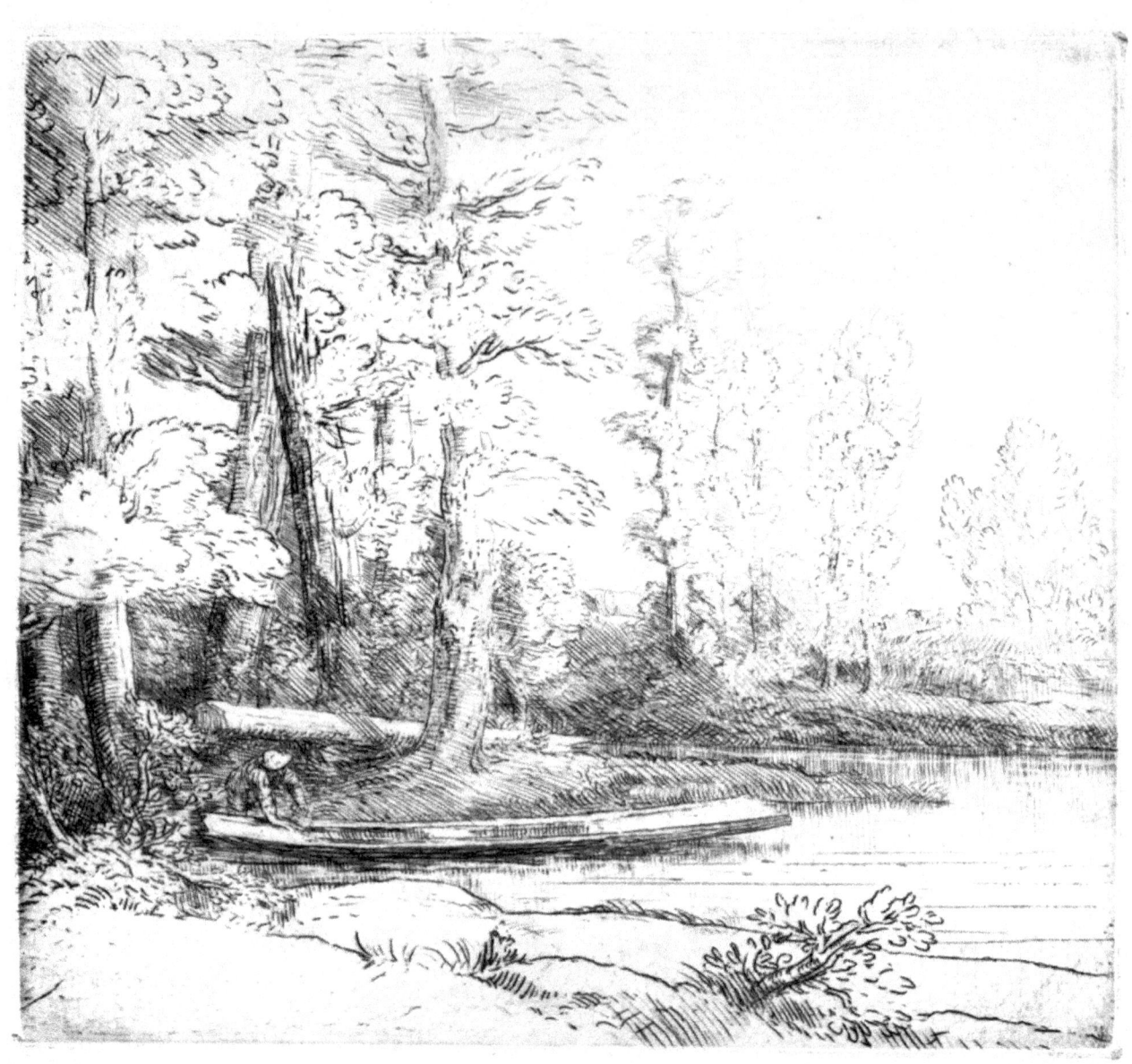

A. Legros

I am being reshaped

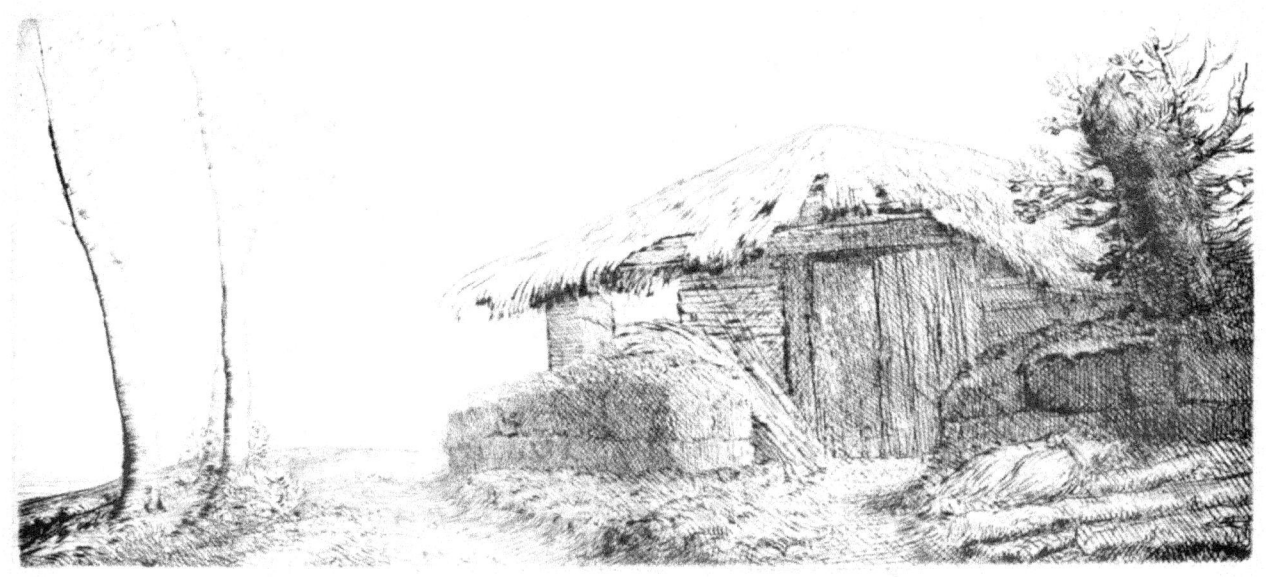

I am a soulful person

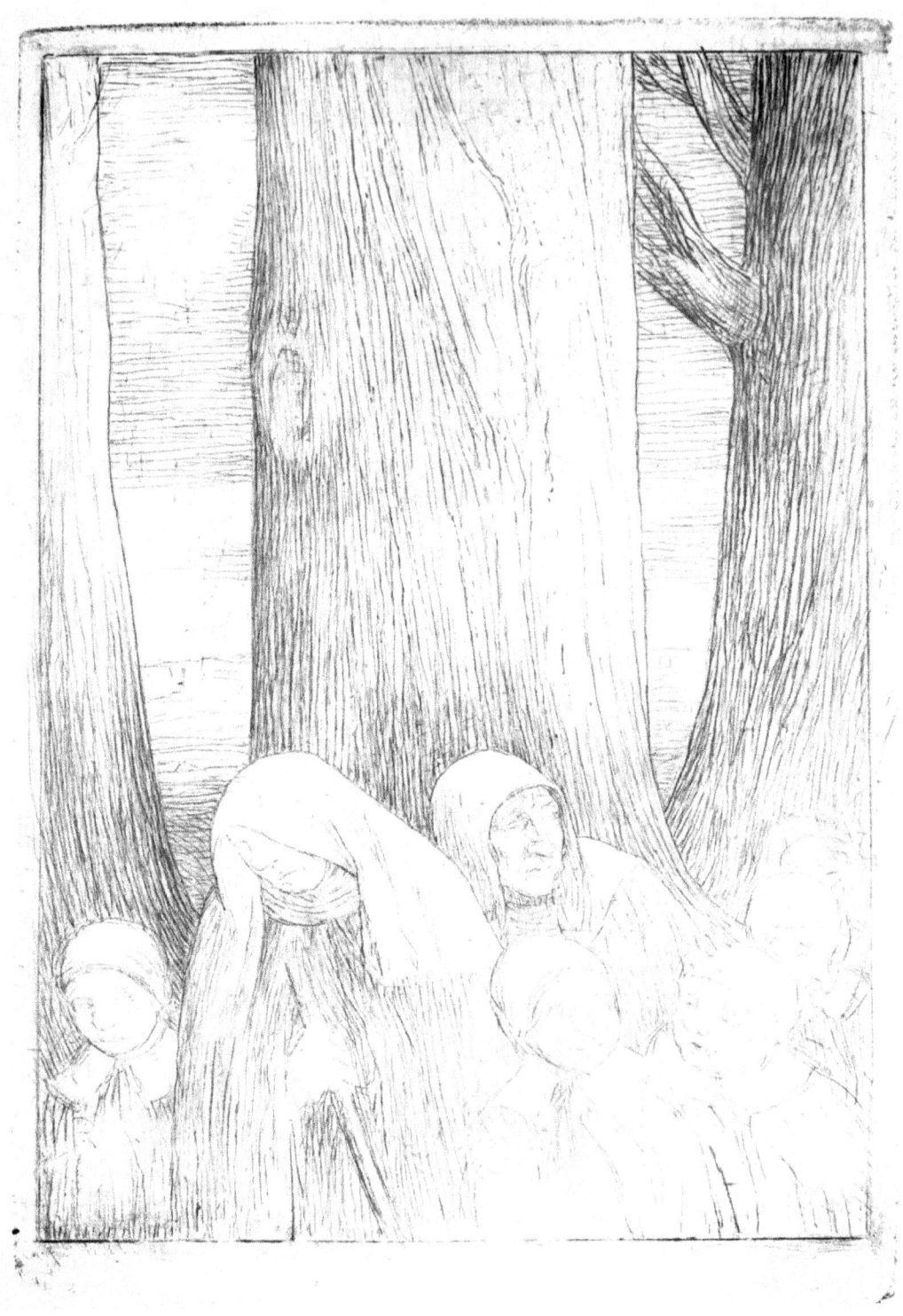

I can be transformed

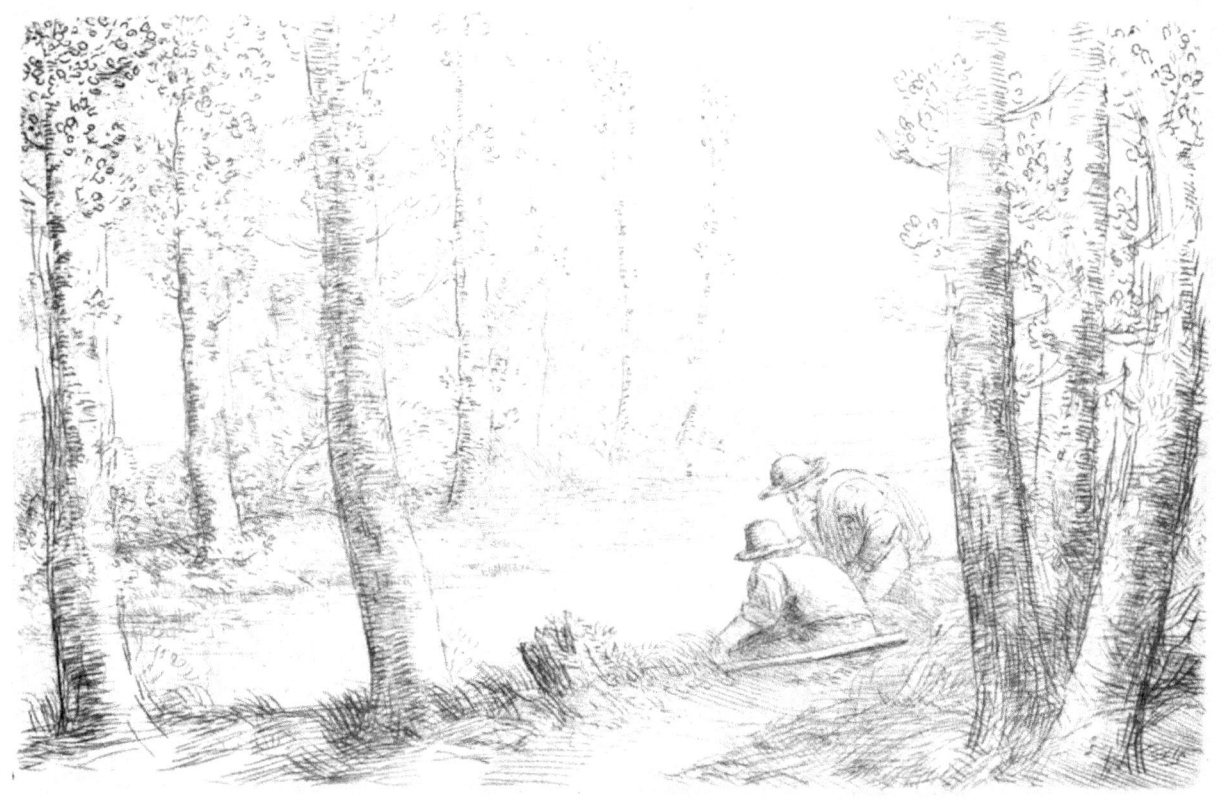

I have a good heart

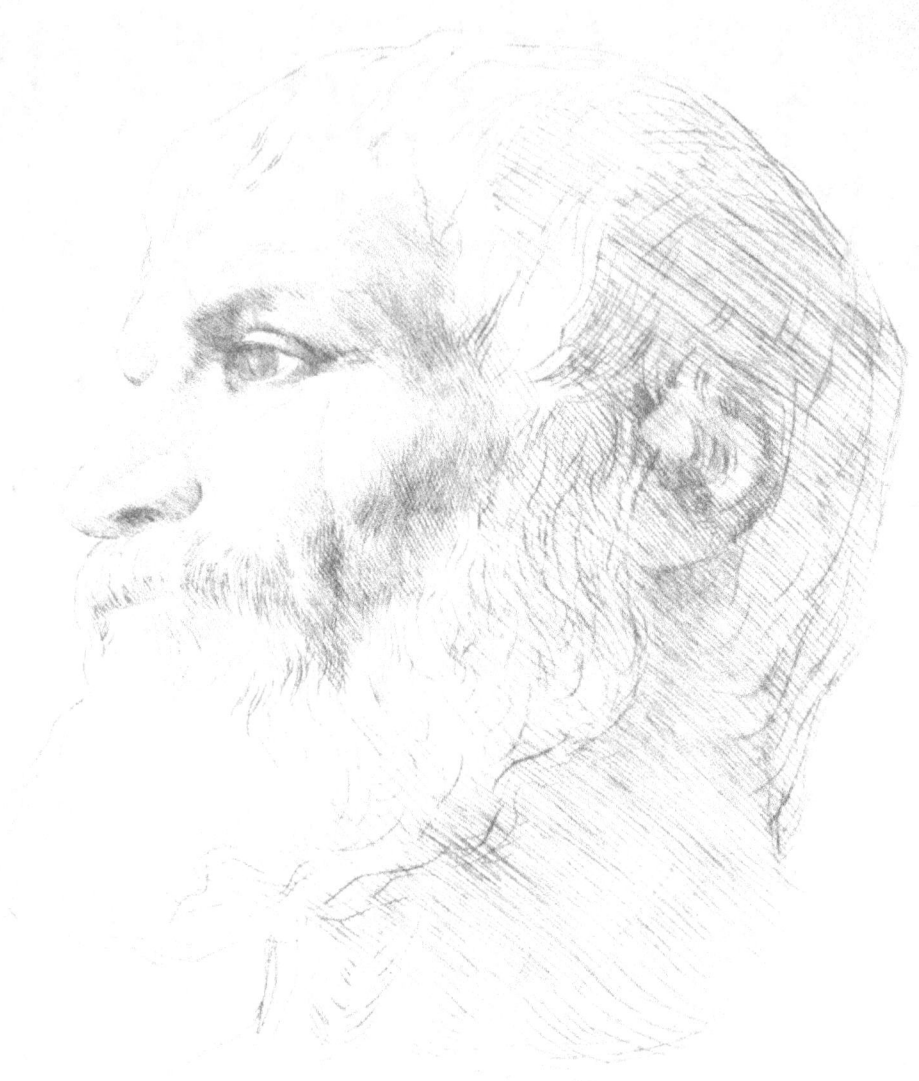

I am calm

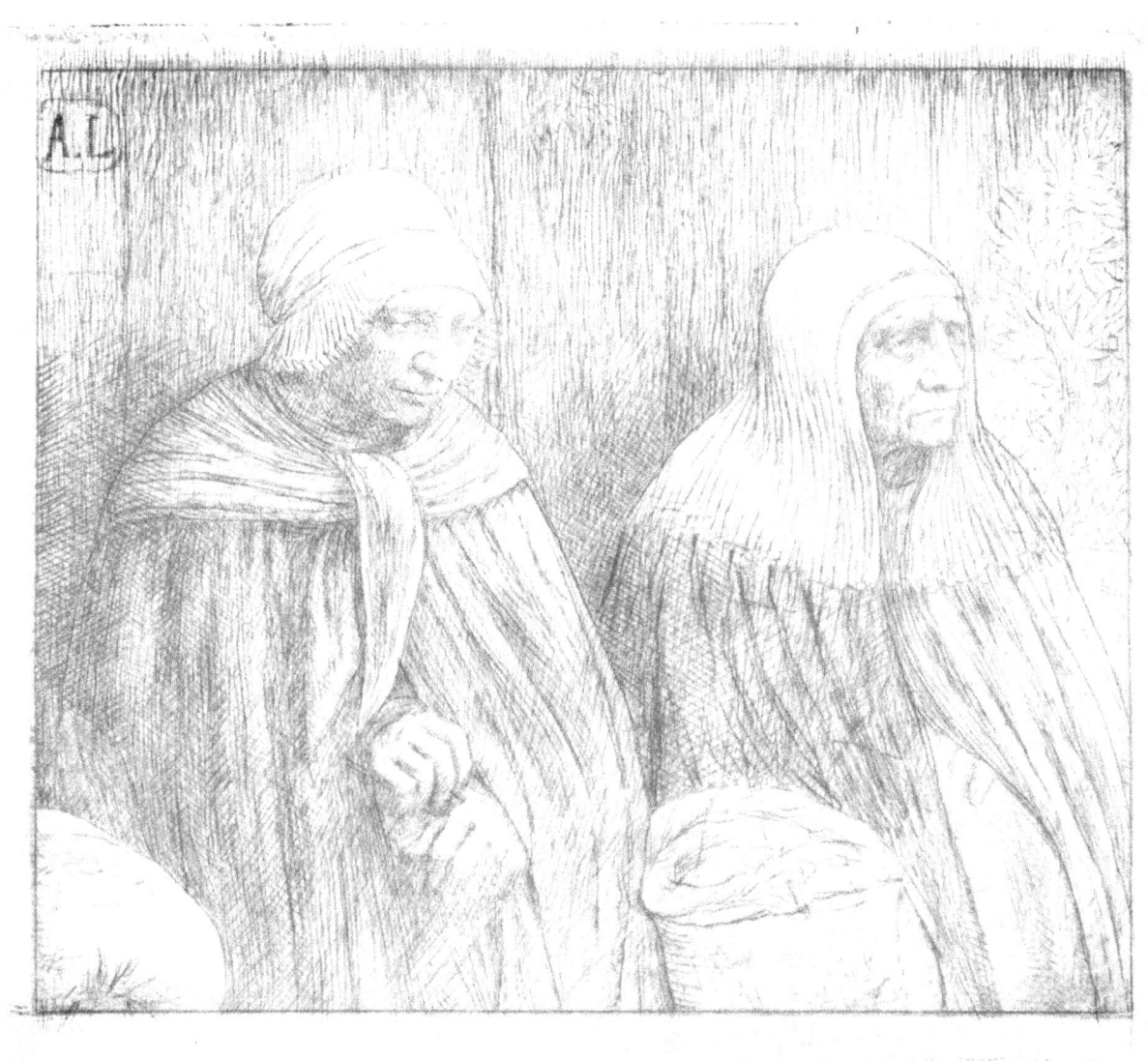

I have soul

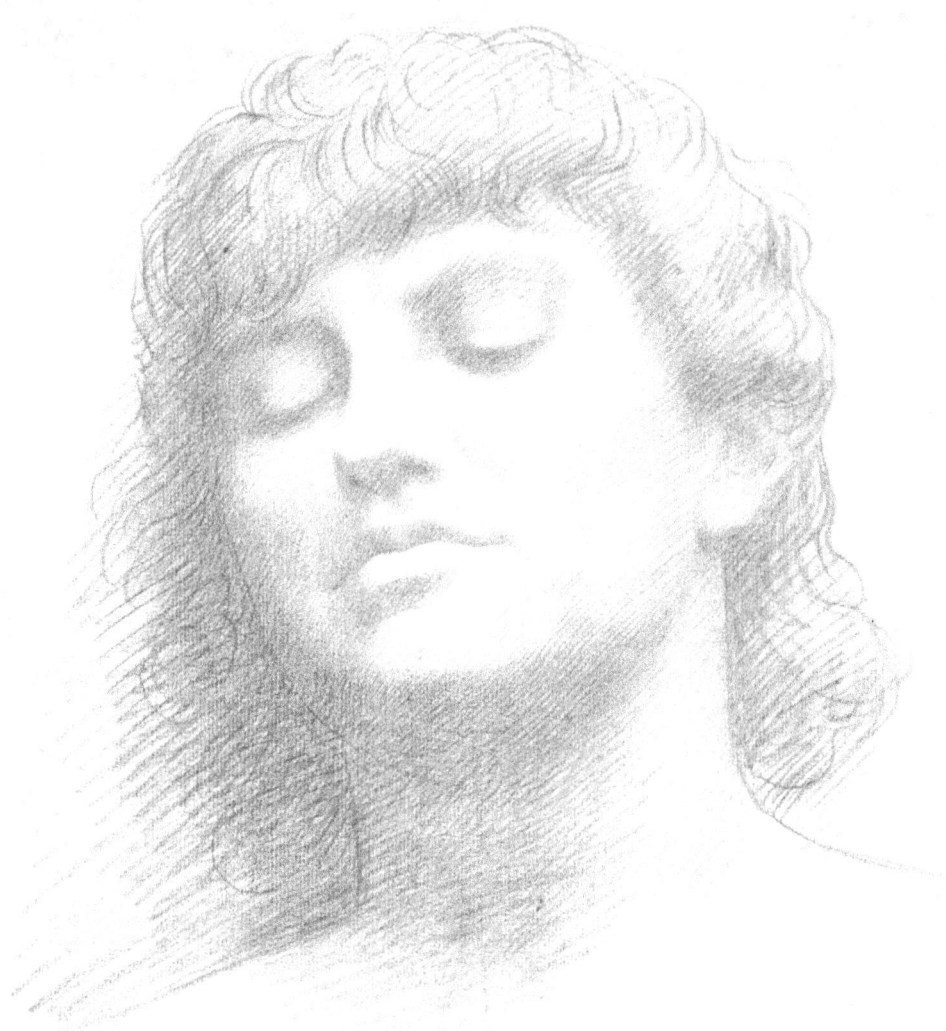

I am able to reach my goals

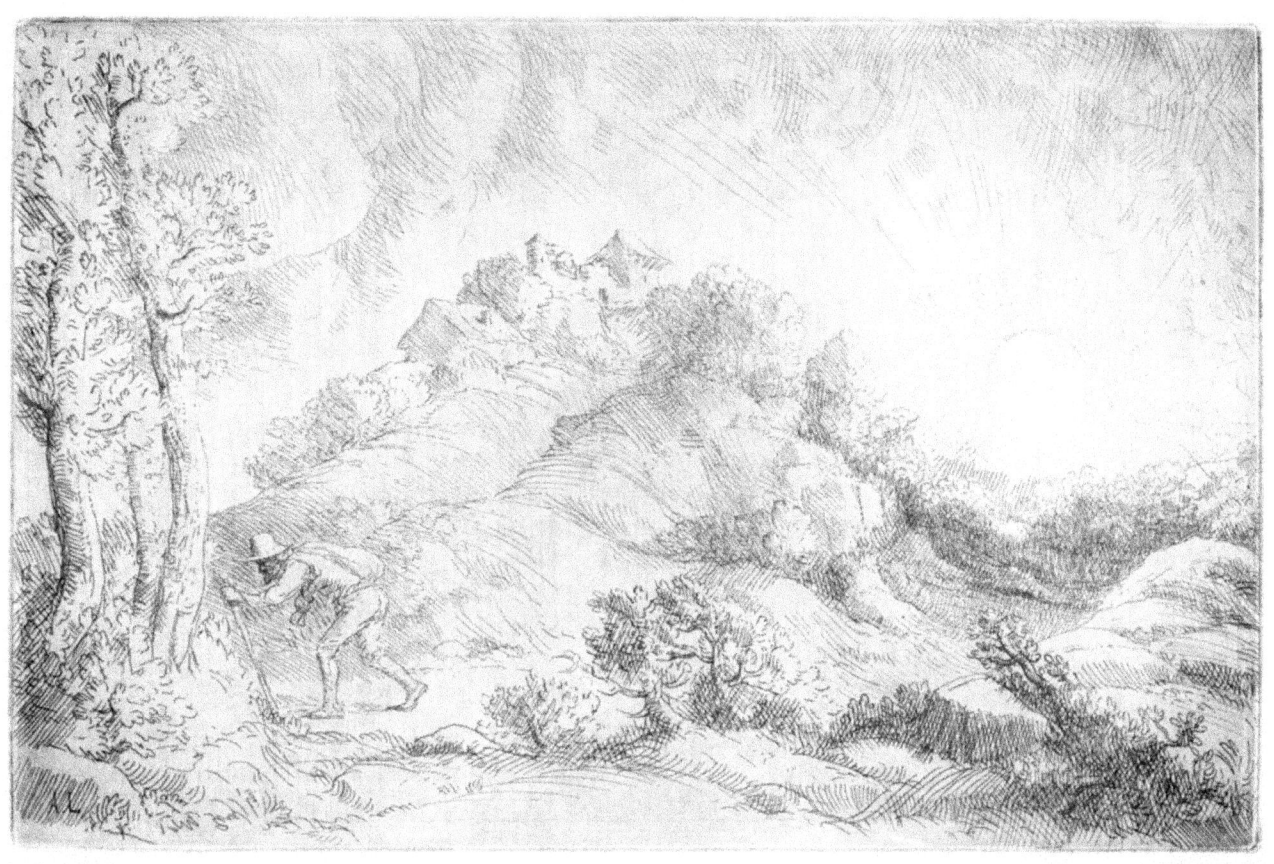

I deserve healthy relationships

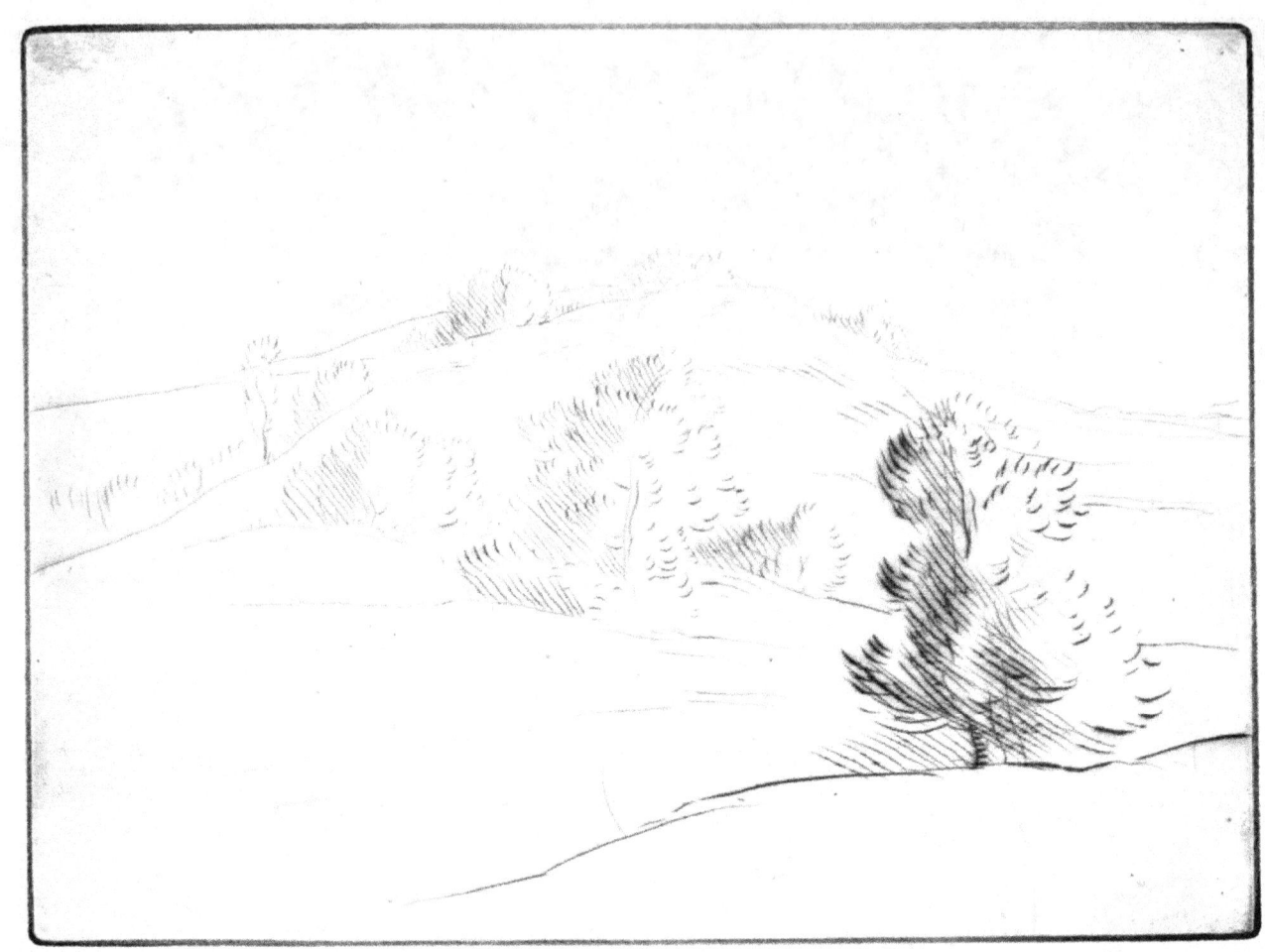

I am valuable the way I am

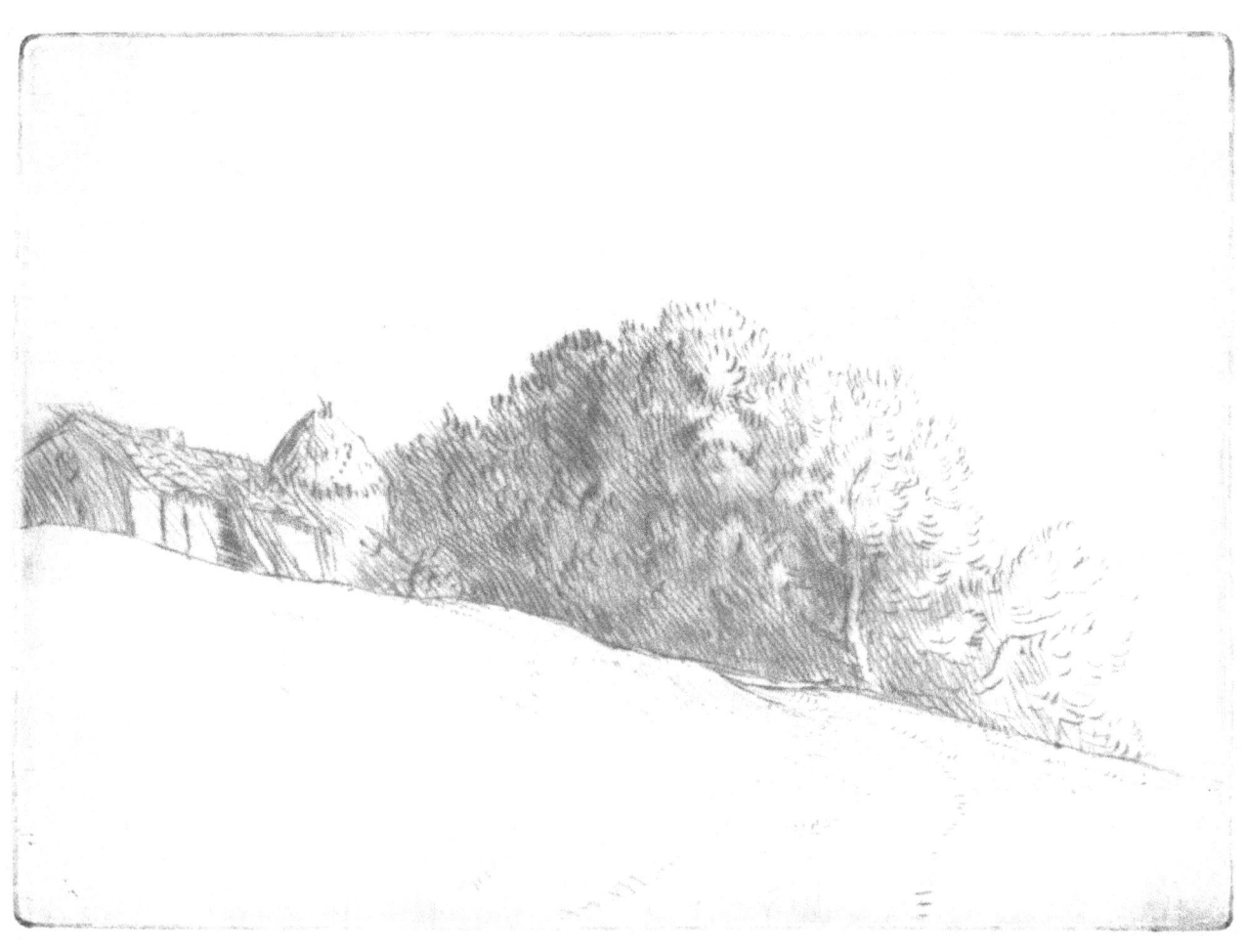

I am a survivor

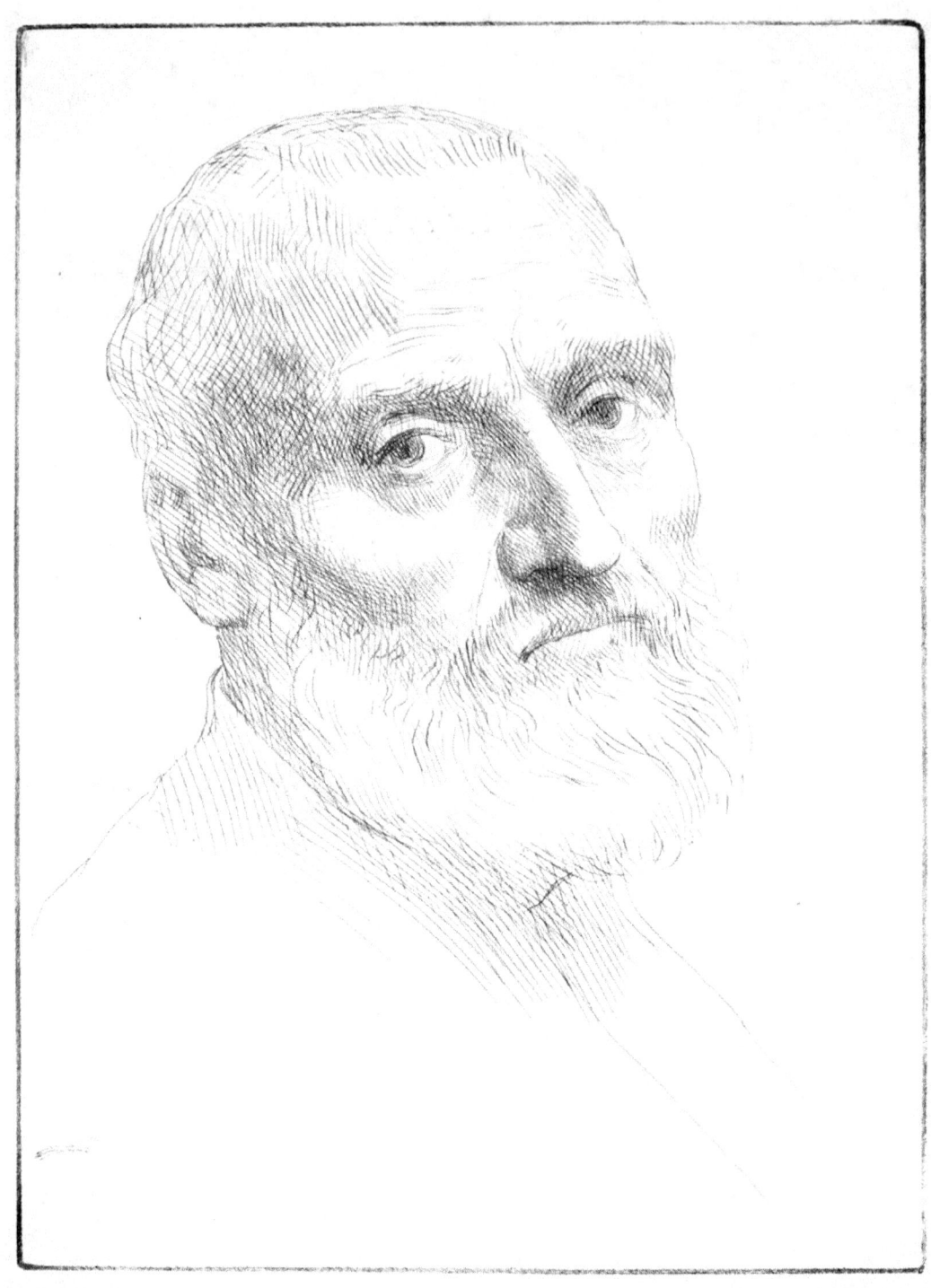

I am not defined by my past

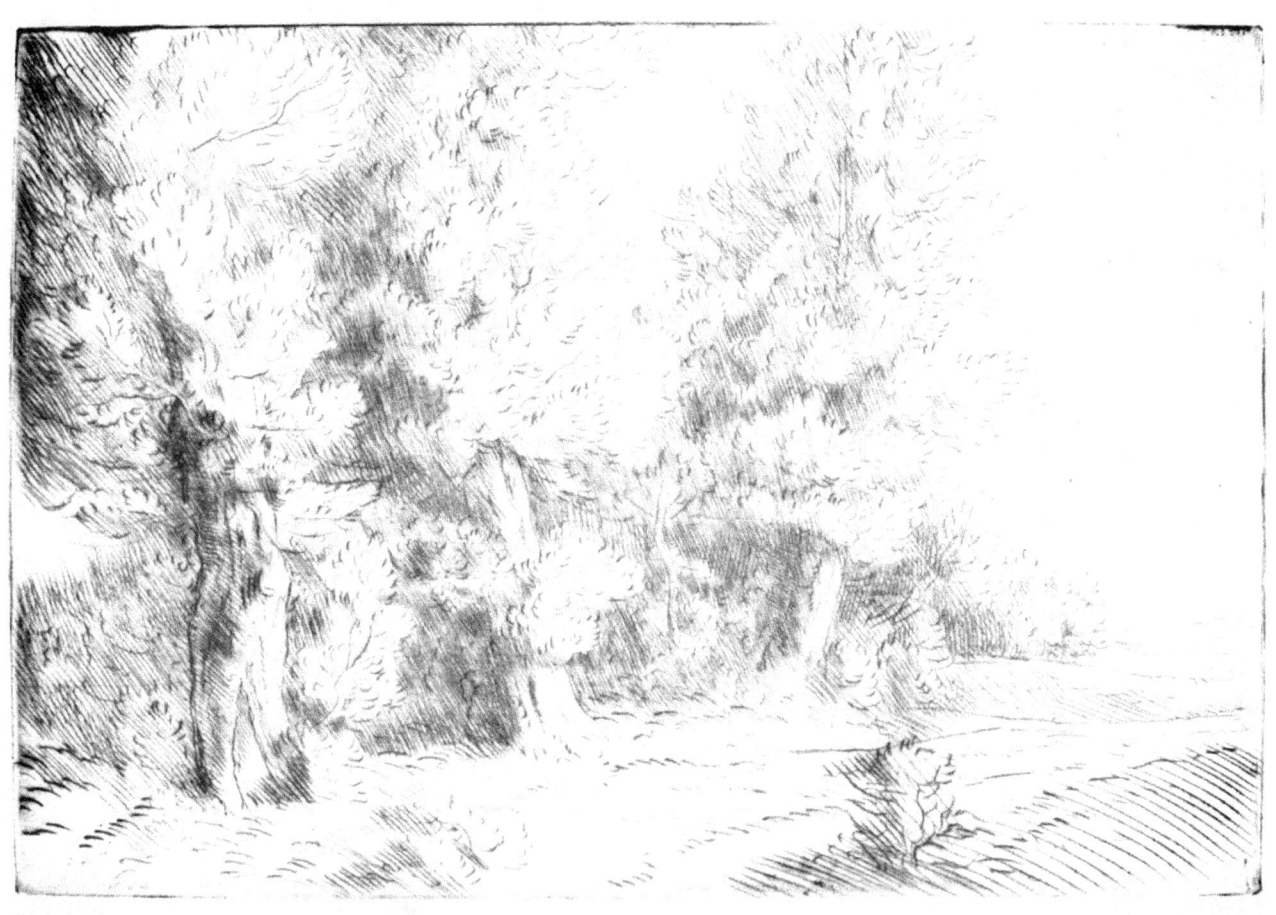

I am acceptable the way I am

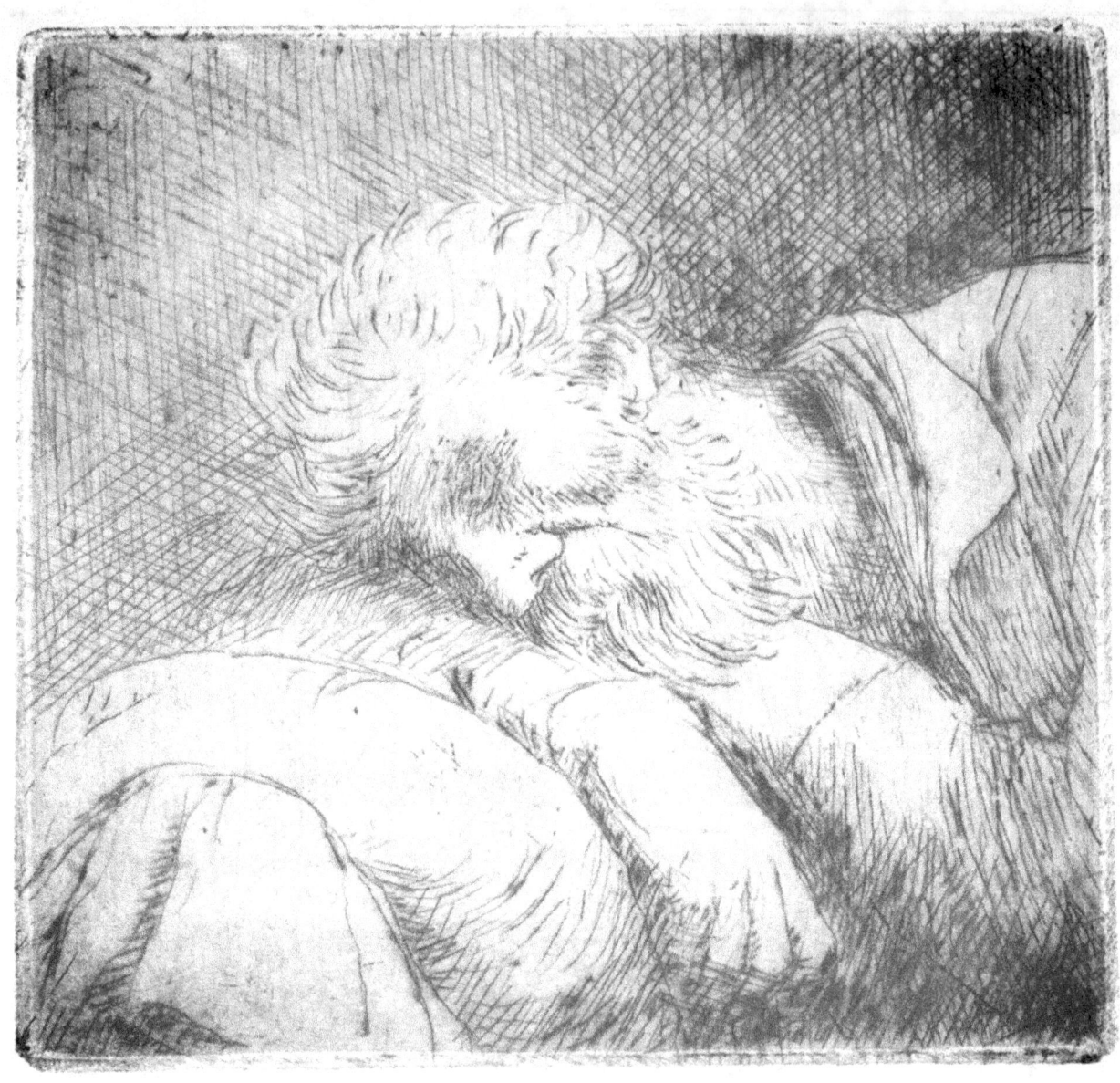

I am dignified

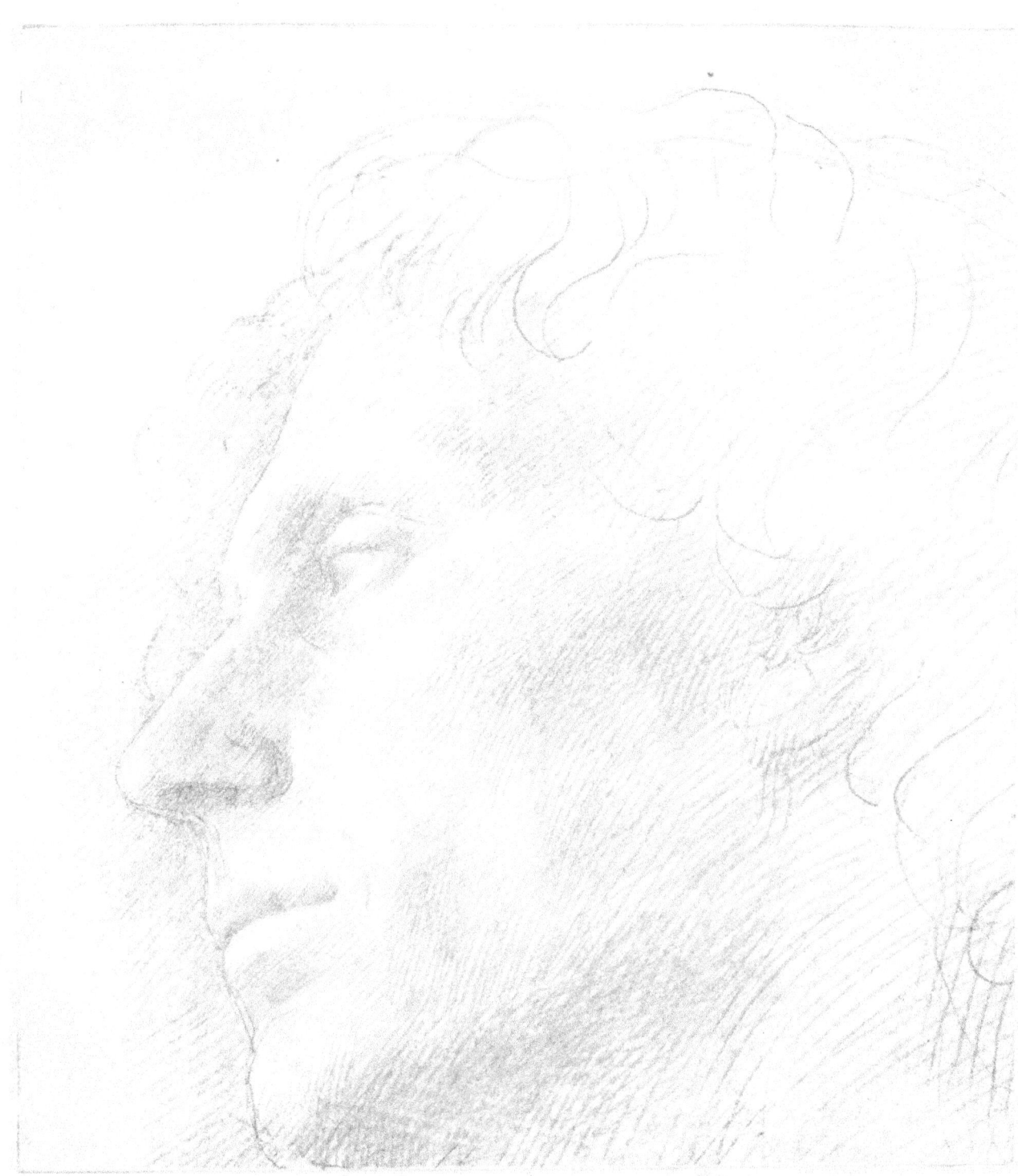

I am able to become healthy

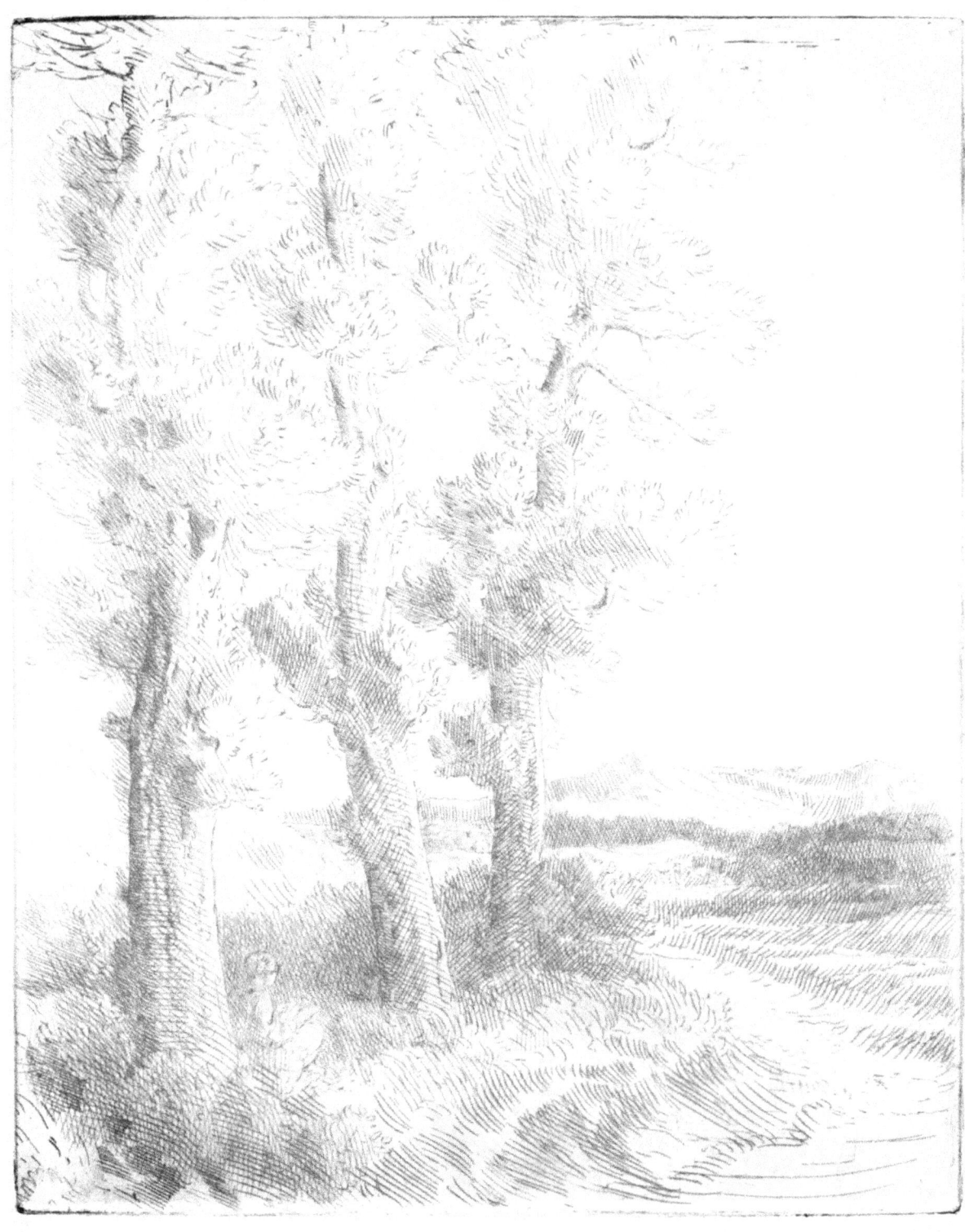

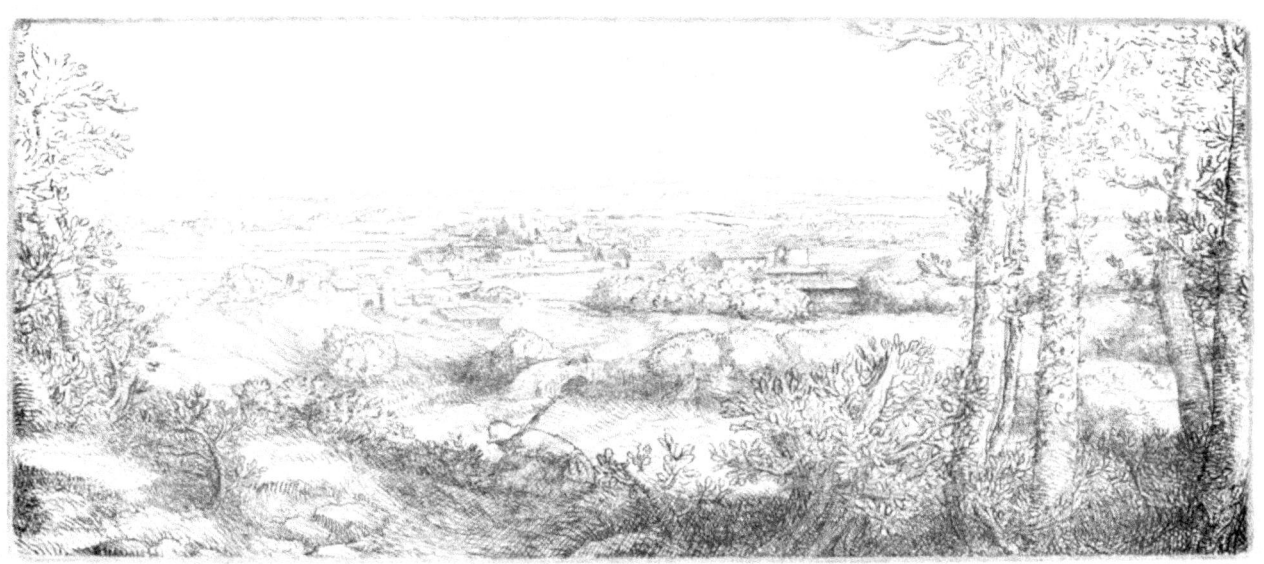

I am stronger now

I am a person of faith

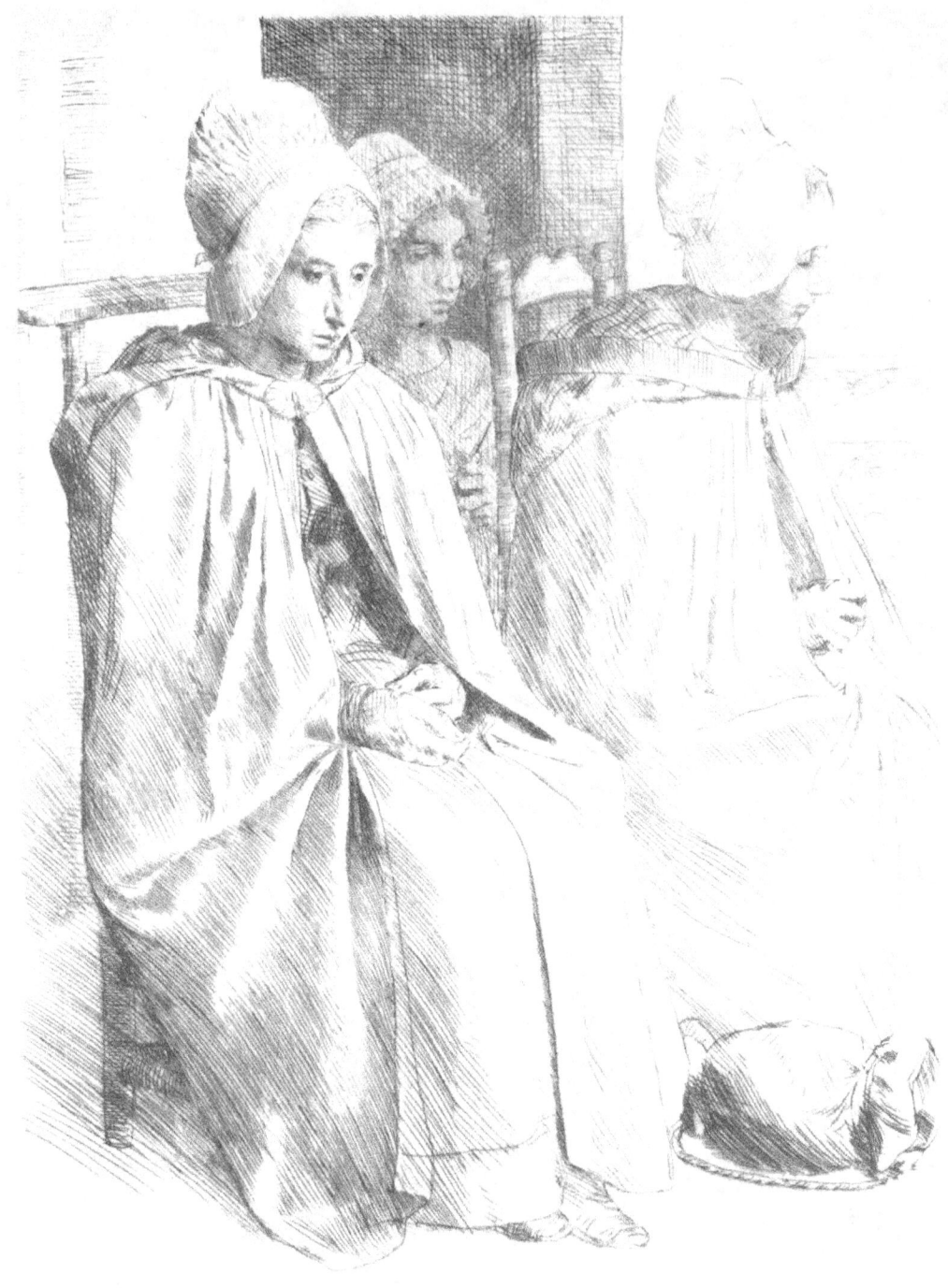

I am resilient

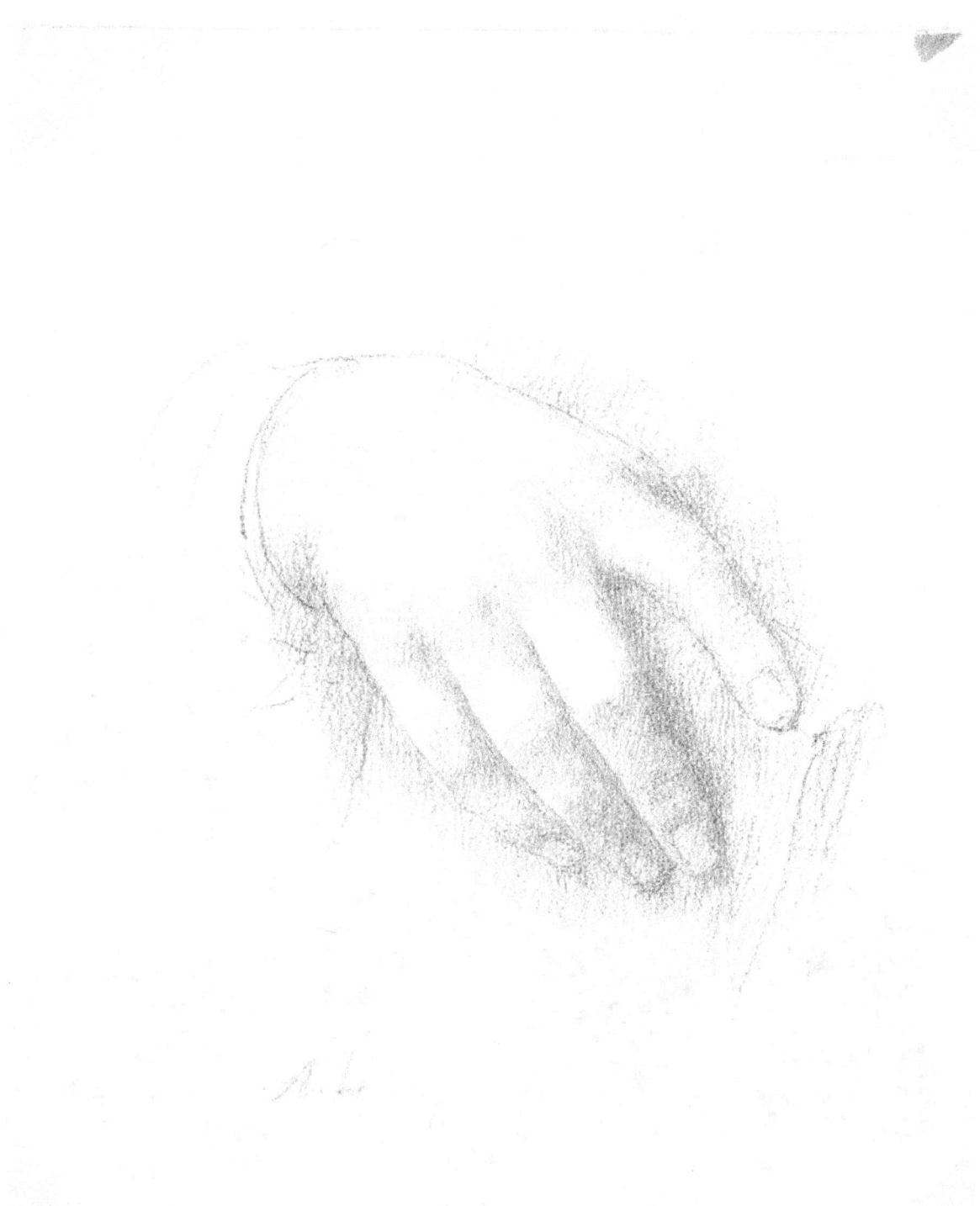

I am safe

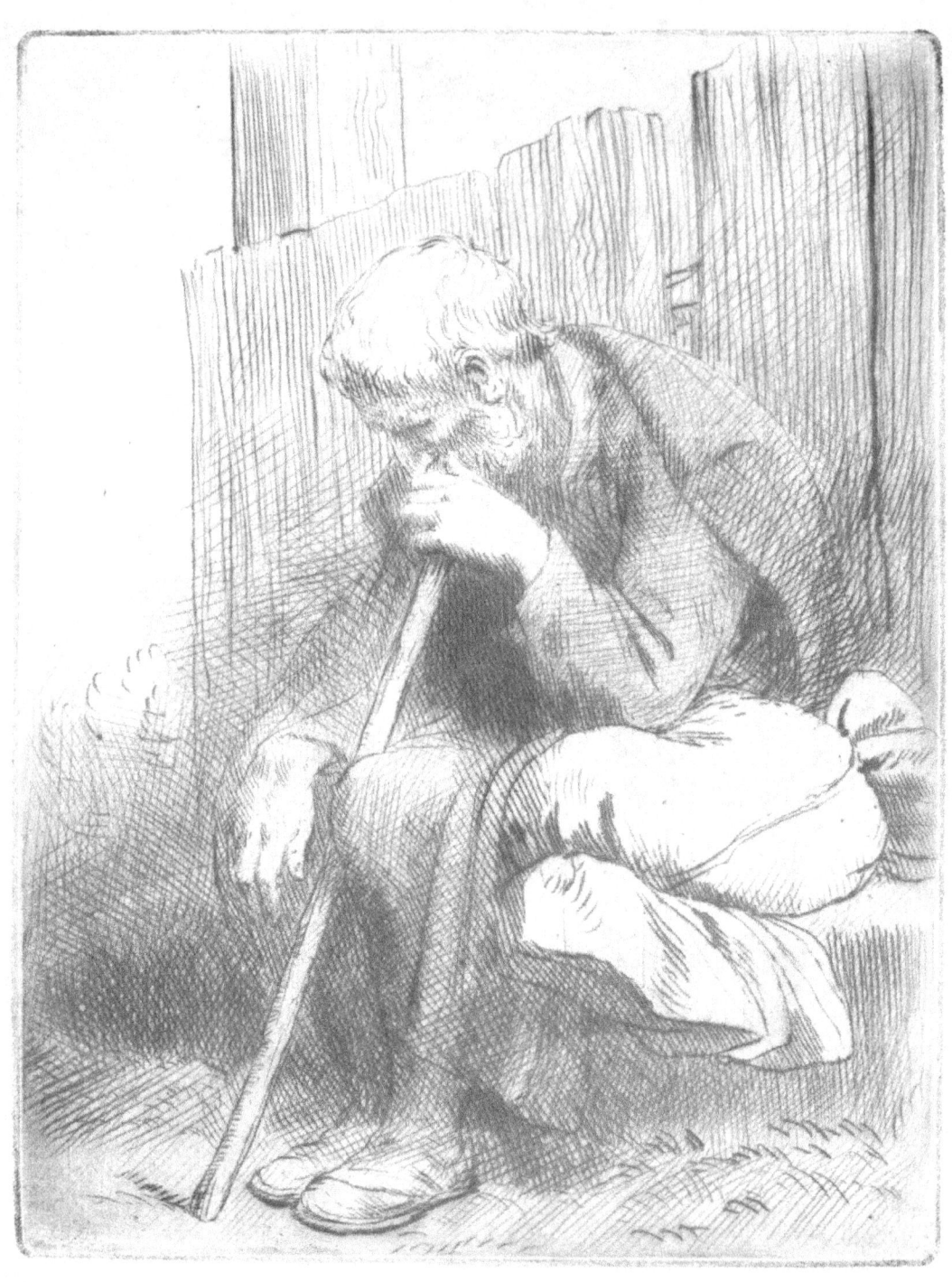

I know more now

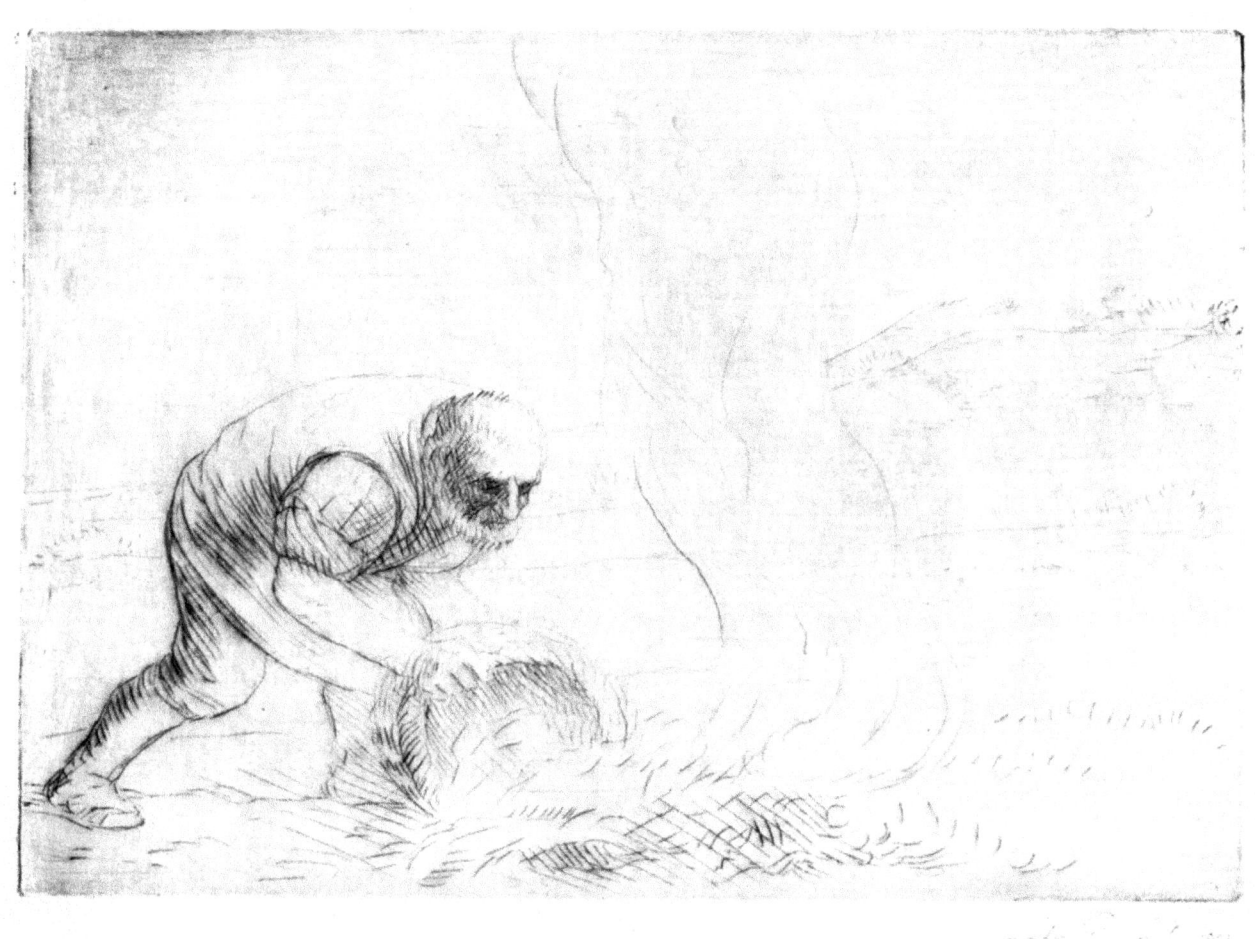

I am a person of strength

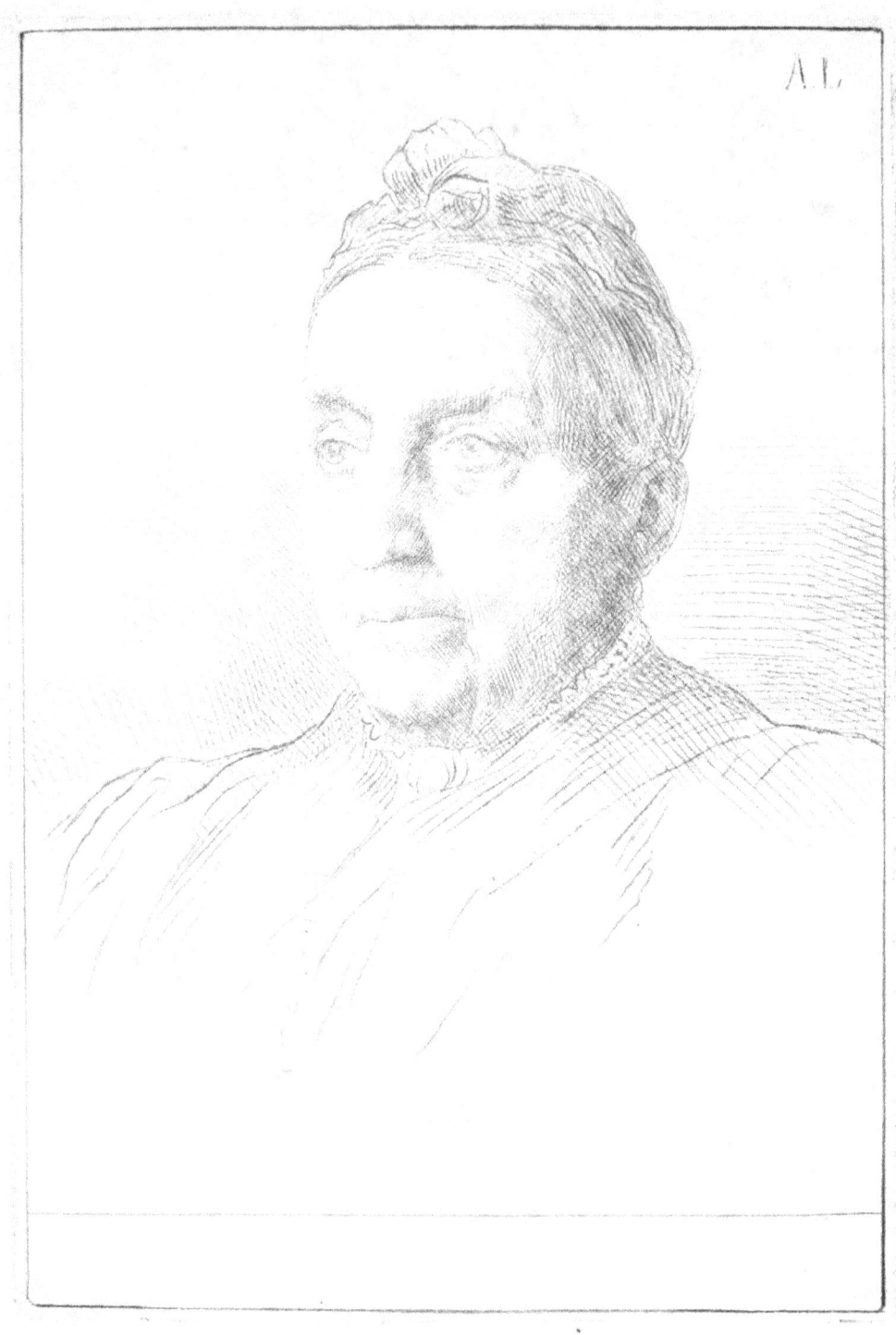

I am redeemed

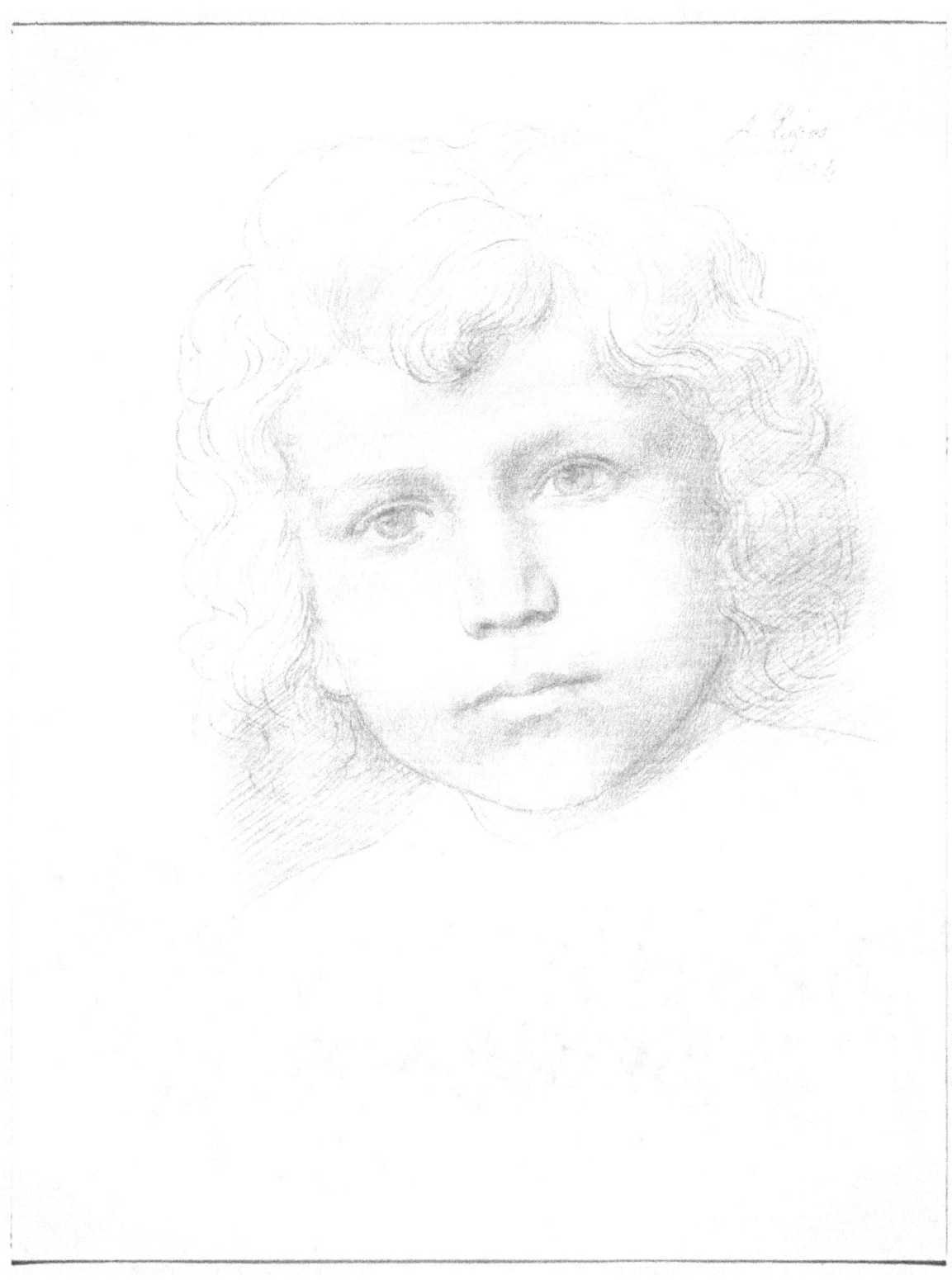

I am worthy the way I am

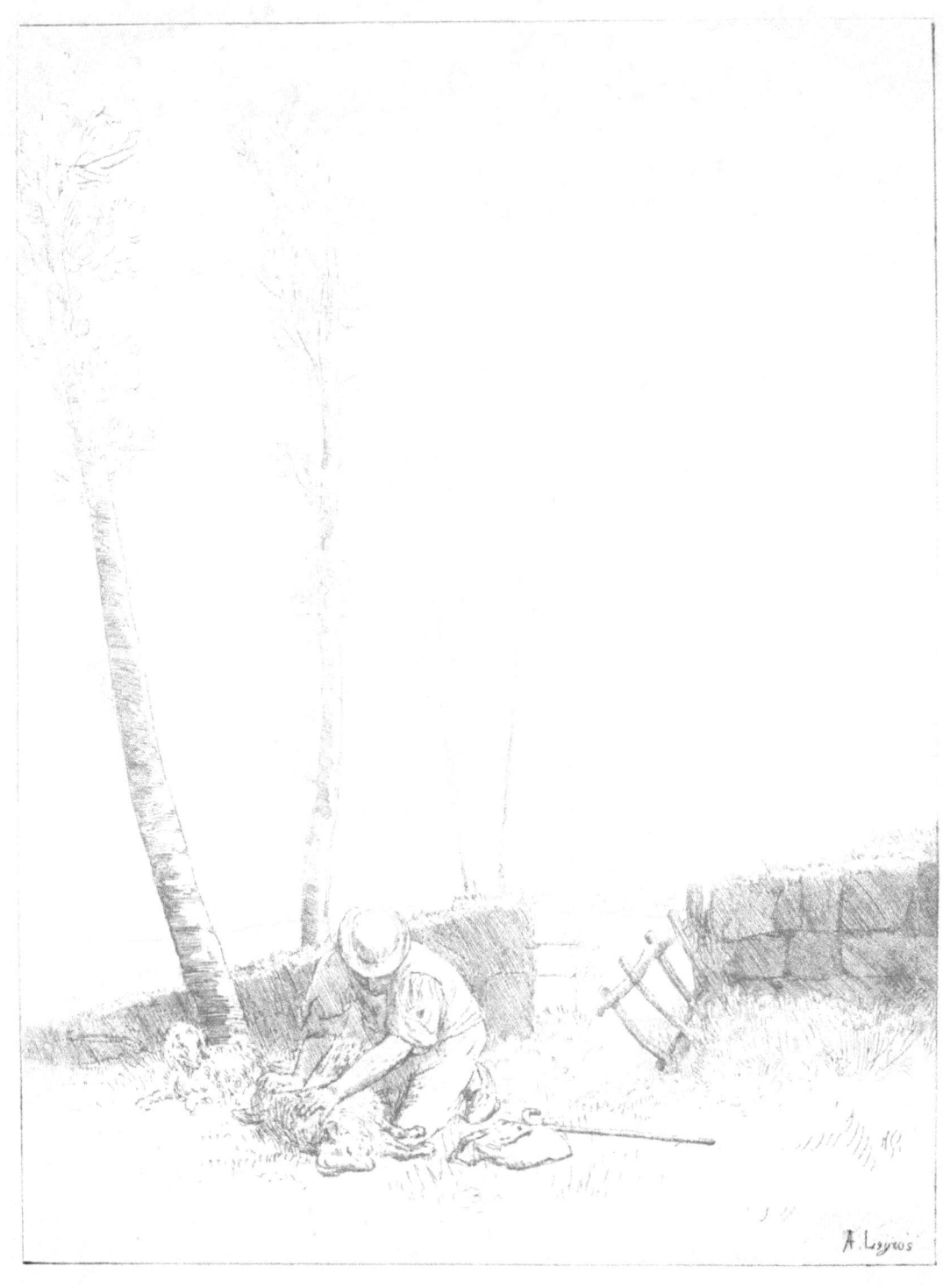

I am a new creation

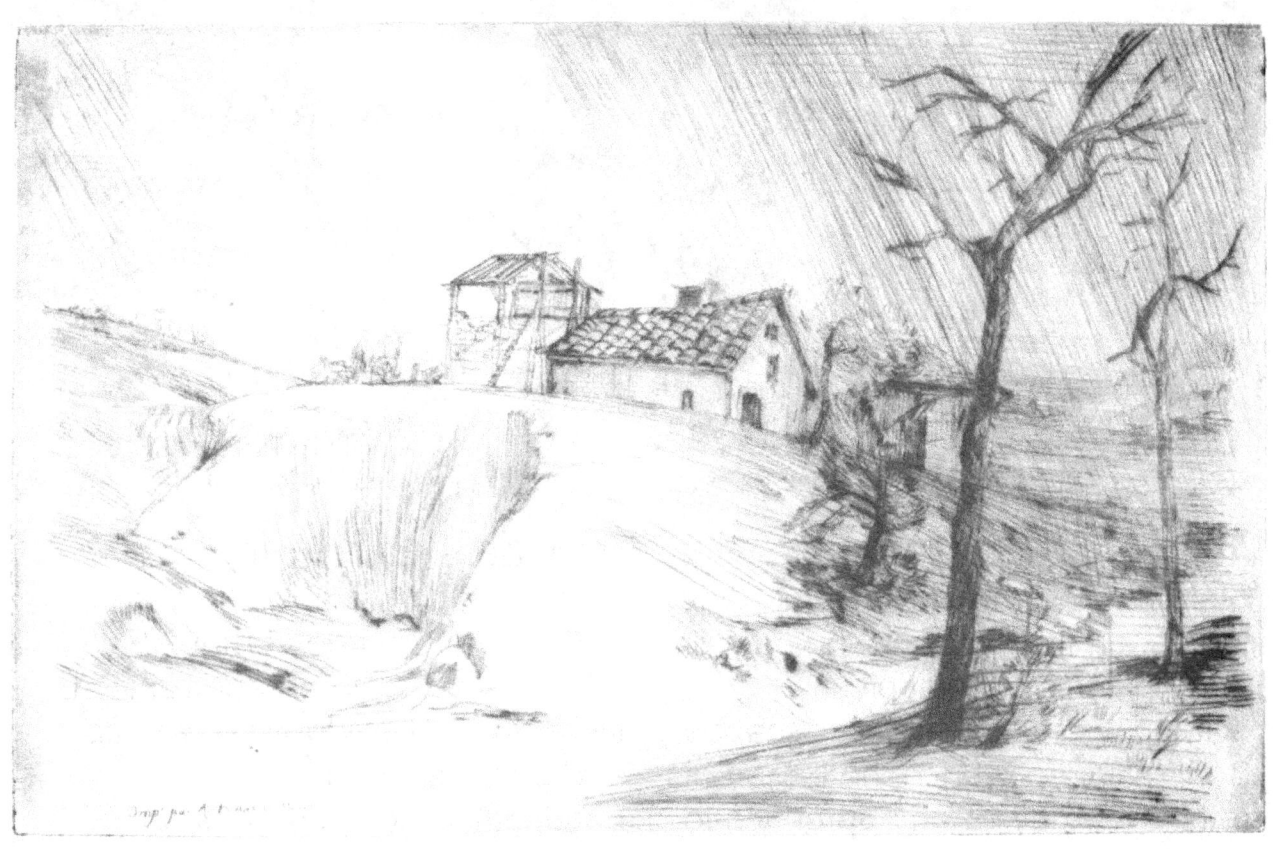

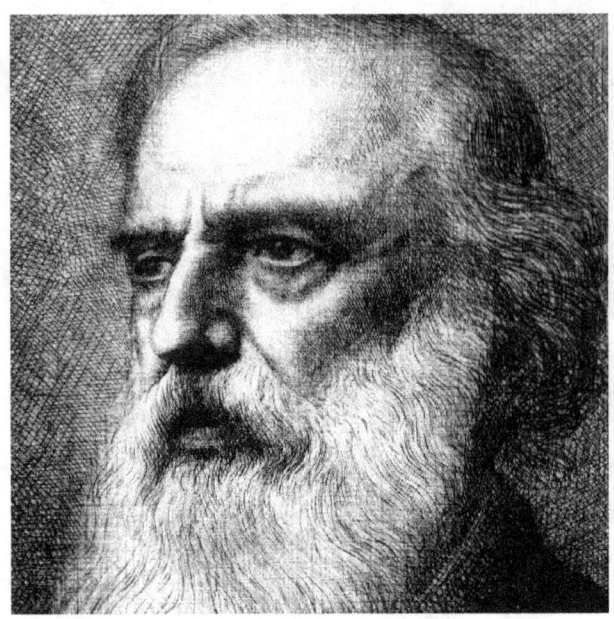

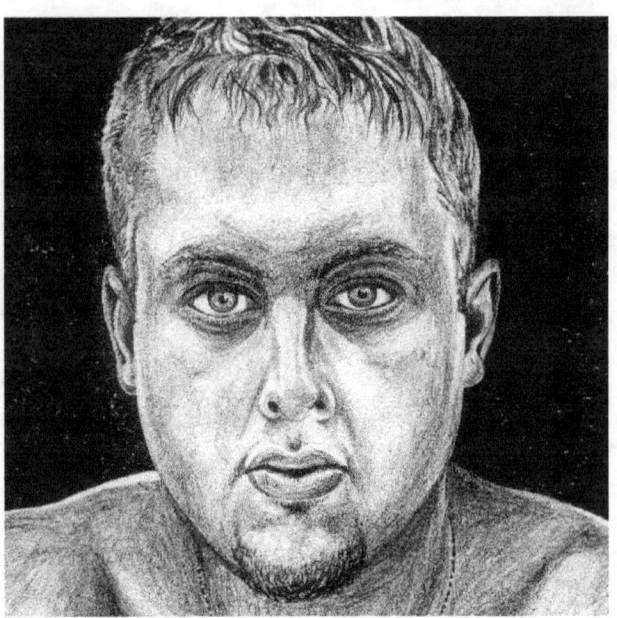

Alphonse Legros (Self-Portrait - etching and drypoint)

Mark Odland (Self-Portrait - lithograph)

Alphonse Legros (Artist)

Alphonse Legros (1837-1911) was an etcher, lithographer and painter who specialized in depicting historical subjects and landscapes. Born in Dijon, France, he began his artistic journey as an apprentice to a builder and decorator. In 1851 he moved to Paris, where he worked as a scene-painter, and studied at the École des Beaux-Arts. In 1863 he moved to London, and a few years later was appointed teacher of etching at the South Kensington School of Art. In 1876 he became Slade Professor at the University College of London (description taken from *Who's Who*. 1911. p. 1193.) Able to convey the simple beauty of nature and the power of human emotion, his artwork has lasted the test of time.

Mark Odland (Editor)

Mark Odland graduated from Augustana College in Sioux Falls, SD, with a B.A. in art and religion. Here he studied drawing, painting, and printmaking under nationally-renowned printmaker Carl Grupp. He went on to earn his M.Div. degree from Luther Seminary in Saint Paul, MN, and his M.A. in Marriage and Family Therapy from the Minnesota School of Professional Psychology in Eagan, MN. An award-winning artist, Mark feels privileged to have his work displayed in various collections around the world. In his work as an EMDR therapist, consultant, and educator, he continues to explore the dynamic intersection between creativity and healing.

CONSULTATION

Mark Odland is able to provide approved consultation for those needing:

1) EMDRIA Certification Consultation
2) EMDR HAP Basic Training Consultation
3) Consultant in Training Consultation
4) Individual Case Consultation

Mark's education, experience, and ongoing training allow him to provide guidance on a variety of issues during consultation sessions. However, he enjoys focusing on the following within EMDR therapy: general practice, spirituality, creativity, childhood abuse and neglect, addiction, and military veterans.

SPREAD THE WORD

If you enjoyed this book, Mark would be grateful if you left an online review at amazon.com and barnesandnoble.com.

PURCHASING BOOKS FOR CLIENTS

If you're an EMDR therapist and would like to purchase more copies for clients, you may qualify to receive a discount for bulk purchases. To find out more, send an email to:
mark@bilateralinnovations.com

CONTINUING EDUCATION

Mark's Odland's continuing education courses are often available as webinars, books, e-books, and audio books. Available to therapists worldwide, his growing list of learning opportunities includes the following subjects:

EMDR and Visual Art

EMDR and Spiritual Trauma

Spiritual Interweaves

Spiritual Resource Building

How to Start a Trauma-Focused Private Practice

PURPOSE

Mark founded Bilateral Innovations with the following purpose:

Bilateral Innovations provides EMDRIA-Approved Consultation and Continuing Education, for the purpose of transforming the world, one client at a time.

To learn more, please visit his website at:
bilateralinnovations.com

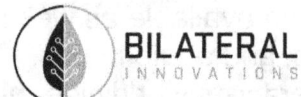